Social Psychology
and Medicine

SOCIAL PSYCHOLOGY AND MEDICINE

M. Robin DiMatteo
Howard S. Friedman

University of California, Riverside

O G
& H
Oelgeschlager, Gunn, & Hain, Publishers, Inc.
Cambridge, Massachusetts

International Standard Book Number: 0-89946-131-x

Library of Congress Catalog Card Number: 82-2123

Printed in West Germany

For David
M. R. D.

For my parents
H. S. F.

Contents

vii

List of Figures and Tables

Note: Listed here are only those figures that are referenced in the text; cartoons and most photos are thus not included.

List of Boxes

(continued)

Preface

This book presents a comprehensive introduction to a new and rapidly growing field. It is intended for college students in premedicine, health psychology, medical sociology, counseling psychology, nursing, and social work. It may also be useful for sociobehavioral science courses in medical schools, and for primary care residents. We have successfully used these materials in courses for both social science and health care students.

This book was challenging to write because it is the first of its kind. Although there have been various attempts to integrate psychology and medicine, such books generally have either a psychobiological or a psychodynamic flavor; in addition, they are usually edited volumes. In this book, we attempt to present a very broad field, but from a unified perspective. We draw freely on sociology, personality psychology, social anthropology, clinical psychology, psychosomatic medicine, and behavioral medicine. Yet our emphasis is very clearly on the influences of *people* on health care, health, and illness. We personally attach the utmost importance to this field, since the proper application of existing social psychological knowledge to medical issues can improve health and save lives.

Students interested in the health sciences receive most of their training in the biological and physical sciences and so sometimes have some difficulty seeing where social psychology fits in. Why learn about such matters as communication among doctors, nurses, and patients when there is so much physiology to learn? Unfortunately, many health students do not fully recognize the value of social psychology until they have finished the bulk of their technical science training and must actually face a patient. However, we have found that the more advanced and experienced a health professional becomes, the more eager he or she is to hear about the topics in this book. To help bridge this educational gap, we attempt to show the real-world applications of our approach whenever possible.

Many, many people helped with the development of this book. Judith A. Hall and Diane Halpern commented on a draft of the whole manuscript. Among the many other psychologists, physicians, and students who helped in some important way were: Ginny Banks, Cecilia Bauernhuber, Cari Baum, Nan Birchall, Terence Davidson, David DiNicola, Deanna DiNicola, Mardi Dornfest, Carol Eckmann, David Eckmann, Kenneth Eckmann, Carl Eklund, Pam Farr, Paul Flandreau, Rhonda Friedman, Marilyn Gregory, Monica Harris, Karen Hartman, Ron Hays, Janet Hinzman, Doris Howell, Louise Prince, Ronald Riggio, Debra Rister, and Dan Takeda. Becky Halt was especially helpful with the referencing, proofreading, and indexing. Kathy Wolff and the University of California, San Diego, Medical Center were very cooperative in providing picture opportunities as was the administration of the San Bernardino County Medical Center. Administrators at the University of California, Riverside—including Robert Singer, David Warren, Michael Reagan, and Marvin Nachman—consistently supported our efforts. Our office staff, including Madelaine Dibler, Dianne Fewkes, Heather Jorgensen, and especially Malinda Fulmer, provided excellent support and clerical services. Finally, we would like to thank our teachers, who inspired and encouraged us during the early stages of our careers, especially Robert Rosenthal, Lucille Palubinskas, Phoebe Ellsworth, Stanley King, Irving Janis, Zick Rubin, and Angelo Taranta.

M. R. D.
H. S. F.
Riverside, California

1
Introduction to Social Psychology and Medicine

In the most dramatic procedure of modern medicine, the human heart of a donor is cut out of the chest of a cadaver and transplanted to the body of a recipient. The recipient awakes from surgery with a new lease on life. This procedure involves many extremely complex biological challenges, but it also raises a number of psychological issues involving relations among people.

Anatomically, the human heart is a hollow, muscular organ that contracts and relaxes to circulate blood throughout the body. It is an efficient pump. Human hearts, however, are inside human beings, people who may have other thoughts and feelings about what a heart is. When a teenage lover speaks of a "broken heart," the reference is not to a malfunctioning valve. In literature and popular mythology, the heart represents the center of feelings. There is a psychological as well as a biological aspect to the heart [45].

This symbolic link between the heart and deep feelings may be important to the ways in which people approach the world. In intimate situations we try to "speak from our heart" and certainly do not want to be seen as "cold-hearted." The links between the bodily organ and the emotional symbol are so powerful that many adults are sure to bring heart-shaped gifts to their "sweethearts" on Valentine's Day. With such emotional meaning invested in hearts, it is apparent that questions about emotional reactions should be considered when a person loses his or her own heart and gains the human heart of another in a heart-transplant operation [66].

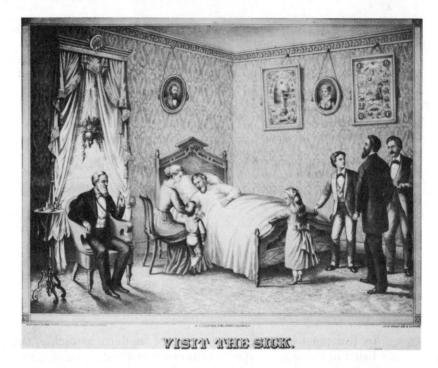

Figure 1-1. The art of medicine. (*The Sick Room* by M. C. Lilley, 1877. Courtesy of the Bettmann Archive, New York.)

In fact, emotional and other psychological reactions are an integral part of physical well-being and the process of medical care. Unfortunately, such processes are often overlooked today. Until the nineteenth century, however, all medicine was an "art." Creative doctors and nurses would talk to their patients, examine them, and, using their intuition, suggest measures that sometimes helped the patients feel better [31]. The interaction between the health practitioner and the patient was very important, but little science was involved [23, 59]. With progress in the biological sciences such as physiology and biochemistry, and the discovery of the link between microbes and disease, medicine became much more of a science. Rules were discovered that described the effective treatment for many diseases.

Scientific medicine has proved extremely effective in combating disease, with seemingly "miraculous" cures performed daily. In fact, medicine has been so successful that, in developed nations, curing disease through drug regimens and surgery is no longer the single major challenge to progress in health care, although of course it is still extremely important. Rather, two other issues have come to the forefront to challenge medicine [64].

The first of these challenges concerns preventive medicine [29, 40]. It is now more readily recognized that a minimally polluted environment and healthy individual habits such as proper nutrition and exercise can have a strong, positive impact on health. The second current challenge to medicine concerns social relations [18, 39]. The ancient concern with the relationship between practitioners and patients is reemerging as a significant medical issue. However, intuition is no longer sufficient. Instead, the study of interpersonal relations and medicine, or "social psychology and medicine," has now become scientific. This new field is the topic of this book.

In this chapter we illustrate and introduce this field by sampling basic social psychological issues involved in medical procedures such as organ transplants. As we shall see, social relations are so much a part of medicine that it becomes difficult to imagine how such factors could not be given a great deal of scientific attention.

Exchange

Friend: Did you visit the doctor?

Grandma: Yes.

Friend: What happened?

Grandma: The doctor feels better.

Friend: What? I don't understand.

Grandma: I wrote him out a big check and so now the doctor feels better.

Exchange is a basic fact of social life. The interpersonal trading of goods and services to satisfy human needs is universal [7]. However, many interpersonal exchanges involve commodities that are not accorded an explicit value. People trade advice, approval, respect, affection, and the like without resort to a cash register. Indeed, as the sociologist Peter Blau asserts, in "social" exchange the terms and obligations of the transactions are not clearly specified in advance [6]. Nevertheless, obligations exist. Social forces insure that some standards for exchange always operate [22].

The Beatles sang that "money can't buy me love," and psychologists have analyzed social commodities to see which are likely to be exchanged. Clearly, a heart surgeon is not "supposed" to be motivated purely by financial incentives. Although surgeons are well paid, people take offense at the idea of exchanging life or health for money. In the medical situation the patient provides many other "social commodities" to the physician besides money. For example, the patient discloses a great deal of personal information to the doctor or nurse, disclosures usually made only to intimates. The patient trusts the practitioner with his or her thoughts, feelings, and body. In return, the practitioner offers a genuine interest in the patient's health [38]. Medical interactions involve very special social exchanges. The subtleties of the practitioner-patient relationship are explored in Chapter 2, "The Art of Medicine." The basic issues raised there are then examined in detail throughout the rest of the book.

Cooperation

In the simplest social interaction, two people exchange fixed commodities. A common example is the exchange of a man's services for pay, which has been extensively analyzed by the psychologist Stacy Adams [1, 2]. Yet even this exchange is not so simple as it first appears. As Adams points out, the worker offers such assets as intelligence, education, experience, training, skill, social status, and of course the effort expended on the job. The worker's benefits or outcomes include such variables as pay, rewards intrinsic to the job, fringe benefits, job status, status symbols, and "a variety of formally and informally sanctioned perquisites, such as the right of a higher-status person to park his car in a privileged location," [2, p. 278]. When health and even life are at stake, the exchange is even more complex, and the social commodities more subtle.

In Western societies at least, the basic rule that regulates exchange is that of proportionality. The ratio of what person A has (or gets) to what he or she deserves (B) must equal the ratio of what person C has (or gets) to what he or she deserves (D). Or, $A/B = C/D$. Aristotle calls this equality "distributive justice" [3]. Issues of justice and fairness enter many medical situations.

The pressures toward justice and fairness have two key influences on the relationship between medical practitioners and patients. First, there are pressures for practitioners to rationalize irrational events; that is, people try to make unfair events somehow seem fair [42, 43, 55, 61]. It does not seem fair that a hardworking young man should develop leukemia, or that a teenager should be struck with epileptic seizures, or that a young married woman should have unsatisfying and painful sexual relations. So people may tend to blame the patient for the illness or to deny that a real problem exists. The social critic Susan Sontag describes how tuberculosis used to be blamed on a weak character and warns that a similar tendency exists today to blame cancer on spiritual deficiencies [61]. Of course, the truth is that many illnesses are tragic and unfair; but it is difficult for practitioners to be both caring about patients and constantly aware of this reality. This difficulty may lead to problems in practitioner–patient interactions.

The second pressure of the desire for fairness involves equity in the practitioner–patient relationship. The rule of distributive justice is, for most purposes, universal. For example, the anthropologist Marcel Mauss analyzed the practice of giving gifts in various "primitive" societies [46]. The *gift* and the demands for reciprocity and equity that go with it were shown to have important legal, economic, religious, aesthetic, and moral functions to many societies. A more modern sociological analysis stresses the *norm of reciprocity* [28]. Patients expect to be able to reciprocate for practitioner help in their care, and patients expect practitioners to return the respect they are given. But the *demands and traditions* of the medical setting often require that the practitioner assume a "fatherly" or "motherly" type of care. Patients are asked to give up control of their health and equity in their relationship. Unfortunately, while this arrangement may promote a sense of "organization" in medical settings, it may have many negative effects on the patient's health [62, 65]. Some of these matters are discussed in Chapter 3, "Patient Cooperation with Treatment," and also in later chapters.

Correlation Versus Causation

A basic concern that has extremely important implications in the field of psychology and health is the issue of correlation versus causation. In understanding illness, we generally want to know what factors cause the illness, for by knowing the causal relationship, we can usually prevent or treat the illness. The most famous and successful causal relationship in medicine is germ theory [10]. When we know that certain bacteria cause certain diseases, we can prevent an illness by avoiding the bacteria or cure a disease by killing the bacteria.

In many types of illness the causal relationship is not clear [19]. Instead, we have only observed associations or correlations between certain attributes or behaviors and certain illness. For example, cigarette smoking is associated with lung cancer, depression with chronic illness, food cravings with pregnancy, anxious behavior patterns with heart disease, alcohol with migraine headaches, and sexual promiscuity at a young age with cervical cancer. The difficulty arises in determining the cause and the effect of the particular illness. The problem is that even though correlation does not necessarily imply causation, we often infer causation. Some of the following examples illustrate this point through exaggeration: People sleep less and less as they get older, but does lack of sleep cause aging? Most teenage heroin addicts were born in hospitals, but does hospitalization at birth cause drug abuse? People who take two aspirins and drink a glass of orange juice often gain relief from headaches, but does orange juice cure headaches?

These examples reveal the nature of the inference problem, but often the nature of the relationship is much less clear. Does jogging help prevent strokes? Do large doses of vitamins prevent the common cold? Do business demands cause heart attacks? Does depression cause cancer? Can the will to live affect the results of surgery? These questions are much more challenging. But the issue of correlation and causation is found throughout medicine. If a doctor prescribes a new antibiotic for a patient with a very bad cold and the patient soon gets better, will the doctor conclude that the medication did the trick? Would the patient have recovered to the same extent without the medication? Such methodological issues can be addressed by well-trained health practitioners. We discuss just such issues at various points in this book.

Perhaps the trickiest problems of causal inference involve the relationship between psychological states and disease states, such as the nature of the relationship between personality and disease, or the nature of pain [11]. The problems of causal inference are further complicated in such matters because most people share some expectations about these relationships. For example, if everyone "knows" that bedrest and calm are good for dealing with the common cold, it is very difficult to evaluate the relationship; the patient "knows" that he or she needs rest and calm to get well fast, and the physician "knows" it as well. With these expectations, such a relationship is almost sure to emerge. The various social psychological factors involved in the relationship between physical and mental states, including the value of placebos and the effects of "quack remedies," are considered in Chapter 4, "The Mind and the Body."

Communication

I was born 40 years ago but I'm three years old.

This puzzling statement was made by the recipient of a heart transplant. The patient dates his age not from the date of his natural birth, but rather from the date he received a new heart and was able to resume many normal activities and so "begin life again."

> Your distention of the rectum and other symptomatology results from habitual neglect of afferent impulses and accumulation of dry fecal masses.

This statement may be confusing to a layperson. It makes perfect sense to the physician who uttered it, however, as a result of years of medical training and constant exposure to medical journals and medical personnel.

Although such statements by physicians are not unknown, most communication between patients and medical personnel involves some shared language and shared expectations. Yet significant misunderstandings are common and widespread [5]. Medical personnel misunderstand patients, and patients misunderstand medical personnel. To make matters worse, both patients and doctors generally *think* they understand each other when many times they actually do not [18].

Ineffective communication is a major problem in modern medicine [17]. Many factors may contribute to the problem, ranging from poor habits to an active desire to withhold significant information [47]. It is clear, however, that significant improvements can be made and that such changes would likely produce great benefits in medical care [34]. Such matters are discussed in Chapter 5, "Communication with Patients: Verbal and Nonverbal."

Although the language of medical interactions is important, we see again and again that the quality, or "social and emotional" aspect, of the provider–patient relationship is a key element of good medicine. The establishment of proper rapport often involves attention to and use of touches, voice cues, facial expressions, and other aspects of nonverbal communication [24]. A transplant patient who claims to be "three years old" is probably expressing his emotional outlook on the event, information that can best be gathered and interpreted through the aid of nonverbal cues. Nonverbal communication is also considered in detail in Chapter 5.

Self-Identify

> To my kidney sister: I think of you whenever I go to the bathroom.

This was inscribed on a picture given by a 17-year-old girl named Maria to her 14-year-old "sister," Laura [56]. These two girls were very interested in each other's health, shared close feelings, and asked to room together whenever they were both hospitalized at the same time. But it was not their close friendship that made these girls consider themselves to be sisters. Rather, it was that each of them had received a kidney transplant from the same cadaver.

Your identity—who you think you are—is an important element of how you cope with the stresses of life. How do you know who you are? Are you your body?

First let us consider where identity begins [32]. Although it is hard to know for sure, it appears that a newborn infant does not have much sense of self. For example, an infant cannot understand the difference between a pain due to diaper rash and a pain caused by a sharp toy poking its foot. With age, the infant learns to move its foot and other body parts in response to environmental stimuli and thus discovers that the body is an important part of its identity. A woman, for example, will find that losing a breast affects her sense of self. If someone receives a kidney transplant from someone else, this person may begin to believe that the organ donor is part of him or herself. Transplant patients often must deal with this new aspect of identity [14, 22].

A much more important part of identity comes from interactions with other people. To understand this point, it is helpful to begin by thinking about animals. Does a dog have an identity? Sure, it will answer to "Fido," but does it really have a self-concept? Does a gold-fish have an identity? Or a cockroach? A psychologist named Gordon Gallup studied this question in primates [26]. Gallup gave primates mirrors to play with. Later, he painted an odorless red stripe above their eyebrows. Higher apes like chimps looked into the mirror, saw the stripe, and reached up to their face to try to pull it off. They thus knew it was them in the mirrors and so at least had some sense of self. Lower primates such as monkeys never developed this ability. Interestingly, chimps raised in isolation (away from other chimps) never did develop this "sense of self."

Now think about a little girl who tells visiting relatives, "I'm very pretty." This statement is part of her identity, but where did it come from? We might think that it came from an objective self-examination in a mirror until we realize that many little tots also proclaim, "I'm very pretty," even if they are not. Such self-knowledge probably often comes from people around the child, especially parents. If Mommy and Daddy continually say, "You're a pretty little girl" or "You're a handsome little gent," the children will often come to believe it. This point was made early in this century by the philosopher-sociologists George Herbert Mead and Charles Cooley [13, 48]. They suggested that identity comes from what people think others think of them. But identity is always changing, especially if people become ill and are cast into the role of a patient. As we will see, patients encounter many communications and expectations from others. If patients think that others around them think they are "ill" or "disgusting" or "pitiful" or "weak," they will often come to believe it themselves [69].

After Chapter 5, where we emphasize the importance of communication to patient care, we focus more directly on the patient's identity and illness behaviors. In Chapter 6, "The Nature of Illness," we examine factors that make patients define themselves as ill, the expectations others have of people who are ill, and the special treatment afforded the ill. The practitioner's and the patient's expectations and explanations of illness are a key part of the health care process.

Dying of a Broken Heart

Heart disease is the number-one killer in the United States [67]. Most people know someone who has had a heart attack. However, when we say that someone has died of a "broken heart," we do not mean that the person's heart has lost its blood supply, has ruptured, or has merely quit pumping. Rather, we are referring to an emotional problem that we believe led to physical demise. The broken heart results from some disruption in interpersonal relations, such as the loss of a loved one, and the emotional trauma is thought to interfere with the process of living.

Does the emotional distress of a "broken heart" really interfere with the body's physical functioning? Can a person die of a broken heart? The scientific answer is, definitely yes. Various aspects of psychological stress and emotional upset produce unhealthy and even ultimately fatal bodily reactions [11, 27, 45, 52, 57, 68]. The psychological and social influences on illness and the pathways through which they may operate are described in Chapter 7, "Psychological Factors in the Etiology of Illness" (see also Box 1-1).

Heart transplants are extremely expensive and very risky. They epitomize the traditional medical approach; that is, wait until something goes wrong, then fix it. Sometimes, as in the use of antibiotics to treat infection, this approach is tremendously successful. In the case of heart disease, however, it seems much more reasonable to *prevent* the development of disease. Fortunately, research has established that the likelihood of developing heart disease can be greatly reduced. Major risk factors include hypertension, diabetes, family history, and smoking. Interestingly, it appears that one set of

---

Box 1-1
Patients' Perceptions and Health

One way in which a patient's perceptions can affect health is through the patient's behavior. A strange but fascinating example comes from the case of a young Florida woman who died from an overdose of water.

Tina's mother died of stomach cancer. Tina soon became convinced that she also had stomach cancer. Doctors told her she did not. But her expectations were more important than the doctor's diagnoses. She did not cooperate with medical treatment.

To cleanse her stomach of cancer, Tina developed a treatment in which she didn't eat, but flooded her body by drinking gallons of water each day. The tremendous amount of fluid intake upset her body's chemical balance. Furthermore, Tina was drinking so much water that her kidneys could not keep up with it. Some of the water drained into her lungs and she drowned. News reports quoted the medical examiner as saying, "It's unbelievable, but it happened."

Information reported in *Newsweek*, March 14, 1977.

---

factors influencing health is social psychological in nature. Chapter 7 also examines the affects of stress, life-change events, and the lack of social support during illness, and the links between a specific behavior pattern—the coronary-prone personality—and coronary heart disease are considered [16, 25, 33].

Giving and Health Care

For an organ transplant to take place, there must be an organ donor. The donor usually faces a significant risk to his or her own health and certainly a period of discomfort [22]. Yet many people donate a kidney to another person (usually a family member) and often feel very gratified for having done so [20]. Similarly, many thousands of people freely donate blood to blood banks each year. In certain situations, people are very willing to contribute to the health and wellbeing of others [4]. Altruism is an important aspect of health care.

Millions of Americans suffer from a chronic illness—some condition such as kidney disease, arthritis, heart disease, or paralysis—that prevents them from engaging in some major, normal activity. Even if they appear "normal" to the casual observer, many people must live daily with one or more serious health problems. They must deal with occasional medical crises, control their symptoms, and manage their daily lives while at the same time avoiding social isolation and other problems in dealing with people [63]. People with chronic illness can often be completely successful if they have the unselfish cooperation of others. Such issues in dealing with chronic illness are discussed in Chapter 8, "Chronic Illness: Psychosocial Aspects of Disability."

Many factors contribute to people's desire to help with the long-term care of others. At the most basic level altruism probably has some basis in biology: In most social animals (including people), parents go to great lengths to care for their young, and members of the species seem predisposed to cooperate with each other. But of course people often do *not* help each other. Helping is influenced by upbringing and by the demands of the social situation.

Most religions and moral codes stress the value of helping others. Such norms or shared expectations are very strong in the field of medicine, where the patient's well-being is seen to be of paramount importance. If doctors and nurses were viewed as mere technicians and hospitals and nursing homes were seen as treatment centers comparable to auto repair shops, the nature of medicine would change dramatically [17]. Similarly, the emphases in the health field on a person's responsibility for helping others, on praise for good care, on setting a good example for others, and on the inner joy of saving lives are integral parts of the "art" of medicine. Such social expectations are rarely explicitly stated and analyzed. But they go a long way toward making a person willing to donate an organ to someone else and toward allowing society to accommodate those with serious chronic disabilities.

Loneliness

The poet John Donne wrote, "No man is an island, entire of itself." People are involved with and dependent on many other people. People are social beings, which is why social psychology is relevant to health and well-being. Loneliness is generally a negative state, even if one has enough "physical" goods such as food, clothing, and shelter. Almost everyone is lonely at one time or another, but people without close intimate relationships, such as college students living away from home and people who have lost their spouses, are especially likely to be lonely.

Illness may promote loneliness [51, 63]. Many of our relationships come from our work and our involvement in the community. If one is confined to bed or to a hospital, these social relationships are disrupted [12]. Furthermore, relationships with health care personnel are built on the basis of social expectations or roles, not usually on the basis of true intimacy. (For example, you are not likely to invite your physician to your home to sip wine and watch TV.) In some cases, loneliness may lead to depression, drug abuse, and even suicide [49].

Loneliness is sometimes caused by the death of a loved one. John Donne's poem continues, "any man's death diminishes me because I am involved in mankind; and therefore never send to know for whom the bell tolls; it tolls for thee." Many people are upset by the death of someone they know, but the effect is especially devastating when the person was someone who provided psychological support and was an intimate friend or constant companion. A bereaved person must pass through various stages of recovery [35]. Knowledge of these reactions can help ease that transition. The death of a patient also has effects on health care personnel, although such factors and stresses were mostly ignored until recent years. Now, however, they are seen as an integral aspect of medicine, and we discuss them in Chapter 9, "Dying and Death."

With many diseases, such as certain forms of cancer, the fact of impending death becomes known to health personnel, to family members, and often to patients themselves. We say "often to patients" because in the past this news was often withheld from the terminally ill patient. The great ambivalence of others about discussing a patient's impending death with him or her illustrates the importance of social psychological issues to this aspect of medical care. Partly out of fear and ignorance and partly out of a desire to protect themselves from becoming too close to someone they will soon lose, people may avoid or distance themselves from a dying patient. If such reactions occur, the patient may of course become extremely lonely [37, 41]. Such loneliness only compounds the lonely feelings caused by the relative social isolation from job and community. Thus loneliness is a major problem facing the dying. It worsens the many other troubling psychological reactions that a dying person may face. These various reactions to dying, and ways in which health personnel and family members can help, are also considered in Chapter 9.

The Heart Surgeons

On December 3, 1967, Dr. Christiaan Barnard of South Africa carried out the first human heart transplant. This operation, a major scientific breakthrough, ushered in a new era of medical technology. However, the timing of the event and the accolades to Dr. Barnard were not purely scientific. It was obvious that the technology for the operation had existed for a long time, for once the first transplant was performed, many others were soon undertaken at various medical centers around the world [66]. Social factors influenced whether the operation was seen as "acceptable." In addition, there was quite a bit of pressure on individual heart surgeons. A successful transplant surgeon could become famous and thus attract a good deal of money to his or her medical center. Furthermore, heart surgeons became "celebrities" and had reputations to worry about. For example, Thomas Thompson wrote a book, *Hearts,* about the exciting personal competition between two famous Texas heart surgeons— Dr. Michael DeBakey and Dr. Denton Cooley [66]. Physicians, like all people, are influenced by the social pressures and expectations of others. In Chapter 10, we examine "The Health Care Professional."

Surgeons are special people. They receive nine, ten, or more years of very specialized training after college, more training than is required for almost any other occupation. Most of this training is very demanding, requiring long hours and both extensive knowledge and a high degree of manual skill. In the operating room, the patient's life is in the hands of the surgeon. Surgeons are also among the most highly paid professionals. They generally are accorded a high degree of respect from the general population. It is interesting to note that very few surgeons are women [21]. Becoming a surgeon is not only a technical scientific process; it is also a social process.

The stresses and contradictions of being a medical intern are dramatized with sardonic humor in *The House of God,* a novel by Samuel Shem [58]. Although the public expects physicians to be wise, knowledgeable, dedicated, hardworking, and selfless, the medical intern may see medical training as a challenge to his or her own survival. There are many contradictions between the goals of helping others according to hospital policy and the necessity of maintaining one's own physical and mental health and one's own personal relationships. These dilemmas create some of the major challenges of modern medical training [8, 9]. An overstressed or an alcoholic physician is not of much help to patients. For example, in the hospital called the House of God, the interns are advised that when there is a case of cardiac arrest, the first thing they should do is take their own pulse. Similarly, Shem writes that a law of the hospital is that "the patient is the one with the disease." Such humorous sayings reveal the unique pressures of medical training, which we also examine in Chapter 10.

Healthy Situations

We touch on the issue of self-image at various points in this book but there is one area where it is likely to be overlooked. This is the *maintenance* of a healthy body. To a large extent maintaining a healthy and attractive appearance is under an individual's control. Overeating, poor nutrition, smoking, and alcohol and drug abuse have dramatic effects on health and attractiveness. And such abuses are often closely tied to problems of self-image. Issues of physical appearance may also lead directly to, or result directly from, problems with sexual relations. Consider the example of obesity, a state in which the body's physical structure and the self-identity are closely related [53, 54]. Obese people tend to think of themselves as "fatties" and "dessert pigs." And they often have trouble attracting members of the opposite sex. Effective treatment seems to necessitate an improvement in self-image: from feeling hopeless, ugly, and fat to achieving a sense of control over one's body [15, 30].

Healthy situations extend beyond the personal to the total health care environment. For example, organ transplants cannot be performed in the doctor's office or in a clinic. Rather, the whole supporting system of a large hospital is required, including assisting doctors and nurses, special equipment, preoperative and postoperative laboratory tests, and a variety of health maintenance procedures. Prior to surgery, a heart patient will have his or her heartbeat recorded by an electrocardiogram, have blood flow studied with cardiac catheterization, be given various blood and urine tests, have chest x rays taken, and so on. The surgery itself may be extremely complex, and postoperative care may require sophisticated monitoring equipment. Yet hospitalization also involves many other changes and procedures that are nonmedical and may at first be overlooked. Patients trade their usual clothes for hospital gowns, are awakened and served food at regular hours, live and sleep in close proximity to strangers, may have their sleep interrupted for testing, and encounter a number of different staff members. In short, the patient's social life is novel, lacking in privacy, and strictly regulated. These social psychological factors in hospitalization may in some cases be just as important to consider when treating the patient as the strictly medical procedures [44, 60, 65].

Disregard of social psychological factors in hospitalization has caused many people to dread hospitals. More importantly, a poor social environment in a hospital may interfere with the patient's recovery. Such problems are not the result of a lack of dedication of hospital personnel. On the contrary, the problems generally result from the nature and structure of hospitals [50]. To combat these pressures, many hospitals have recently instituted a "patient's bill of rights," which is designed to improve the social and physical environment of the hospitalized patient. We consider the reasons for such interventions in Chapter 11, "The Health Care Environment."

Hospitalization is a special problem for the elderly, who are more likely to have chronic conditions requiring constant care [36]. Although we touch on the special problems of various age groups throughout this book, we give special attention to the elderly in Chapter 11.

Medical Ethics

Several years ago, the case of a man with aplastic anemia made headlines. This often fatal disease of the bone marrow can sometimes be helped by a bone marrow transplant. In the case in ques-

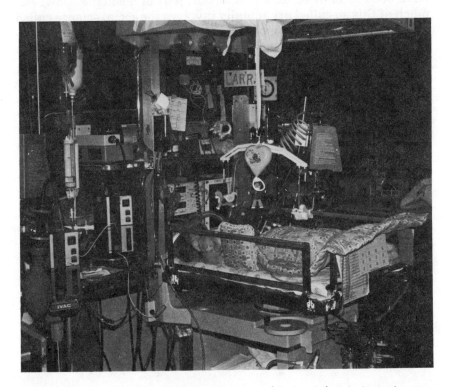

Figure 1-2. The colorful mobile hanging over this tiny infant in intensive care adds a human dimension to highly sophisticated technical care. (Photo by Howard S. Friedman, © 1982)

tion, the only known perfect "match" for a tissue transplant was the patient's cousin, who refused to agree to the relatively safe procedure.

The patient went to court, asking the judge to order the cousin to agree to the procedure. However, the judge ruled that such an operation could not be forced on an individual, even to save another's life. Needless to say, the family relations involving these people became quite strained.

Modern medical procedures like transplants raise many questions of ethics. Sometimes the ethical challenges grow directly out of a biological issue such as whether a dangerous but promising new drug should be tried. Often, however, the problems involve a significant element of interpersonal relations. We touch on such ethical issues throughout this book.

In sum, most of medicine, even including such technical procedures as surgical organ transplantation, involves a significant element of interpersonal relations. Traditionally, "art" and "intuition" have been recognized as an important part of medicine. However, much of this so-called art actually involves the social science called social psychology. This book applies the findings of social psychology to medicine for the student interested in the field of health care.

2

The
Art of
Medicine

In all cultures, certain individuals are designated caretakers of the sick. In traditional Mexican culture, for example, the *curandero* treats patients with religious symbols and herbal remedies. In American Indian cultures, medicine men have traditionally treated illness with a variety of techniques, including dancing, shaking rattles, and beating drums. American evangelical religious leaders may include singing, prayer, and other religious rites in their approach to healing. These diverse individuals play the role of healer [36].

In mainstream American society, on the other hand, the healing roles are filled by physicians, nurses, and allied health personnel such as pharmacists, medical technicians, and social workers. These healers possess many attributes that are not logically required by their work. For example, unlike Soviet doctors, who have relatively low status, American physicians have a great deal of prestige and power. Americans do not value their leaders, their workers, or their craftsmen as much as they value their physicians. In fact, surveys have shown that the job of physician ranks second in prestige only to that of Supreme Court Justice. In exchange for this prestige, most Americans expect their physicians to be wise and professional, caring and sensitive, and generally deserving of respect. They expect this of nurses and other health care professionals as well. The job of the health professional is thus in many ways special in terms of the expectations of others [8, 28, 36, 45].

The Role of the Health Professional

Respect and power are accorded physicians for three major reasons. First, the job of a health professional requires a high degree of technical competence. Physicians, nurses, dentists, and physicians' assistants are extensively trained: their formal education may continue up to ten years beyond college. They differ from other skilled individuals, however, in that they have access to a body of knowledge that is difficult or impossible for a person who is not a health professional to acquire. A person with a severe sore throat and earache finds it nearly impossible to make an accurate diagnosis and obtain treatment without help from a health expert. Health care professionals have access to necessary knowledge and resources that the lay public cannot easily obtain.

Even if the knowledge and resources of health professionals were generally available, health professionals probably would still be held in awe. Automobile mechanics, for example, have a distinct body of knowledge that is not generally available to most untrained individuals. So do the computer programmers in a bank who diagnose and repair problems in monthly bank statements. But the car mechanic and the computer programmer are dealing with problems that have limited impact on the individual who must deal with them. People can forget for a while that their car does not work or that their bank statement does not match the checkbook total. But it is difficult to forget a very painful sore throat and earache when continually trying to swallow. Problems with body functions are problems central to the person; they are not easily ignored and are usually accompanied by strong emotion [43]. The health care professionals who can solve these problems find themselves endowed with great respect and awe, for they deal with issues of life and death.

Second, the power and respect accorded health professionals is hinted at by the following questions: Should physicians devote a great deal of their time to financial investments? Should physicians be involved in elaborate real estate sales deals or in owning convalescent homes? Should nurses demand higher wages and go on strike, leaving hospitalized patients unattended? Many professionals invest their money, and many union members strike. Should health professionals be any different?

These questions illustrate the point that the health professional is expected to show a high degree of commitment to serving people. That is, the health professional is supposed to be concerned about the welfare of others and to focus primarily on helping people. It is expected that nurses, paramedics, and physicians chose the health profession primarily because of their desire to serve others. Money, status, power, and intellectual challenge are expected to be secondary considerations. Whether this assumption is realistic or not, the primary goal of health professionals is expected to be caring for *people,* and not financial gain. Health professionals are respected partly because they are presumably less concerned with their own financial gain than are other workers in society. For this reason "transgressions" by health care professionals receive very negative responses from society.

Third, the awe and respect given to health professionals may be because they are viewed as nonjudgmental and emotionally neutral. Health professionals learn a great deal of intimate information about patients. For example, a physician might ask a patient if he or she has had regular bowel movements or ask about the most intimate details of sexual functioning. Patients in fact often disclose their thoughts and feelings more readily to physicians and nurses than to their thoughts and feelings more readily to physicians and nurses than to their closest friends or spouses. Therefore the physician or nurse is put into a position that requires objectivity. It would not be appropriate for a nurse or doctor to be judgmental toward a patient, for example, by giving a lecture on religious morality. The health professional's role involves simply learning as much as he or she can about the patient, avoiding negative judgments about the patient as a person, and helping the patient to engage in healthful behaviors.

Sociologists and psychologists who theorized about the relationship between health care professionals and patients originally proposed that emotional neutrality and objectivity also meant cold detachment [45]. It was assumed that because health professionals deal all day long with such traumatic events as patients' dying, they must remain emotionally detached from their patients. The assumption was that they needed to treat the disease and ignore the person with the illness. But research on physician–patient relationships such as described in Renée Fox's book *Experiment Perilous* and other works has shown that detachment is really not possible for physicians and other health care professionals [25]. They become acutely aware of the patient as a person and are strongly affected by the human side of medicine. Health professionals are personally touched when their patients suffer, and they strive to learn as much as possible about the patient as a person in order to best help the patient (see Chapter 3) [58]. Studies of the job satisfaction of physicians show, for example, that the human communication found in teaching and caring for patients is the most rewarding aspect of the physician's role [24].

Emotional detachment is not only very difficult for health professionals to maintain, but it is also not good for patients. For a variety of reasons, which are discussed in Chapters 3, 4, and 5, patients need to be treated as individual people. The manner in which health professionals treat patients—their caring, concern, kindness, and understanding—can have important implications for patients' health. We will find that patients' willingness to cooperate with recommended treatments (e.g., to take medication) is highly influenced by the manner in which the regimen is prescribed during the course of the professional-patient relationship. Furthermore, a patients' level of anxiety can be considerably reduced if the health care professional is not cold and emotionally detached but rather is concerned enough to speak openly and empathetically with the patient.

Thus, patients' expectations about their doctors' behavior are very specific, and these expectations need to be fulfilled in order for doctors to command their patients' respect. In exchange for prestige and power, all health professionals are expected to develop a significant degree of technical expertise, be totally oriented toward serving people (often at cost to themselves, such as overwhelming fatigue), and in a nonjudgmental manner be caring and concerned with the feelings of patients [11]. This is a tall order for anyone to fulfill.

The Role of the Patient

There are also demands made on patients. When people become ill they occupy what the sociologist Talcott Parsons called "the sick role" [46, 47]. Considered briefly, the sick role involves certain expectations people share about the rights and obligations of the person who is ill. The sick individual is relieved of normal social responsibilities such as going to work and taking care of others. He or she is allowed to refrain from contributing to production in society [39]. In return for this right, the sick person is expected to seek competent medical help and to profess a desire to get well. The individual who is ill has an obligation to seek the advice of a medical expert and to follow that advice [41, 46, 47]. We will discuss this concept in more detail in Chapter 6 as we consider the meaning of illness.

A Historical Perspective

From the earliest times in the history of medicine, physicians such as Hippocrates (the fourth-century B.C. Greek physician, called the "Father of Medicine") recognized how important it is for health care professionals to deliver care to their patients with understanding and sensitivity [32]. Hippocrates wrote about the interpersonal

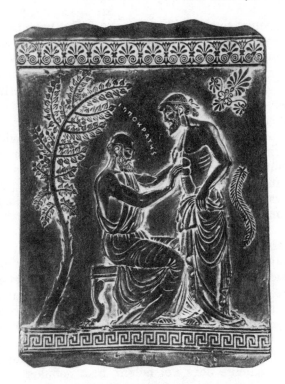

Figure 2-1. Hippocrates examining a patient.
(By permission of Professor L. J. Bruce-Chwatt,
the Wellcome Museum of Medical Science,
London, England.)

transaction between health professional and patient, stating that
while the health care professional should not allow the patient's
sentiments to lead him or her to deliver care that is inappropriate,
the health care professional should practice a science of effective
human relations. The health professional should learn to modify the
negative sentiments and fears of patients with hope and positive
behavior.

In this century the prominent medical educator Frederick Shattuck
wrote in 1907 that a serious problem in health care would occur if the
gap between the science of medicine and its actual practice were to
grow [52]. Shattuck suggested that the gap could be bridged by the
art of medicine. We must remember that disease is one phenomenon
whereas the diseased *person* is another. Shattuck wrote of the importance of sensitivity and genuine concern for patients' feelings
when taking a history, for much can be learned about patients from

the way in which they tell their stories. Another prominent educator, Sir William Osler, in 1899 recommended that a health care professional *listen* to the patient, for the patient may actually reveal the diagnosis [44]. The early physicians were, in sum, suggesting a certain sensitivity on the part of the health care professional in dealing with patients.

Hippocrates also spoke of the importance of the health care professional's manner in dealing with patients. He suggested that "the patient, though conscious that his condition is perilous, may recover his health simply through his contentment with the goodness of the physician." How is this goodness communicated? He suggested that the health care professional monitor his or her behaviors and always be in control, communicating calmness and positivity to the patient.

Many writers have assumed that relating to patients in an artful manner involves simply good manners, respect, and compassion [12, 30]. Physicians often see the art of medicine as "common sense." As we will see, however, these behaviors are far from simple. There are many pressures from within the structure of the health care delivery system to treat patients as objects and to attend to the disease and not the patient. Many factors operate to reduce communication between health care professionals and their patients.

The art of medicine does not belong in a nebulous, ill-defined realm, however. In order to enact successfully the art of medicine the health care professional needs to understand many key social psychological issues [17, 23, 56]. These include verbal and nonverbal communication of the patient, the sociocultural context of behavior, and the effects of the physician's own verbal and nonverbal communications to the patient. The health care professional also needs specific information regarding the problems in social relationships that are faced by patients with problems like cancer. Specific information is necessary for effectively dealing with patients and for developing the art of medicine [23, 33]. It involves both a positive attitude toward the patient and a *knowledge* of what to do in specific circumstances. Complete, effective care of a patient is not an accident. It comes from fully acknowledging the psychosocial factors in the care of patients [8].

THE SIGNIFICANCE OF THE
ART OF MEDICINE
IN CARING FOR PATIENTS

Mr. Pratt is a coronary patient whose rehabilitation requires a salt-free diet, weight loss pills, and engaging in an exercise program. His doctor is an excellent physician, but too busy to give Mr. Pratt the reassurance he needs. Mr. Pratt suffers from anxiety about his heart condition, but his doctor does not know this. Although he may not recognize it, Mr. Pratt's lack of faith in his doctor makes it hard for him to maintain his difficult rehabilitation regimen.

Mr. Warner, on the other hand, has the same condition but feels quite satisfied that he is being taken care of completely and effectively. His confidence in his doctor helps him face his difficult treatment regimen. When Mr. Warner started to become anxious about his heart condition, he told his doctor and felt better after their discussion. The art of medicine has important implications for health care.

Patient Cooperation

The most important factor contributing to patient cooperation (compliance) is the art of medicine in the health professional–patient relationship [31, 33, 48]. The multidimensional character of the art of medicine as it affects patient compliance tells us a great deal about the importance of various aspects of the art of medicine. That is, there are many different kinds of behaviors by health professionals that can affect patients' compliance. Analyzing these behaviors tells us a great deal about what the art of medicine is and why it is important.

Communication. The importance of clear and free communication between the health care professional and the patient has been discovered again and again in research. One series of studies was conducted in Children's Hospital in Los Angeles by Dr. Barbara Korsch and her colleagues [26, 38]. In these studies, researchers tape recorded conversations between pediatricians and the mothers of their patients. These tape recordings were analyzed carefully, and it was found that physicians whose patients were noncompliant were often vague in communicating with the mothers. They tended to use medical jargon often (e.g., "We have to watch the Coombs titre") and did not take time to answer questions thoroughly or to determine whether each mother understood what was wrong with her child and exactly how to carry out the prescribed treatment. Noncompliance can be the direct result of poor communication, because the patient never learns, understands, or remembers the treatment regimen [4]. We discuss these communication issues more thoroughly in Chapter 5.

A physician who takes time to collect information from the patient and gives little or no information back *to* the patient suggests that the patient's concerns are being avoided; the patient probably feels that he or she is not being treated as a valuable person [15, 54]. When the disclosure of information about illness is one sided, with the patient telling a great deal to the health care professional and the professional simply collecting the information from a superior position, showing little or no reaction, the patient is likely to be uncooperative.

In fact, social psychologists have consistently found in research on human interaction that "reciprocity" (give and take) is necessary in order to maintain a relationship and to continue it in a mutually satisfying manner [7]. Reciprocity in self-disclosure requires disclosure by the health care professional as well the patient. Self-disclosure is important to the development of a respectful and caring health professional–patient relationship.

Rapport.   The *quality* of the interaction between the health care professional and the patient—involving, for example, caring, concern, respect, and understanding—is critical in its influence on patient cooperation [15]. If these components of the art of medical care are missing, patients tend to be less likely to comply. For example, in one study researchers found that patients who were most likely to fail to keep their appointments in an outpatient referral clinic were patients who felt that they had no doctor with whom they could talk and that doctors in general were not interested in their patients [2]. When anger and hostility felt toward patients are communicated to them by health care professionals, noncooperation results [42, 49].

Responsiveness.   Patient cooperation is also affected by the provider's responsiveness to the patient's needs as a person [31]. As discussed in Chapter 3, many psychological, environmental, and social factors in patients' lives exert significant influences on the tendencies of patients to cooperate with their medical regimens [16]. Their attitudes, health beliefs, and intentions to cooperate are also important [1, 3]. Health care professionals must learn about the social psychological and cultural facets of their patients' problems as well as the physiological characteristics and become sufficiently aware of the norms and values to which the various patients subscribe in order to be sure that the health regimens prescribed can be realistically followed [14, 19]. If a diet prescribed for a patient with a strong religious orientation or cultural identification is not easily compatible with the religious dietary prescriptions or cultural habits of the patient, this patient is unlikely to follow the diet.

Thus the art of medicine as it affects one of the most important aspects of patient care—patient cooperation—has many facets. Research has shown that the important elements of the health care professional's treatment of patients include (a) establishing effective communication with patients, (b) developing rapport with the patient, and (c) understanding the patient's social, psychological, and cultural environment [31]. The goal of much of this book (especially Chapters 3, 5, 6, 7, and 8) is to prepare the health professional to deal with these issues effectively so that the patient can be helped to cooperate.

In the examples of Mr. Pratt and Mr. Warner we observed two heart patients who may or may not cooperate with their treatment depending on the quality of the professional-patient interaction—the art of medicine. However, there are two other important reasons why the art of medicine is crucial to proper medical care. First, the art of medicine may directly affect the outcome of treatment; the expert use of biological science is not sufficient. Second, the art of medicine affects patient satisfaction with medical care. A dissatisfied patient can be both dangerous and expensive, in various ways. We now examine these topics as they occur in the art of medicine.

The Outcome of Treatment

Early in the history of medicine it was recognized that the health care professional personally can be a therapeutic agent who is just as effective as a drug or therapeutic procedure. Although we consider this notion in Chapter 4, when discussing placebos, we mention it here in connection with the art of medicine. The manner in which care is delivered—the positive expectations that are communicated to the patient—may at least in part be responsible for the patient's getting well. It has been suggested that the history of medicine is in fact the history of the communication of comfort and positive expectations from physician to patient [50, 51]. When treatment administered by health professionals had no scientific basis and no specific positive pharmacological effects, health professionals, particularly physicians, remained in high esteem because they actually could cure their patients' symptoms with surprising frequency. The art of medicine, particularly the interpersonal behavior of the health care professionals—their warmth, humanism, and enthusiasm—has been shown to affect the outcome of treatment.

Surgical Patients. Four researchers from Massachusetts General Hospital in Boston demonstrated the importance of good anesthetist-patient communication [20, 21]. In this study almost 100 surgical patients were randomly divided into two groups, an experimental group and a control group. The experimental group patients were told about the postoperative pain they would experience and how to relax in order to reduce the pain. The anesthetist gave these patients both information and a pep talk about how to deal with the impending surgery. The other patients, from the control group, were not told about their postoperative pain, and they received the usual preoperative preparation. While the experimental and control groups did not differ on the first postoperative day, after that time the group of patients given the special anesthetist visit and information required significantly less pain medication than the patients from the control group. Furthermore, their surgeons decided that some of these patients were well enough to be discharged from the hospital earlier than the control group patients. The surgeons were "blind" to the condition in the experiment in which the patient had participated; that is, they were unaware of which kind of preoperative preparation the patient had received. The patients in the experimental group were discharged an average of 2.7 days earlier than the other group of patients.

The results of this study demonstrate that a good relationship between the health care professional and patient in which the health care professional makes an effort to reach out to his or her patient with reassurance and information can influence the outcome of a purely technical procedure such as surgery. Similar research by the same authors has shown that visits by an informative, caring anesthetist relaxed patients and made them as calm and drowsy before surgery as did phenobarbitol. Patients who are drowsy and calm before surgery require less anesthesia during the surgery—a distinct positive therapeutic effort contributing to the patient's more immediate postoperative recovery as well as his or her greater chances of surviving surgery.

Heart Attack Patients. The interpersonal behavior of health care professionals toward their patients can actually influence the patients' observable physiological condition. Studies have shown that a physician's behavior can affect the stability of the hearts of patients who have suffered coronaries [34]. In one study, it was found that a significantly large number of cardiac patients who had been stable and recovering from their heart attacks in the hospital actually suddenly died of a second heart attack during or very shortly after ward rounds. Ward rounds are generally very stressful for patients, often because physicians behave in a very formal, aloof manner and frequently discuss the patient's illness in front of him or her. Patients may respond with fear, confusion, and distress to such formality and to the use of unintelligible technical jargon regarding their own bodies and malfunctions. Other researchers partially explained the sudden deaths by showing in their research that human contact can have a major effect on the cardiac rhythm and the electrical impulses of the hearts of cardiac patients [40]. These matters are considered in detail in Chapter 7.

Patient Satisfaction

A final important consequence of the concerned communication, rapport, and respect shown by the health care professional involves the patient's satisfaction with the medical care received. When rapport is missing, patients tend to turn from the medical profession to nonmedical healers, or bring medical malpractice suits against physicians and hospitals.

The health care professional–patient relationship has been shown to be seen as very important to patients—the consumers of health care. Surveys have revealed that patients' greatest criticism about health care tends to center around the nature of the doctor–patient relationship [10, 27, 37, 53]. A majority of patients feel that the technique-centered medical practice of today lacks human warmth. Patients feel that in addition to medical competence, the delivery of effective medical care requires taking an interest in the patient as a person. Knowledge, skill, intelligence, and training must be accompanied by kindness, understanding, sympathy, interest, and encouragement.

Doctor-Shopping. Each time a patient changes doctors, it is an expensive and time-consuming event. The new primary care physician must repeat a medical history, conduct a physical examination and systems review, and also perform the necessary diagnostic tests. Sometimes it is necessary for a patient to change doctors, for example, if the physician or patient changes location or if the physician retires or dies. But many times patients end the physician-patient relationship simply because they are displeased with the interpersonal behavior of the physician [29, 35].

Studies of the phenomenon of doctor-shopping reveal that few patients terminate the relationship with their physician because they believe the physician is incompetent technically [5, 6, 8, 68], but rather it is because of the way in which health professionals have behaved toward the patients. In fact, most patients probably cannot effectively judge the technical competence of their physicians or other health care practitioners. Patients instead tend to judge technical competence and base their trust in the physician on what is referred to as the "socioemotional" aspects of care—the components of the art of medicine that we discussed earlier [8].

Patients of course care about the technical quality of the health care that is delivered to them but tend to assume that a certain basic level of technical expertise can be expected. Beyond that they focus on the interpersonal side of care—that is, how their health care professionals treat them. Patients in one study changed primary care physicians almost exclusively because of what they called inadequate interpersonal treatment and attention. When questioned further, they revealed that their dissatisfaction was with the socioemotional dimension of care. Patients were most likely to terminate the physician–patient relationship if their physician was too busy to talk with them or appeared to be uninterested in their welfare [29]. In another study, it was found that doctor-shopping was significantly increased if patients disliked the doctor as a person, were dissatisfied with the amount of time spent in health delivery, or if they felt the physician was not interested in them as people [35]. Finally, in another study it was found that patients' intentions to return to a particular physician were dependent upon the patients' feeling that the physician listened to them, cared about them as people, explained their medical condition to them, were accessible, and took enough time with them [18]. The patients' perceptions about their physicians' degree of intellectual capability and seriousness, as well as their specific technical performance, were less important.

Rejection of the Medical Establishment. Another distressing result of patients' dissatisfaction with their medical care that sometimes occurs leads patients to inflict serious harm on themselves. Patients who discover that they are seriously ill need, as one might expect, much sympathy and understanding and also attention to their feelings, concerns, and fears. If their health care professionals do not provide these important aspects of care and give patients both reassurance and information about what will be done for them, seriously ill patients can easily feel abandoned by their physicians. They then are likely to reject the medical establishment and seek nonmedical cures.

Beatrix Cobb examined the reasons why some cancer patients reject the medical establishment (with its low but nevertheless existing cure rate for the disease) and seek nonmedical cures (usually religious healers or nonmedical [e.g., herbal] cures) [13]. From Cobb's many interviews, she learned that these patients felt they received little understanding and reassurance from their physicians and other health personnel and were not sure that all that could possibly be done would be done for them. The patients felt that because their illness was very serious and had a low cure rate, their health professionals treated them as terminal cases. Therefore the patients turned to nonmedical healers.

Malpractice Litigation. Malpractice insurance rates have skyrocketed in recent years, and the entire health care system appears to be alarmed at the extensive patient retaliation against physicians, hospitals, and even nurses and other health professionals. Nearly all patients tend to recognize and acknowledge that objectively there is a risk attached to any medical procedure and that medicine is not foolproof and the results of care may not meet with their expectations. After a failed treatment, this objective analysis does not always occur, however. In actuality, patients sometimes become distracted from an objective analysis. Often their emotionality and anger result from a breakdown in the health care professional–patient relationship.

In the ideal situation, the health care professional, usually the physician, carefully explains the medical procedure to the patient. All of the attendant risks are described, the expected results considered, and a trust is built up between the physician and the patient. A joint decision is then made, and if the treatment does not go as expected, the patient is informed and takes part in the additional decisionmaking.

In this ideal case, the patient can rely on the health care professional for continued support and for respect, care, and concern for him or her as a person. The patient is an active, rather than a passive, participant. Under these conditions, patients deal relatively well with problems that arise in their health care—even with physicians' errors. Cases have been reported in which after surgery a sponge was found to have been left in the patient, or a serious, correctable condition was missed in reading an x ray. Surprisingly, the health care professionals were not sued. Communication with the patient had been so open and honest that a solution to the problem was found without calling in a third party (i.e., a lawyer). Such is not the case, however, when the health care professional–patient relationship has gone awry. A psychological researcher and a lawyer have both written about the overwhelming influence of the health care professionals' behavior toward patients as an influence on the patients' decision to sue if the results are not completely satisfactory [9, 57].

It is important to note, however, that we are not suggesting that "malpractice"—the actual practice of medicine with negligence in which the health professional makes serious errors—does not exist.

Box 2-1
Ways to Minimize the Risk of Suits

(The following material is reprinted, with permission, from a pamphlet prepared by the Task Force on Professional Liability, American Academy of Family Physicians.)

Most physicians do practice good medicine.

The majority of awards paid out in professional liability claims are to patients dissatisfied with alleged missed or delayed diagnosis or with results of therapy, or to those who incur permanent minor or major injuries during the normal course of medical therapy.

Many "malpractice" suits against physicians have been initiated by patients improperly informed concerning the procedures to be carried out or the risks involved.

Other suits have been brought because once the patient develops a complication the physician appears to be less than honest and acts in a secretive or "guilty" manner, suggesting to the patient that the doctor really is at fault.

Claims may arise because physicians undertake procedures beyond their competence and, once having a complication, hesitate to get early and adequate consultation.

Here are a few things an individual physician can do to decrease the risk of professional liability claims and suits ...

In Your Practice

Know Your Abilities
Be sure you know your abilities and stay within your capabilities. You should be willing to refer or consult early when needed.

Participate in CME
Participate actively in continuing medical education including participation in risk management programs. A significant percentage of suits have been for misdiagnosis or failure to use an acceptable new form of therapy or diagnostic procedure.

Keep Thoughts Private
Keep your thoughts private concerning other physicians' capabilities or adequacy to manage a case. Discussions on such topics should be held only under appropriate circumstances, and should be handled in a positive way instead of a negative one.

Establish "Risk Management Committee"
Encourage your hospital to establish a risk management committee of the hospital medical staff to investigate all incidents and maloccurrences, to make sure that the patient is helped in the most aggressive, concerned and sympathetic manner and to prevent similar occurrences in the future.

Nofity Carrier Early
If you feel that an untoward incident or event is likely to cause a claim or suit, notify your insurance carrier early. Sometimes their early inter-

vention can head off an escalating chain of events and settle a problem with minimal expenditure of time and money. Insurance companies are doing more aggressive claims management, but to be most effective you need to notify them early.

With Your Patients . . .

Involve the Patient
Give your patients an adequate explanation of risks and possible complications and frankly discuss the fees involved before initiating treatment. Involve the patient in treatment and diagnostic decisions and document this involvement.

Avoid developing parent-child relationships with patients. Don't accept "You're the doctor, do what you think best." Such patients are escaping and want your omnipotent cure, but if things don't go well they also want you to have all the blame.

Second Opinion
Give all patients having major surgery or serious diseases the opportunity of a second opinion and document it in the record. With any medical high-risk or unusual procedure, such as hysterectomy in a woman who wants children, insist on a second opinion.

Be Completely Honest
If your patient develops complications or if there are untoward events, be completely honest. Be aggressive in management and get early consultation, if indicated. Be sure you keep good records of the events and your advice to the patient and family.

Confront Disgruntled Patient
If you feel that a patient is disgruntled, confront him as soon as possible and discuss the apparent concerns. Try to settle differences reasonably. This will usually defuse the problem.

Beware of Doctor Shoppers
Patients who talk down every physician they have seen prior to you will probably put you in that same group in the near future. Be wary of "doctor shoppers."

Likewise, if you find you are beginning to feel antagonistic toward a certain patient, you should refer that patient to another physician. Encourage good doctor–patient relationships.

Serve as Patient Advocate
If your patient has an untoward incident while hospitalized, such as an injury caused by falling out of bed, serve as his advocate and approach the problem aggressively with the hospital administration. Be sure the patient is cared for and financial differences settled before he leaves the institution.

And Finally
Remember . . . there is no substitute for care with caring. An honest, concerned, sympathetic attitude is your number one preventive measure—develop it.

Court cases are tried daily in which physicians and other health personnel are responsible for doing harm to their patients. There are many other cases, however, in which health professionals have practiced standard acceptable medical techniques. Yet, because of some unfortunate circumstance, the results were less satisfactory than expected. The patient then brings a lawsuit against the physician (or at least attempts to do so, consulting a lawyer to determine the strength of the case). Under which conditions do patients decide to attempt to file a malpractice suit, regardless of the actual degree of "malpractice"?

The analysis by a lawyer [57] and the research data by a psychologist [9] suggest that it is the nature of the health care professional–patient relationship that determines the patient's behavior more than any other factor. Physicians who become involved in malpractice litigation tend to be unwilling to communicate with their patients and to lack the skills of communication. They do not listen to patients, failing to explain treatment details and attendant risks to patients as well as to talk with them about their dissatisfactions. In fact, when something did go wrong, the physicians who were prone to being sued were unable to admit their own limitations. When faced with a poor treatment outcome they punished the suffering patient with indifference and rejection, and the patient responded with a lawsuit. A lawsuit was especially likely when the physician ignored the patient's complaints and sent the usual bill.

Physicians and other health professionals can help prevent malpractice litigation by acquiring the skills and orientation described in this book. With the medical malpractice problem as serious as it is today, this approach is certainly worth trying [55] (see Box 2-1).

SUMMARY

"Bedside manner" is an attribute of the successful health care practitioner. But what is it? In this chapter we have seen bedside manner described as practicing the art of medicine and *not* as something that happens automatically. Even with good intentions, health care professionals are not naturally endowed with the skills and knowledge to meet successfully all the requirements of effective, artful care. For example, it is one thing for a health care professional to acknowledge that he or she must *listen* to patients, but it is quite something else for the health care professional to acquire the skills of effective listening. That is, health providers must *learn* to communicate to the patient that he or she is understood,

Box 2–2
Patients Teach Doctors

An interesting innovation that may improve doctor–patient relationships involves the use of patients as instructors. Physicians-in-training usually do not receive any direct feedback from their patients as to how well they are conducting themselves. Patients are often expected to remain silent unless asked a direct question. However, certain patients with chronic illnesses are in an excellent position to evaluate how well a young doctor is doing both technically and interpersonally, and they may be able to help him or her improve.

A patient-instructor may be someone suffering from multiple sclerosis, emphysema, a heart murmur, or other chronic condition. After some basic medical training, such patients are made available to medical students. They are encouraged to respond to and instruct the students. Such patients are also willing and able to tell medical students such things as: their hands are too cold, they forgot to wash their hands, or certain mannerisms are anxiety provoking. In this way, medical students can quickly learn through experience to correct various difficulties.

to monitor his or her own cues, to observe the patient's cues, and to understand the social and psychological conditions (e.g., culture, religion, family, past experiences, and social expectations) that affect the ways in which the patient presents him or herself and which affect the patient's response to illness and medical care [22].

In the following chapters we consider these issues in detail, providing information that is currently available in the research literature and outlining ways in which this information is applicable to the care of patients and the delivery of effective health care. We provide information about the complex sociocultural influences on patients' responses to illness and medical care. We discuss the social psychological phenomena that occur in the health care professional-patient interaction, for example, the verbal and nonverbal aspects of listening to patients. We show how the health care professional can learn about patient anger, dissatisfaction, and pain by observing the patient's expressions and body movements, and how the health care professional can help the patient to feel cared about as a person. We consider such issues as the effect of stress on patients' health and the factors that contribute to patients' varying reactions to pain and illness.

Recent research strongly supports the notions of earlier physicians like Hippocrates, Shattuck, and Osler, who wrote of the importance of the interpersonal quality of the health care professional-patient relationship. There is a growing awareness that a scientific, rational approach to the teaching and practice of the *"art"* of medicine is indeed possible. Research on patient satisfaction strongly suggests that physicians and other health care professionals who hope to satisfy their patients must learn to communicate concern as well as learn to listen to and educate their patients (see also Box 2-2).

3
Patient Cooperation with Treatment

Mr. Castiglione, a 46-year-old husband and father of three teenage children, is a truck driver. After a few weeks of experiencing chest pain and discomfort, Mr. Castiglione went to his family doctor. After a series of tests Dr. Johnson confirmed his suspected diagnosis; Mr. Castiglione had angina and high blood pressure. Over the span of the next few visits, Dr. Johnson followed the usual course of treatment for such cases. He prescribed the antihypertensive medication methyldopa, a diuretic (water pill), and a salt-free diet. He told Mr. Castiglione to "take it easy," to stop smoking, and to lose weight. Dr. Johnson's recommendations were sound medical advice.

Mr. Castiglione stopped taking the methyldopa when, to his dismay, it seemed to cause him to be impotent. He kept forgetting to take the diuretic. Because he was on the road so often in his job, the salt-free diet was almost impossible for him to follow. He eliminated desserts from his diet and was able to lose a few pounds. Driving his truck at all hours of the night, however, tempted him to smoke and to drink a great deal of coffee. Mr. Castiglione could not take it easy because he was determined to save the money required to send his children to college. When Dr. Johnson saw Mr. Castiglione on a followup visit, he reprimanded his patient for not following medical advice. Dr. Johnson labeled Mr. Castiglione an "uncooperative patient."

Patients usually face many obstacles in their search for advice from their health professionals. They have to make advance appointments and obtain transportation to their clinic or private physician. They must fill out forms and disclose information about themselves, wait long periods of time, explain their conditions to the health care professionals, and then submit to a physical examination and diagnostic tests. Finally, the patient is usually required to pay directly or indirectly (through insurance) for the service. After all this, many patients fail to follow their doctors' orders. About one-third of all patients do not cooperate with the medical recommendations given to them [4, 14].

Patient noncompliance with medical regimens seems at first glance to be clearly irrational behavior. It is certainly costly and a waste of medical expertise and the resources of health care. The noncompliance of patients with medical regimens is also dangerous to patients, for they may remain uncured or develop serious complications from their conditions [40]. In spite of these dangers, lack of cooperation is widespread. How can we explain it? How can we prevent it?

A key problem in the issue of compliance is reflected in the terminology traditionally employed. The matter is usually referred to as patient *compliance* with medical treatment. This term tends to reflect and perpetuate the image of patients as passive, submissive, and unable to make their own decisions. It creates expectations that providers of health care are all-knowing and all-powerful, and can decide what is best for the patient. The term tends to imply an attitude held for a long time by the medical profession—that if recommendations are not followed, it is the fault of the patient. As we shall see, noncompliance usually results from particular aspects of the practitioner–patient relationship and the way in which health care is delivered. Patients often fail to follow recommendations for good reasons or reasons beyond their control, as in the case of Mr. Castiglione.

Throughout this chapter, we emphasize that when patients are *told* what to do by their health care practitioners, noncompliance may ensue. Having the patient and health care practitioner work together as a team may be the most effective approach in patient care. The term compliance tends to emphasize an approach to patients that is one sided instead of a mutual endeavor. Therefore we will try, whenever possible, to use the term *cooperation* (or participation). Throughout this chapter, we emphasize the "give-and-take" that is characteristic of all social relationships. Perhaps it should be also characteristic of the health care professional–patient relationship.

In this chapter we examine the extent of the problem of nonco-operation, the many forms that it takes, the ways in which it is measured, as well as some of its causes. We look at noncooperation as a consequence of social psychological factors. Finally, we demonstrate some of the ways in which patient cooperation with treatment can be improved.

THE PROBLEM: NONCOOPERATION

The failure of a patient to follow precisely the recommendations of the physician or other health care professional constitutes lack of cooperation. (In the case of a child, of course, noncooperation involves the failure of the parent or guardian of the child to carry out specific recommendations for the care of the child.) Noncompliance has traditionally referred to the failure of the patient to carry out the recommendations as the health care professional *intended* they be carried out [18]. This is an important distinction, and it should be kept in mind, for it brings up a number of important questions. The obvious question is: Did the patient understand the regimen when it was described? In many cases, the assumption that the patient understood what to do is premature and unrealistic.

Noncooperation can occur in many ways and take many forms. For example, a patient may fail to keep an appointment for followup care. Or when sent to a specialist-consultant, the patient may fail to follow through with the visit. In such cases, the patient has not followed the recommendation of the physician (or other health care professional) to invest time, energy, and money into yet another health care encounter.

Patients' lack of cooperation can occur in relation to primary prevention measures (which are designed to prevent illness from developing, such as measures to reduce patients' weight and help them to be more active) or secondary prevention measures (such as measures designed to lower blood pressure to prevent stroke). Patients may also not cooperate with therapeutic measures, which are designed to alleviate symptoms such as pain and fever.

Patients can fail to cooperate with treatment by deviating from their physician's exact prescriptions for medication. They may vary the size of the dose of medication that is taken, the number of doses taken, and the number of days (the amount of time) over which the therapy is continued. A patient with a urinary tract infection may be instructed to take an antibiotic four times a day for ten days. The patient might take a pill only once or twice a day, for example, or take two pills at once after skipping a number of pills scheduled, or fail to evenly space the four pills taken over the day. The patient might discontinue taking the pills after five days, when the symptoms have subsided. (The patient's health is endangered by failing to follow the instruction of the physician to take the medication for ten days, since the infection can recur if it is not totally eradicated.) *Any* deviations from the recommended treatment are examples of noncooperation. This analysis points out to us that what is termed "noncompliance" or lack of cooperation on the part of the patient could easily involve *lack of understanding*. If a patient is supposed to carry out recommendations for appropriate dosage, temporal spacing, and duration of medication ingestion, the patient needs to understand fully what is to be done and the reasons for it [20]. With several aspects of the medication regimen to be carried out, the patient has many opportunities to make errors.

Noncooperation with treatment can also involve a patient's *unwillingness to make major changes in lifestyle for the sake of health*. Recommendations to change diet, to engage in exercise, or to avoid smoking often require major changes in the living patterns of patients. Most such preventive health behaviors are very difficult for patients because they require significant behavior change in the face of only possible future dangers [35].

The Extent of Noncooperation and Its Measurement

One-third of all patients fail to cooperate with their medical regimens according to the results of many studies. In some situations the percentage of noncooperation is as high as 50 percent. When we consider the many negative consequences that could result from noncooperation (which we examine later) we see that noncooperation is indeed a very serious problem [37].

Estimates of the degree of noncooperation depend upon the specific measure that is used [15, 16, 40]. The estimate has been found to be positively related to the objectivity of the measure. That is, the more patients' or health care professionals' own subjective reports are relied upon, the higher the estimate of cooperation; the more objective the measure, the lower the rate of cooperation. Let us consider this finding in more detail. An example of a subjective estimate of patient cooperation is the opinion of the health care professional (the physician or nurse) regarding whether or not the patient has followed orders. The impressions of the nurse, physician, or other health care professional concerning patient cooperation tend to be inaccurate, however. This is probably because health professionals do not like to face their own failure at influencing the patient. Health care professionals desire to see themselves as effective providers of care who are fully aware of the health behaviors of their patients and in touch with what changes are necessary. But evidence suggests that health care professionals are not very good at recognizing noncooperation when it exists [10, 22]. Patients' reports of their compliance behavior—whether or not they have taken their medication for example—are also low in reliability. Because they do not want to disappoint or even be scolded by the health professional, or because they are reluctant to admit that they have not followed the advice of the expert whom they have sought out, patients overestimate the extent to which they have cooperated with treatment [17].

More objective measures of cooperation with treatment include the checking of medical records to determine the patient's faithfulness in returning for visits or in seeking consultation visits. Objective measurements become somewhat more complex, however, when we try to assess cooperation with prescribed medication. Some researchers have tried to examine pharmacy records to determine whether patients have had their physicians' prescriptions filled, but there are many problems with this method. First, the many patients of one physician may use a variety of pharmacies to fill their prescriptions, and the assessment could quickly become unwieldly. Second, we can never be certain that because a patient has filled the prescription that this patient will take the medication as prescribed. Most noncooperation with medication treatment consists not in the patient's failure to fill the prescription, but rather in the patient's taking too little medication or taking it at the wrong times [37].

Some researchers have suggested that practitioners should use "pill counts" to determine the extent of patient compliance with medication regimens. If the health care professional asks the patient to bring the pill bottle to the health care setting, and then counts the remaining medication, the practitioner may be able to determine whether the correct amount of medication was taken. Of course, it is still impossible to know for sure whether the medication was taken at the proper time or even whether the medication was taken at all (i.e., whether the patient actually removed the appropriate number of pills in an effort to avoid being reprimanded). It is a more objective measure than simply asking the patient, however.

Perhaps the most objective measure of patient cooperation with medication regimens is the direct measure of the medication in the patient's body by means of a tracer or the medication's metabolic byproduct. For example, if a patient is taking penicillin, it is possible to test for urinary excretion of the antibiotic. Patient reliability in reporting is often measured against this objective criterion. Studies have shown that patients state that they have taken their medication much more often (close to 40 percent more often) than their objective tests corroborate [17, 40].

At least two experts, however, have noted that pill counts and direct-assay measures are not needed if the relationship between the health professional and patient is a partnership. If the patient feels comfortable admitting difficulties in cooperation to the health professional, and if those difficulties are accepted with understanding, the reports of patients may be the least expensive as well as most useful and accurate of all measures of cooperation [36, 40].

On the whole, however, it is clear that noncooperation is a serious problem. Research shows that about 30 percent of patients do not cooperate with taking therapeutic medication, while over 60 percent do not cooperate when lifestyle changes are required [37].

The Consequence of Noncooperation

If patients do not follow recommended courses of action for the treatment of their medical conditions, the result is clearly a waste of valuable health resources. Such a loss may be irrelevant to the condition of the patient, however. Of greater immediate consequence are the health problems that patients encounter when they are derelict in carrying out the terms of their medical treatment [40].

The specific consequences of noncooperation vary with the nature of the medical regimen. Recurrence of symptoms or inability to stop the progress of disease in the patient may result if medication is not taken regularly, or if it is terminated too soon. It is also possible for the health care professional to prescribe for the patient an overdosage of a drug believed to be having no effect at a lower dosage. For example, suppose the patient has been given 2 milligrams (mg) chlorpheniramine for allergy symptoms, and the patient reports no improvement. The physician might raise the dosage to 4 mg, using the patient's nonresponse to 2 mg as a gauge of the patient's tolerance. Because the patient has not taken any of the 2-mg tablets of the drug, the patient's sensitivity is still high and 4 mg may be too much. In another case, a physician might prescribe two drugs that must be taken in conjunction with each other in order to be safe and effective. If the patient takes only one of these medications, a detrimental reaction might occur.

Finally, diagnoses are often made on the basis of the responses of the patient's symptoms to a particular medication. If the patient has not actually taken the medication that was prescribed, whereas meanwhile the physician believes that the medication is not working, a misdiagnosis might occur. It has been suggested, too, that when new drugs are tested, researchers should obtain estimates of the compliance of the patients in the study. Although a new drug may appear to work much better than an old drug in eradicating an illness, its efficacy might be brought about solely because patients take the new drug and do not take the old drug.

REASONS FOR LACK OF COOPERATION

Many health care professionals have incomplete knowledge about patients' lack of cooperation with medical regimens. For example, many physicians believe that noncooperation occurs only in the clinic setting. Physicians tend to believe that in their own private practices their patients cooperate perfectly with treatment. This is not true. Noncooperation can occur in any setting in which recommendations are offered [37].

A second misconception is that noncooperation is limited to patients who are uneducated, or of low social class. As we shall see, there are few sociodemographic variables that are consistently related to compliance.

Another misconception of health care professionals regards the extent of the noncooperation problem. Studies show that physicians and health care professionals grossly underestimate the rates of noncooperation in their practices [10]. Health care professionals wrongly tend to assume that their patients follow their advice. In addition, health providers are not very accurate in identifying which patients are not cooperating with treatment [22]. This lack of knowledge and understanding is one of the key obstacles to reducing the incidence of noncooperation.

First we compare personality and situational influences on rates of cooperation and then we examine the influence of the illness. Finally, we consider the practitioner–patient relationship as it affects cooperation with treatment.

Psychological Attributes of the Patient

Many health care professionals believe that lack of patient cooperation with treatment can be attributed to the "uncooperative personalities" of their patients [12]. In fact, few if any personality characteristics are clearly related to compliance among patients [20].

Box 3-1
The Problem Patient

Certain patients arouse strong negative emotions in physicians. The psychiatrist James Groves labels these patients "hateful." These patients create problems for their physicians, but can be dealt with by a well-trained practitioner. These patients necessitate special attention to the nature of the doctor–patient relationship so that effective medical care can be provided. Groves claims that there are four basic types of problem patients.

The first type of troublesome patients is called the *dependent clinger.* These patients need repeated attention, reassurance, explanation, and affection. Their dependency will eventually exhaust the doctor. Such patients must be dealt with by a firmly enforced schedule of followup appointments.

A second group of problem patients consists of *entitled demanders.* These patients also ask for excessive service, but they do not flatter or cooperate with the physician. Rather, they threaten and control the physician's behavior. For example, they may withhold payment, threaten malpractice suits, and appeal to the physician's guilt. Such patients may actually be terrified by their illness. Hence, the physician should reassure the patient of his or her rights, help the patient deal with his or her fear, and endeavor to rechannel the patient's energies into coping with the illness rather than the doctor.

Groves's third category of problem patients involves *manipulative help rejectors.* They are commonly known as "crocks." These patients believe that no treatment will help them. When some symptoms are cured, others often develop. These patients may undergo a series of operations. They fear losing their medical care. It is unlikely that the pessimism of these patients can be quickly eliminated.

The fourth type of problem patient is called the *self-destructive denier.* Self-destructive deniers are very dependent and frequently suicidal in some sense. For example, an alcoholic patient may keep drinking even when told it will soon kill him. He cannot give up the pattern because it serves a purpose for him. Physicians may become very upset or even angry at such patients. They may be tempted to abandon such patients. However, all the physician can usually do is provide normal service and try to help the patient find the reason behind the self-destructive behavior such as alcoholism.

When patients can evoke hateful feelings in doctors, problems in diagnosis and treatment are not far behind. It does no good to blame or dislike patients. Instead, physicians should try to understand the patient's needs and maintain a friendly orientation and positive expectations. Even when the practitioner–patient relationship is a good one, some patients will continue to be a problem.

For further reading: J. Groves, Taking care of the hateful patient, *New England Journal of Medicine*, 1978, *298*, 883–887.

By personality characteristics, we mean traits that are measurable and stable. Labeling patients who do not comply as "uncooperative personalities" without further explanation is uninformative and unscientific.

It has been suggested that patients who do not comply are dependent people, and while attracted to the authority of the physicians, seek their independence by rebelling against it [14]. In this conception, noncooperation stems from the active resistance of the patient prompted by unconscious fears and conflicts. This hypothesis is interesting in that it reveals the possible complexity of the processes motivating noncooperative behavior. However, this characterization has not been supported by research evidence. (See Box 3-1 for a discussion of the extremes of patient personality in health care.)

Some psychological characteristics, namely characteristics that are not personality traits but rather relate more to the way people think and what they believe, do have some relationship to compliance behavior. These factors are part of the *Health Belief Model* [3, 5, 33]. For example, it has been found that patients who do not cooperate with their medical treatment believe themselves to be less susceptible to and less threatened by their illness (or possible future illness). To these patients, the physician's assessment of the danger of their illnesses does not matter very much. Rather, to them it is their own perception of the severity of the illness that is important, even if this estimation is not correct. In addition, it has been found that patients who do not cooperate with their medical treatment regimens tend to be generally less concerned about their own health than patients who do cooperate. Noncooperators also tend to believe less in the efficacy of modern medicine (i.e., in the ability of modern medicine to have any impact on treating disease) and believe the costs of treatment are too high.

Finally, the anxiety level of patients can influence the extent to which they can remember and act on what their physicians have told them [26]. Intermediate levels of anxiety are best. When patients have very low anxiety, they do not remember what they have been told and therefore cannot comply adequately. If their level of anxiety is too high, patients are so afraid of what is happening to them that they cannot process information, and hence do not follow their recommended treatments.

Environmental and Situational Factors

As R. F. Gillum and A. J. Barsky have suggested in their literature review on patient compliance, each patient has limited resources—limited time, money, and energy. Health care is only one of their concerns. Very often, patients who have limited resources (e.g., because of poverty) cannot comply with their prescribed medical regimens [14]. In a study of mothers of pediatric patients who did not keep their clinic appointments, for example, it was found that the three most common explanations were lack of money, lack of transportation, and other pressing problems at home (such as other children to take care of). Other studies have shown that mothers with fewer opportunities for *help* in the home were less compliant with regimens designed for the care of their children. In general, if people have a great many factors in their lives competing for few resources, they may find it difficult to channel resources into their own (or a child's) care [1, 11, 27].

Since adopting a medical regimen usually requires changing habits and developing new patterns of behavior, cooperation may be very difficult. Changing patterns requires the encouragement and reinforcement of family and other intimates, as well as assistance [9]. Behavior change requires social support. Thus, as one might guess, when patients are faced with disharmony in their families, family instability, or social isolation, they are less likely to cooperate with their medical regimens [2, 31].

Cultural factors also affect cooperation with treatment. Sometimes patients fail to follow the recommendations of health care practitioners because of religious or cultural restrictions. In Chapter 6 we consider the influence of culture on reactions to illness, to medical care, and on health behaviors. However, here we consider these factors as they are related to compliance. First, ethnic, cultural, and religious factors influence cooperation by affecting the restrictions placed on the person's actions [29, 34, 38]. Few patients are willing to cooperate with behavior that goes against what is prescribed by their cultural group. If they do, they will face social rejection. Second, the symbolic meaning that patients attach to various behaviors are affected by ethnic, cultural, and religious values. To individuals from cultures that value the importance of food (where food is equated with love and attention), restrictions on food intake are very difficult. These restrictions will necessarily be bound up with emotional meaning [6, 23]. Third, ethnic and cultural factors are important in influencing the attitude of patients toward responsibility for their health. Some cultures are more fatalistic than others. The individual's belief in self-efficacy *versus* the random influence of fate is likely to be influenced by the culture. This belief in turn will affect the person's willingness to assume responsibility for care. The influence of the family is also a function of culture and ethnicity. Few patients will cooperate with a regimen easily if that regimen goes against family requirements, responsibilities, and values [28, 43].

In examining the evidence so far, we see that it is extremely important for the health care professional to know what the relevant circumstances are in the life of the patient and to examine how those circumstances influence the patient's ability and willingness to follow recommended behaviors. The health professional should be able to adjust the requirements of the regimen if necessary.

The Influence of the Characteristics of the Treatment

A patient's ability and willingness to cooperate with medical treatment depends to some extent on the nature of the illness and on the nature of the treatment. When a patient has an acute illness with painful symptoms that are directly alleviated by the medication and the medication is prescribed for a short period of time (say, ten days), the probability of compliance is high. When the medication brings prompt relief from distressing symptoms, the taking of medication is strongly reinforced. Even when the symptoms are alleviated, but the medication must be continued for a few more days (such as in the case of a urinary tract infection for which the patient must take medication for ten days although the symptoms disappear after five days), cooperation is likely to occur *if the patient understands what is expected of him or her and the reasons for continuing the medication for ten days are explained* [19].

However, in the case of chronic illness requiring treatment of long duration, patient cooperation is comparatively poor [37]. For example, in a study of diabetic patients, 30 percent errors were found in insulin dosage among patients who had the disease one to five years. Moreover, when patients had the disease for more than twenty years, the dosage errors occurred in about 80 percent of the cases. Taking a medication that may be troublesome, time-consuming, or associated with side effects (and without any immediate discernable positive consequences) is difficult for patients. If the disease is subclinical like hypertension (i.e., it exists but presents the patient with no symptoms), then social rewards must be introduced in order to substitute for the physical rewards that would result if the medication were alleviating symptoms such as pain [9]. We discuss how this can be done in Box 3-2.

The more complicated the treatment regimen, the less likely it is that the patient will follow the regimen precisely as prescribed. Among patients with diabetes or congestive heart failure, errors in medication were found to increase as the complexity of the treat-

Box 3–2
Compliance and Social Support

Cooperating with medical regimens may be very difficult sometimes, but family support can make it considerably easier. This was a finding of the research on patient education and social support done by Robert Caplan and his associates at the Institute for Social Research at the University of Michigan.

Medical studies of the drug treatment of hypertensive patients have shown that if patients are *perfectly* adherent to their drug regimens and *consistently* restrict their salt intake by maintaining a low-sodium diet, they can produce an impressive drop in their blood pressure and considerably reduce the chances of stroke and heart attack. Adhering to hypertension regimens is difficult for patients, however. They usually have no symptoms and they feel fine. They must deny themselves salted foods and remember to take their medication every day, while they continue to feel quite well. In fact, taking the medication can sometimes precipitate negative side effects. There may be muscle weakness with diuretics or impotence from methyldopa (though the physician will usually withdraw this latter drug or give it only intermittently if impotence does occur). Certainly the avoidance of salty foods is difficult when there is only a less-than-certain probability that one will develop some trouble in the future. The treatment of hypertension represents a situation in which the person is "at risk" and must deny present gratifications to produce a possible future well-being. Treating hypertension is a lifelong enterprise. There must be some immediate rewards to maintain the behavior.

Understandably, perfect cooperation with regimens for hypertension is rare. Only about half the people in the United States receiving treatment for hypertension are under effective control. However, since cooperation can be so efficacious (i.e., the hypertension can be controlled), investigation of the factors that determine cooperation and adherence is important.

Caplan and his colleagues found (in a literature review) that a number of social psychological factors contributed to the extent to which a person can follow a physician's recommendations. A very important factor in adherence to the many different regimens was *social support*. Caplan defined social support in this case as encouragement from family and friends (also see Chapters 7 and 8). Encouragement from loved ones can help the patient to carry out the regimen, and increase his or her feelings of self-competence and motivation. In this research, the factor that made a large difference in adherence was support to the hypertensive from his or her spouse. Support from the spouse was associated with low levels of depression, with higher motivation to adhere, and with greater knowledge of the regimen. Social support was also explored in a field pilot experiment done by Caplan.

A special patient education program was set up in which some patients received information in lectures while others were assigned to social support groups with their spouses. Patients in the social support experimental groups were involved in sharing their thoughts and feelings with other hypertensive patients and their spouses at the periodic meetings. These patients were more likely to achieve and maintain a clinically controlled level of blood pressure than were those who were not in the social support experimental group.

Interestingly, in the experiments done by Caplan in which social support groups were set up, patients and their spouses found that getting together with other couples, one member of whom had hypertension, was very beneficial. It helped them to share problems that they encountered, and to gain social reinforcement. They also dealt with everyday problems such as learning to cook good-tasting, low-sodium foods.

For further reading: R. D. Caplan, E. A. R. Robinson, J. R. P. French, Jr., J. R. Caldwell, and M. Shinn, *Adhering to Medical Regimens: Pilot Experiments in Patient Education and Social Support* (Ann Arbor: Research Center for Group Dynamics, Institute for Social Research, University of Michigan, 1976).

---

ment increased. For example, the error rate (or nonadherence) was only 15 percent when one drug was prescribed and 25 percent when two drugs were prescribed, but it exceeded 35 percent when three drugs were prescribed [21].

Relatedly, the greater the interference with patient's usual habits, the more difficult it is for a patient to cooperate with treatment. Taking oral medication one, two, or even three times a day is a relatively minor change in habit for a person. However, if the patient must totally restructure his or her usual routine (e.g., lose weight, stop smoking, and exercise), the likelihood of total adherence to the entire routine is low. The health care professional must recognize the difficulties patients face in making major changes in their lifestyles and thus give patients some leeway in adjusting to the regimen. Interestingly, some studies have shown that patients adopt only a portion of their therapeutic regimen if it is particularly difficult. They pick and choose the parts of the regimen that are least difficult for them [14].

Treatment influences on patient cooperation are easy to understand when examined; but they are not obvious. In practice, they are often ignored by health practitioners. Interestingly, while they are important, these factors are not the *most* important influences on cooperation.

The Health Care Professional—Patient Relationship

A factor that has consistently been found to be very strongly related to patient cooperation with medical regimens is the quality of the relationship between the health care professional and the patient [40]. There are two different aspects of the health care professional–patient relationship. One is the degree and quality of the communication of information between the patient and the health care professional. There must be open communication between the health professional and the patient and they must understand each other. The second aspect of the relationship is the rapport between them, which is also referred to as the "socioemotional component." As we considered in Chapter 2, the effective quality of the relationship between the physician and patient is called the art of medicine [30, 40].

There is a strong relationship between the quality of communication of information from the health care professional to the patient and the patient's degree of adherence to the therapeutic regimen. This relationship is not surprising, for patients need to know what recommendations have been made and what is expected of them before they can conform to the treatment. Health care professionals should not take for granted that their patients completely understand what has been explained to them. The vocabulary, ways of thinking, and expectations of health care professionals are often very different from those of their patients [26].

Numerous studies have documented extensive communication problems between health professionals and their patients. In one study over 60 percent of the patients actually misunderstood the oral instructions given by their physicians for taking medication [7]. Another study found that more than 50 percent of the patients made at least one error when they were asked to describe their physician's recommendations for their treatment only a week after their visit to the clinic [41]. Writing instructions down for patients sometimes helps, but these written instructions must be clear and unambiguous in order to be useful [40]. It is often true that physicians' written instructions are sufficiently ambiguous that patients cannot understand them without a complete explanation beforehand [41]. In addition, an explanation that involves giving information one sidedly from the health professional to the patient is not sufficient to be effective. There has to be a give and take of information between the health care professional and patient so that the health professional can obtain continual feedback from the patient about what he or she understands and what needs to be made clearer [39]. Communication is discussed in detail in Chapter 5.

Studies of the art of medicine show that when patients are satisfied with the way in which they have been treated as people, they are much more likely to follow recommendations. Studies at Children's Hospital in Los Angeles found that acceptance, appreciation, and respect were requisite for mothers of pediatric patients to follow recommended courses of care for their children [24, 25].

A theory proposed by psychologists Judith Rodin and Irving Janis states that the art of medicine is a necessary factor in the development of *referent power* [32]. Because of the nature of the physician-patient relationship, only a few sources of *social power* are available to the physician or other health care professional [13]. The physician or health care professional actually has no way to guarantee control of the behavior of the patient. Reward power (the ability to withdraw rewards for noncompliance) is limited because the physician controls few of the patient's needs, except perhaps for caring and esteem. Expert power is part of the professional–patient relationship, because the health care professional is seen as an expert in matters of health and illness. Patients follow advice partly because they know the health care professional has more knowledge and expertise than they do. But for the most part, the greatest influence that the health care professional can have on the patient's health behavior is by using referent power, the process of forming a social unit with the patient. Through mutual caring and respect patients come to trust the health care professional and to model themselves after the health care professional as someone who values healthy, responsible behavior. The quality of the health professional–patient relationship is thus critically important for the care of patients and for building patient motivation (see Box 3-3).

In the remainder of this chapter, we examine how patient cooperation can be enhanced through development of the practitioner-patient relationship.

TREATING NONCOOPERATION

Even when noncooperation is recognized, physicians and other members of the health care team may ignore the problem or deal with the problem using inadequate means. In one study 67 percent of the senior attending physicians interviewed stated that noncooperation was due to the patients' uncooperative personalities [12]. Only 26 percent of the physicians believed that the physician personally could be responsible. Forty percent of the doctors in the study blamed noncooperation on the patients' inability to understand recommendations. They placed the responsibility for understanding

Box 3-3
The Ultimate in Patient Cooperation

Many patients do not lose weight or take pills as the doctor prescribes. Such failures to cooperate with treatment can, of course, lead to serious problems. However, if the proper patient attitude emerges, tremendous cooperation can result. A prime example concerns dialysis patients.

Tens of thousands of Americans stay alive because of artificial kidneys. They must be hooked up to a dialysis machine several times a week and have their blood filtered of waste products. The procedure may take several hours, and discomfort arises. Leg cramps can occur and the needles can be painful. Dialysis patients may feel weak, may itch, and may be on a severely restricted diet. Nevertheless, most patients willingly and precisely cooperate with treatment. When the right circumstances exist, the degrees to which patients will help themselves are truly remarkable.

For further reading: H. S. Abram, Survival by machine: The psychological stress of chronic hemodialysis, *Psychiatry in Medicine*, 1970, *1*, 37–51.

the instructions on the patient, not on the health care professionals. When faced with noncooperation, many physicians and other health care professionals (if they are not aware of the complexity of the problem) usually take the following steps: First, they explain the regimen to the patient and then they try rational arguments to persuade patients. After that, physicians and other health care team members resort to threat tactics. Finally, they withdraw from the case. Of course, communicating knowledge about the disease to the patient or even changing the patient's attitudes in no way insures that the patient's health behavior will change as desired. The arousal of fear in the patient might bring about the patient's denial of the problem altogether, or else bring about behavior that is the opposite of that desired. Fear tactics work only if the patient is shown very specific behavioral steps to take and is convinced both that they will work and that he or she is capable of carrying them out. For obvious reasons, the withdrawal of the health care professional from the case is highly undesirable [4].

We next consider methods for dealing with noncompliance that take into account the great complexity of the problem and the individuality of each of the patients concerned.

Models of the Practitioner-Patient Relationship

The role of the health care professional can be conceptualized in various ways. The framework of three models of the practitioner-patient relationship provided by Thomas Szasz and Marc Hollender allows us to examine the appropriate role of the health care expert in trying to bring about patient cooperation [42]. As we consider various methods that have been developed to enhance patient cooperation with medical regimens, the questions of responsibility and patient control are systematically considered.

There are three basic models of the practitioner-patient relationship. The first is the *Activity-Passivity* model. In this relationship the health professional does something to the patient but the patient is totally passive. An obvious example of this model is when the patient is unconscious during an emergency or while undergoing surgery. In this case something is done to the patient and the patient has no control or responsibility. The practitioner has absolute control and absolute responsibility. On occasion, this model is applied to a conscious patient, for example, when the patient is too sick or old to be a participant in the care. Of course if the physician or other health care professional ministers to the patient as if the patient were not a living, thinking human being (as some do at times), this activity-passivity model may be used inappropriately with a conscious and capable patient.

The second model is very common in medical practice and is accepted as the norm. It is the *guidance-cooperation* model, and it typifies the relationship that exists when the illness is not very serious. The patient is aware of what is happening and is capable of following instructions. The practitioner tells the patient what to do and the patient is expected to cooperate. In this model the health practitioner *decides* what is best for the patient and makes the recommendation. The patient is expected to follow the recommendation because the "doctor knows best." This is typical of many physician-patient interactions.

In the guidance-cooperation relationship health professionals try to be supportive. But the practitioner assumes responsibility for deciding what is the right treatment. In this situation the patient is simply expected to follow the rules. These rules, however, are set up by the physician who does not experience the problems of treatment that arise. The physician cannot be with the patient to deal with problems, and also cannot determine whether the patient is cooperating. Cooperation may be unlikely in this situation because the patient is merely following someone else's recommendations about how to behave. The patient may choose to reject those orders at any time. Social psychological theories of "reactance" indicate that patients are in fact likely to reject the recommendations because they tend to act to restore their lost freedom in the situation [18]. For example, the patient might rebel against the "fatherly" guidance of the physician, whose restrictions are troubling.

The third model of the practitioner–patient relationship is *mutual participation*. Szasz and Hollender state that in modern medicine this model is still rare unfortunately, although things have been changing in recent years. This model is based upon the belief that the physician and the patient are pursuing common goals of eliminating illness and preserving the patient's health. The practitioner and patient have equal power in the relationship; they need each

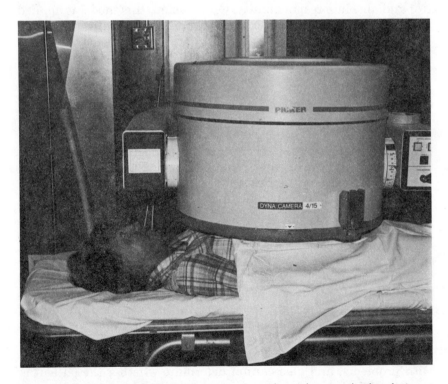

Figure 3-1. Whether patients will cooperate with modern medical techniques such as nuclear medicine depends heavily on the quality of doctor-patient rapport. (Photo by Howard S. Friedman, © 1982)

other (i.e., are mutually interdependent), and their behaviors must be mutually satisfying in order for the relationship to continue.

In the mutual participation model the patient's dignity and respect are maintained. In this model there is a true sharing of responsibility. While it avoids a false sense that patients and the physician are equal socioeconomically, in knowledge, or in education, this model provides the opportunity for patients to maintain freedom of control over their lives and the decisions that are made concerning their bodies. The patient's input is included in medical decisions before they are made. The model suggests an open and responsible partnership. Perhaps because of assumptions that patients are not capable of taking responsibility for their care, or perhaps because health professionals are reluctant to consider themselves in equal power positions with their patients, this model has not so far become the standard practitioner–patient relationship. This model may be the best for everyone concerned, however.

The Health Transactions Model: Solving Problems with Patients

Cooperation with medical regimens is the positive result of a succesful transaction between the health care provider and the patient. Patient satisfaction with the health professional's concern and understanding may be one of the most important determinants of patient cooperation. Here we consider this issue in the framework of the relationship between the health professional and the patient.

Following the model of health psychologist George Stone, which is called the health transactions model, we suggest that health care professionals must look carefully at the question of whether their recommendations really address the client's problem adequately and whether the suggestions that are made (the health care professional's "orders") are necessary steps for the patient to follow [40].

A helpful way of looking at the health care professional's delivery of medical care to the patient is in three stages: (1) the statement of the problem by the patient and the exploration of symptoms by the physician; (2) the development of the diagnosis and the decisions regarding treatment; and (3) the implementation of treatment. In the traditional model of health care, where concepts such as "doctor's orders" prevail, limited views of patient compliance lead to the inappropriate placement of responsibilities for each of the three phases of health care.

In the first stage of the health care transaction the patient brings a problem to the physician. For example, the patient describes a set of symptoms and notes when they occur, explaining something about their personal meaning. The expert usually questions the patient extensively about the symptoms and history, most often confining the discussion to purely medical issues. While the patient probably describes the problem in common behavioral terms, the medical expert usually redefines the problem in purely medical terms [39].

An example of this kind of transaction is the patient who describes feeling faint and dizzy and having difficulty breathing while walking outside. The physician will probably define the problem in terms such as "shortness of breath upon exertion." It is possible, of course, that the patient is having heart trouble, but it is also possible that the patient is having an anxiety reaction. The health provider also needs to explore the possibility of "agoraphobia" in the patient. (Agoraphobia is the fear of going outside, and can involve fear of meeting people.) Take another example of a patient with a sharp pain in the stomach area. The physician will most likely be concerned with gathering information from the patient to explore the possibility of a tumor or the possibility of a gastric ulcer. Most likely, questions will center completely on the physical aspects of the case. In fact, however, it could be equally important in the care of the patient to know something about the patient's lifestyle, beliefs, family or other support systems, coping mechanisms, and general emotional health. These are critical pieces of information for the diagnosis of the patients with shortness of breath and stomach pain. Combinations of physical and emotional data are needed in order to be able to make an accurate diagnosis. The described symptoms could occur in many different conditions. Thus if the patient with a shortness of breath describes a hesitancy in dealing with others or the patient with stomach pain describes a very hectic, unsatisfying lifestyle in addition to the pain, the health professional is alerted to a particular explanation. Knowledge about the social and psychological aspects of the patient's life can be critically important in the planning and implementation of treatment as well. As we have seen these factors may profoundly affect the patient's ability to cooperate with medical regimens.

During the second stage of the health care transaction, the health professional makes a decision about the diagnosis and chooses the treatment to prescribe for the patient. The health care professional, according to psychologist Stone, has a great deal of knowledge about the intricate details of various treatments—for example, how much each costs, what the side effects and restrictions are, what degree of pain exists, and what the duration of the treatments will be. But a rational selection among these possible treatments demands some knowledge of the values assigned by the patient to the various complicating factors and outcomes. For example, suppose one treatment requires the patient to remain sedentary for a few weeks to relieve back pain. A physician may decide upon this remedy, placing a particularly low value on mobility. Suppose, however, that the patient is an athlete; the prescription of a restriction in movement is likely to be very distressing for the patient's social, psychological, and physical health. A better treatment may be available for this patient.

The health transactions model maintains that although traditionally health care professionals have made the sole decisions about treatment, such unilateral decisionmaking is inappropriate. The health care professional can never completely know or anticipate the values of the patient, the meaning of various outcomes, or the problems the patient would face in trying to cooperate with the therapeutic regimen. Rational selection of a course of treatment that the patient can follow requires that the patient take (and the health professional give) some responsibility when the treatment course is being selected. The fact that traditionally all the responsibility has fallen upon the health care professional has probably contributed significantly to low compliance. The responsibility must be shared. The health care professional must be willing to take advice from the patient, who, after all, is the only person who really knows what manner of treatment he or she will be able to follow. The patient must take responsibility for deciding on the treatment plan and also for providing information that is representative of his or her wishes and needs.

The third and final stage of the health care transaction is implementing the treatment. Traditionally, total responsibility has been placed on the patient for carrying out the treatment. If full responsibility for carrying out the treatment—say, taking medication for high blood pressure and controlling or losing weight—is borne by the patient, both parties to the health care encounter may be reluctant to admit the patient's inability to carry out the treatment regimen. The health care professional is likely to avoid the fact that he or she has not explained the treatment adequately or convinced the patient to follow it. The patient may be reluctant to admit an embarrassing inability to carry out the regimen. The health care professional probes half-heartedly for noncooperation, and the patient hides it as much as possible. Everyone plays a social game, and the patient fails to benefit from treatment.

If, on the other hand, the entire health care transaction is considered the shared responsibility of the health professional and the patient, no fault is assigned when difficulties arise. Difficulties are

Box 3-4
Iatrogenic Illness

Should a patient always cooperate with a doctor's advice? Is compliance necessarily in the best interest of the patient?

Countless examples of iatrogenic illness suggest that the answer may be "NO." *Iatrogenic illness* is illness that is caused specifically by medical intervention. It can be the result of problems occurring in surgery (e.g., perforation of the bowel with resultant peritonitis during abdominal surgery). Or it can be the direct result of the side effects of drugs or the dangerous interaction of two drugs administered by the physician. Iatrogenic illness also commonly involves infections contracted during hospitalization.

This problem is complex. Can the occurrence in a patient of an improbable but still *possible* side effect of a drug be considered an iatrogenic illness? Probably, since the side effect would not have occurred without administration of the drug. But this does not mean that the physician was incompetent or negligent, or that the patient should have refused to take the drug in the first place. But what if the physician has not told the patient that the side effect might occur? Is the illness as well as the resulting anxiety of the patient then the fault of the physician? On the other hand, what about the patient's anxiety that results from knowledge of what might happen if a certain drug is administered?

The issue is complicated still further by the fact that the medical management of a patient might never be questioned because the patient remains unaware of the role of the physician's treatment in the exacerbation of this medical problem. It is easy to hide iatrogenic illness, disguising it as the normal course of the patient's problem.

Thus, some have argued that patient noncompliance may sometimes, in fact, be adaptive. Fortunately, such issues usually disappear when the practitioner and patient have an open and trusting relationship, with knowledge of each other's special strengths and weaknesses.

For further reading: Ivan Illich, *Medical Nemesis: The Expropriation of Health* (New York, Random House, 1976).

---

expected naturally to occur, and noncooperation is addressed by the provider and by the patient, who work *together* to alleviate the problem. They design or redesign a treatment program that the patient can follow successfully—a program that fits the patient's social, psychological, economic, and cultural situation.

In summary, the health transactions model recommends that in the initial stage of the health care interaction, the health professional explore the situation of every client, examining their beliefs about their illness and symptoms, and their willingness to receive and carry out recommendations. In the second stage, the health care professional should examine the patient's values and engage in open communication with the patient about them. The health care professional should explore the patient's expectations about treatment and outcome and examine expectations regarding the rights, duties, and responsibilities of the patient. Finally, in the stage in which the patient is charged with carrying out the regimen, the health professional should share in the responsibility by remaining an integral part of the treatment. The practitioner should continuously check the patient's compliance progress and discuss the regimen and its modification. The health care professional must listen carefully to the patient, provide an accepting atmosphere in which the patient can admit mistakes and ask for help, and explain the many aspects of the treatment regimen, its purpose, expected effects, side effects, and expected duration. The health professional must educate the patient. Specific information about these topics appears throughout this book.

Finally, it is important to recognize that not all patients will benefit from treatment with the health transactions model. A different approach is necessary with patients who insist on being totally cared for by the health professional and who refuse to participate in discussions of their illnesses.

SUMMARY

Despite the time and expense patients put forth in obtaining medical advice, a large number of them fail to follow it. Although many health professionals believe that patients' failures to cooperate are the result of "uncooperative personalities," extensive research on this topic has shown that patient cooperation is dependent upon a number of social psychological factors—many of which can be directly changed by the health professional's intervention. In order to cooperate with their treatment regimens patients must believe they are susceptible to serious disease, they must trust in the efficacy of the treatment, and they must believe its benefits outweigh its costs. They also must have clear, open communication with the health professionals, who provide understandable explanations to them and prescribe regimens compatible with the patients' social and cultural norms. Cooperation may also be enhanced by support and help from the patient's family and network of close friends.

4

The Mind
and
The Body

Whereas some people make remarkable recoveries from serious, and even life-threatening, diseases or dangerous surgery, other seemingly similar people succumb—they become more debilitated or die. In many cases it seems that the only major difference between success and failure is an abstruse quality of the patient known as the *will to live*.

A famous case of the will to live is Norman Cousins, the former editor of the *Saturday Review*. Cousins developed a degenerative disease that was progressively paralyzing him. His doctors told him that he had one chance in 500 of recovering. Cousins checked himself out of the hospital and into a hotel room. He devised his own treatment: laughter. He watched old Candid Camera films and read humorous stories, and he recovered [10]. Can laughter relieve pain or cure certain diseases? If so, how?

Each year millions of sick people visit the healing shrine at Lourdes, France. These pilgrims have tremendous faith in the possibility of cure. They pray, and sometimes medical miracles occur. People who were paralyzed walk again; people with tremendous pain are suddenly relieved of it. While biological impossibilities do not occur at Lourdes (e.g., people do not grow new arms or legs), some who are crippled get up from their wheelchairs, and others with serious illnesses recover despite the poor odds given them by their doctors. Why?

Jerome Frank, of the Psychiatry Department of the Johns Hopkins University Medical School, studied American soldiers who were infected with a parasite during World War II. Hundreds of soldiers surprised their doctors and failed to recover on schedule from this disease despite adequate medical treatment. Their symptoms continued; they were weak and had cramps and headaches. Purely medical explanations failed, but as Frank discovered, negative expectations seemed to contribute to the soldiers' problems. Confused and hopeless about their recovery, these soldiers were demoralized by seemingly conflicting reports from doctors. They believed they would die, and despite recommended treatment, their symptoms continued [17, 18].

In the early 1950s medical researchers reported discovery of a new drug called Krebiozen, which was believed to be a cure for cancer. When the news was made public, a panic was created as thousands of cancer patients tried to obtain the drug, which was not generally available. Some patients did obtain it, and in many cases the drug was dramatically effective [16]. Some patients who were very ill and bedridden with cancer were given Krebiozen and soon were out of bed, their tumors shrinking miraculously. However, when later research showed that Krebiozen was ineffective, patients who had been helped by the drug suddenly had relapses and died of their cancer.

Researchers who have studied pain, as well as doctors, dentists, and nurses, marvel at the differences among people in their ability to tolerate pain. After surgery, for example, some people cry out for more and more pain medication, while others lie quietly or become ambulatory soon after surgery. Likewise, some people insist on taking pain killers after dental work, while others go on with their daily business in spite of having been treated by the dentist. Studies of these differences in people suggest a pattern, for social and psychological factors affect the perception of pain.

In this chapter we consider the relationship of the mind and the body. We include such topics as faith healing, expectations, placebos, and pain. We attempt to understand such phenomena as "miracle cures," and in doing so, we apply a social psychological framework to achieve a scientific understanding of some of the most fascinating phenomena in medicine.

THE CARTESIAN DUALISM

The seventeenth-century French philosopher René Descartes proposed that a human being has a mind that exists in the spiritual realm and a body that exists in the realm of physical matter. Descartes saw the mind and body as separate, although very closely related [13]. However, this separation or dualism led subsequent thinkers to maintain a mind–body distinction. When they tried to merge the two, some argued that the body could think. Others proposed that the body existed *in* the mind. But no one was easily able to conceive of the mind and the body as one entity. This is still true for many people today.

In modern medicine, "mental" problems are almost always distinguished from "physical" problems. Many physicians focus on physical problems such as bacterial infections, broken bones, and blocked arteries. Matters such as depression, anxiety, unexplained pain, and the lack of a "will to live" are usually labeled mental problems and referred to mental health experts. But this false dualism is actually so inaccurate that it leads to serious errors in the approach to many important illnesses [19].

First, as we have seen in Chapter 3, the patient's cooperation with treatment often depends on proper interpersonal relations. Ignoring a patient's mind while trying to cure his or her body may result in a patient who does not cooperate with treatment. More generally, many health problems result from a poorly regulated lifestyle—too much smoking, drinking, eating, and too little exercise. A doctor who focuses only on the physical results of such behavior—cancerous lungs, cirrhotic livers, and diseased hearts—is surely being shortsighted and inefficient.

Secondly, the mind–body dualism incorrectly assumes that the mind and body operate independently, whereas, in fact, mental and physical factors are almost always closely intertwined. A prime example is pain, which is discussed later in this chapter. Pain can be caused by physical problems but also by mental difficulties. Furthermore, pain can be controlled through mental means as well as through drugs or surgery, and it is misleading to consider pain and illness to be either exclusively physical or exclusively mental. Although we can emphasize one aspect or the other, in truth the mind and the body are parts of one system. In Chapter 7 we present a detailed analysis of the relationship between psychological factors and illness. First, however, we need a more general analysis of the relationship between the mind and body.

PSYCHE AND SOMA: PSYCHOSOMATIC MEDICINE

One area of medicine in which the mind–body relationship has been explored is *psychosomatic medicine*. However, the term psychosomatic medicine at present has too many meanings to be of much value. Sometimes psychosomatic medicine refers to the use of principles of psychology in understanding and treating illness. (This broad definition applies to all of this book.) At other times psychosomatic medicine refers to medical problems that are caused by psychological states. This latter definition encompasses three different but important areas.

First, as it is often pointed out, a significant proportion of patient complaints made to physicians are social psychological in nature and have no significant physical counterpart [31]. If the social psychological problem is resolved all symptoms disappear. For example, a patient may complain to a doctor about vague symptoms such as headaches or weakness for which no physical explanation can be found. These symptoms may result purely from tension in an unhappy marriage or reaction to a problem child. Recognition and resolution of these problems are part of the art of medicine.

Second, psychosomatic illness sometimes refers to organic disorders that are directly *caused* by psychological and emotional problems [1, 14]. That is, people with certain psychological difficulties are much more likely to develop specific, definable, and detectable physical problems. For example, a person with excessive worries who does not cope well but constantly experiences tension may develop ulcers. In this second type of psychosomatic illness, the physical symptoms have a physical explanation such as tissue damage as well as a relationship to underlying psychological difficulties. The physical as well as the psychological problems must be treated. Other examples are allergies, skin disorders, hypertension, colon disorders, and even heart disease. Some of the important factors in this type of problem are considered in more detail in Chapter 7.

Third, psychosomatic medicine sometimes focuses on the body as an *environment* that may be changed by psychosocial factors. In this sense illness is caused by outside agents invading the body, the defenses of which are affected by psychological factors. The psychological factors do not cause the disease but rather weaken the body's resistance. For example, it is theoretically possible for all people to contract bacterial pneumonia. But certain psychological difficulties make some people more susceptible than others. This use of the term psychosomatic is gaining wider popularity as medical researchers increasingly focus on immunology (susceptibility to disease) and as psychosocial researchers focus on the notion of "wellness" (preventing disease) [15] (also see Chapter 6). While all these aspects of psychosomatic medicine are important to proper medical treatment, we should be more specific in defining the phenomenon of interest in any particular analysis.

HOLISTIC MEDICINE: ONE APPROACH

There is a growing modern movement to bring the mind and body together in medical treatment that is known as *holistic* medicine. This approach involves treatment of the person as a whole human being with the mind always affecting the body and vice versa.

There is a problem with the holistic movement, however. While its basic goals are worthy, unfortunately the term and the concept are sometimes used in highly *unscientific* approaches to medical treatment. For example, imagination or hypnotism may be used as therapies without first establishing their therapeutic value for a given illness through controlled experimentation.

Holistic medicine *can* be scientific. There is an enormous amount of evidence that thoughts and feelings are inextricably tied to physical processes. Furthermore, the social psychological aspects of patient care are as important as the physical aspects. In fact, it is unscientific to ignore the so-called mental aspects of general health. In this chapter we point out some key benefits of a truly holistic approach but will refrain from calling our approach holistic.

BELIEF AND ITS FUNCTION IN CURE

Faith Healing

In converted theaters or under tents, thousands of people gather each week, and they may sway with the music, writhe and shout, or close their eyes and hold hands. Many are in pain or have some disability. On the front stage is a charismatic figure urging the followers to believe. These people are at a faith healing gathering.

There are dozens of prominent healers in the United States, many of whom are religious zealots who call on a higher power beyond themselves. Famous faith healers include Kathryn Kuhlman and Jimmy Carter's sister Ruth. Goals and techniques vary; some attempted cures involve the development of a quiet inner peace while others involve dramatic attempts to raise the handicapped from their wheelchairs. Although such healing is shunned by modern medicine as unscientific, faith healing often works [21]. Belief can materially affect the outcome of treatment. The principles of faith healing are very powerful and it is critical that we understand them; they deserve a place in medicine.

Quackery

The word *quack* might bring to mind a thin man who curls his black waxed mustache while selling snake oil. He is hard to find these days, but health quackery is rampant in America. Part of the reason is that medicine displays insufficient attention to psychosocial factors.

With an emphasis on beauty in America, fad diets (and faddish nutrition therapies) are a preoccupation of many people. There is no scientific evidence that they work, and often they do harm. Diet books proposing medically dangerous diets are often best sellers in the bookstores. Many Americans gulp enormous quantities of vitamins and other diet supplements. Like snake oil, these supplements are often touted to prevent baldness and increase sex drive. The self-care movement is thriving. In part, fads represent a rejection of the health establishment's separation of the mind from the body. People are increasingly dissatisfied with physicians, most of whom solely focus on "fixing" bodily malfunctions while mostly ignoring the whole person (including diet) and paying little attention to the psychosocial influences on health [28].

Earlier we mentioned the drug Krebiozen, which was extracted from the blood serum of horses. The main evidence for its effectiveness was the testimonial of cancer patients. Patients given this new miracle drug in the 1950s felt less pain, had improved appetite, and lived longer than expected. The U.S. Food and Drug Administration was dubious about claims for Krebiozen for years, although it was not until the early 1960s that interstate dealings in Krebiozen were banned. The drug was eventually found to be ineffective against cancer, but even after its official ban, some congressmen were calling for Krebiozen to be given another chance [35, 46].

Several interesting observations can be made about Krebiozen. First, evidence for the drug's effectiveness came from individual case studies, not from controlled experiments. Second, the drug was claimed to cure cancer, a fear-provoking and poorly understood disease. Third, there was secrecy associated with the development of the drug, with one scientist proclaiming the need to protect the drug from falling into Communist hands. Fourth, the drug soon acquired an almost mystical or religious significance. And finally, bitter charges of fraud and counterfraud against its developers were involved. These factors are familiar to the medical scene.

A surprisingly similar set of circumstances has surrounded the development of another so-called cancer drug, Laetrile. Laetrile is an extract of apricot pits, although there is some doubt about what the chemical structure of "true" Laetrile is. Although it was developed many years ago, Laetrile did not become a public issue in the United States until the 1970s. Since Laetrile has not been shown to be safe and effective, many legal disputes exist over its use. Many Americans travel to Tijuana, Mexico, to Laetrile clinics [36, 47].

At its core, the controversy over Laetrile (like that over Krebiozen) results from the social and emotional issues in medicine that are at the heart of this book. Many patients turn to unestablished therapies like Laetrile because of disenchantment with their own physicians, out of anger at the impersonal care they receive from the medical establishment, or from a need for emotional support [8, 52].

Many people proclaim the catchy argument that patients should have the right to choose their own therapy. However, there are very real dangers that may result from the promotion of fraudulent substances. Government regulation of drugs and medical treatment does help to protect consumers from dangerous substances as well as from the use of ineffective substances that might be taken in place of the available effective drugs. Patients who ignore conventional, effective cancer treatment and instead take unproven cancer drugs may incur enormous costs for themselves and also for their family, the community, and society as a whole.

These drugs and the belief that people have in them dramatically illustrate the importance of faith and expectation, which are crucial to all medical treatment. Through a variety of mechanisms, the proper beliefs can promote cures. Fortunately, the healing power of faith can be studied scientifically; the key concept is expectation.

Expectations

Phenomena such as faith healing, the will to live, and the power of fraudulent drugs can be understood in terms of people's *expectations,* most of which arise in interactions with other people [24, 25]. People are social beings and their actions are heavily influenced by the actions of other people. Many times the expectations of others are very subtle (being communicated by nonverbal communication). The nature of expectations is considered here (nonverbal communication is considered in detail in Chapter 5).

At the turn of the century many scientists were interested in the special powers of the horse named Clever Hans [37]. Hans was a very smart horse, and when asked questions, he would tap out the correct answer with his right forefoot. Hans could perform various mathematical functions, including multiplication and finding the factors of a number. Hans was also able to analyze music and seemed able to read German. Trickery on the part of his owner was ruled out.

It was some time before a psychologist, Oskar Pfungst, figured out the key to Hans's success. Pfungst determined that the horse could not answer questions correctly if the questioner was not visible to Hans or if the person asking the question did not know the correct answer. Hans, it turns out, was detecting cues from people about when to start tapping the answer with his hoof and when to stop tapping. After systematic investigation, Pfungst found that when observers leaned forward to watch Hans's hoof, he would start tapping. When Hans neared the correct answer, the observers would change their posture; this was the clue to Hans to stop tapping. Hans would respond to a lifted head and even the observers' raising their eyebrows. Hans was not an extremely intelligent horse but he was an extremely astute observer of nonverbal communication.

Hans did not intend to appear to be a very smart horse and behave according to his observers' expectations. Similarly, many patients do not intend to behave according to the expectations of their physicians, family, and friends. Nevertheless, people do pay close attention to the subtle expectations of others.

In the early 1930s social scientists investigated the productivity of employees at the Western Electric Company's Hawthorne Plant in Chicago [39]. These researchers were attempting to identify specific influences on production but stumbled on an important general social psychological effect. The researchers expected certain changes such as increased lighting to raise productivity and other changes to lower productivity. To their surprise they found that everything they did resulted in greater productivity. The workers were producing more because someone was paying attention to them. Thus the term the *Hawthorne effect* refers to the phenomenon by which production rises when special attention is paid to the workers, independently of changes in the working conditions.

The Hawthorne effect has important implications for doctor-patient interactions. Patients often appear at a doctor's office and want a doctor to do *something*. It is likely that as long as the doctor pays attention to the patient, anything the doctor does will have at least some beneficial effect in many cases. Interestingly, when medical treatments were few and ineffective, doctors counted on their very presence to have a positive effect on the patient. Of course, any treatment must be considered in light of the medical injunction to "first, do no harm."

When we are in the presence of certain people, we sometimes find ourselves behaving in ways in which we might not normally behave. For example, a very assertive superior may make us feel uncharacteristically anxious or inferior. An illustration of the strength and subtlety of this phenomenon is provided by a study of nonverbal communication [50]. In this study college women were videotaped while chatting casually with a partner of either the same sex or the opposite sex. It was found that the nonverbal behavior of the women who were with a male partner was significantly related to their partner's personality. Women were submissive when with dominant male partners and dominant when with submissive male partners. They molded themselves to the personality of the male.

If college students could quickly but unknowingly adjust their own behavior to fit the personality trait of their male partner, we can easily imagine a similar process occurring in the medical setting. If some practitioners make it clear that they are in charge and are going to dominate the situation, many patients may in turn act submissively. The patients then communicate this orientation to the practitioner through their nonverbal cues, and the practitioner decides that it is necessary to behave dominantly—after all, the patient is so submissive!

In this way subtle mutual expectations arise between the practitioner and patient. Because of the central importance of medical interactions to most patients, these expectations can dramatically affect health. They have been studied under the rubric "placebo effects."

Placebos

"The placebo effect is a neglected and berated asset of patient care" [3].

Throughout the history of medicine up to the twentieth century, almost all medical treatments had no specific biological foundation. Yet physicians were able to retain respect, and they sometimes even produced cures. This happened because of what is known as the placebo effect. Arthur Shapiro defines a *placebo* as any therapy that is without specific activity for the condition being treated. The effects of placebos may be psychological or psychophysiological. Placebos may be "drugs" such as sugar pills, but they can also be surgical procedures, physical manipulations, prescribed diets, exercises, or other regimens [41, 42, 43].

Placebo effects are sometimes dismissed in medical circles because it is incorrectly assumed that they do not have physiological effects. But a number of studies indicate that placebos can induce symptoms such as weakness, nausea, rashes, and pain. Similarly, placebos can produce beneficial physiological changes like improvements in skin condition, increased activity, and recovery from fever [26, 51]. However, many people are surprised to learn that placebo effects can induce the body to produce substances called Endorphins, which help the body control pain [29].

The psychological state of the individual can either enhance or inhibit the individual's reactions to specific drugs. Human beings are active biological organisms that respond in complex ways to the introduction of foreign agents. Just as the body may be more or less susceptible to various diseases at various times, the body will also react to various therapies and treatments in different ways at different times, depending on the psychological and emotional state of the person [28].

Throughout the history of medicine, every imaginable substance and treatment has been used in the attempt to cure disease. Drugs ranged from crocodile dung to the spermatic fluid of frogs. Sometimes the reasoning was that "like cures like." For example, parts of a hairy animal might be given a patient in an attempt to cure baldness, or muscles of a strong animal be eaten in an attempt to cure muscle disease. Some of these treatments were actually very destructive, such as the well-known treatment of bleeding or leeching. Nevertheless, because of the placebo effect, these treatments were also sometimes helpful [41, 43].

The use of similar substances to cure disease developed into a separate discipline in the early 1800s. This field, which is still in existence, is called *homeopathy* [20]. However, since many of the prescribed substances were actually harmful, a clever theory was developed that asserted that very minute quantities of a substance were needed for a cure. In fact, the more diluted the substance, the more effective it supposedly would be. Hence homeopathic treatment often involves administering water or ethyl alcohol with a minute quantity of an additional substance, for example, plants or herbs. At the very least traditional homeopathy does no harm. (That is, no direct harm, because the patient might be diverted from seeking another kind of treatment, which might be beneficial.) Often it seems to help because of placebo effects. Homeopathic medicine, which is still used in the United States today, illustrates the importance of expectations to healing. The placebo effect deserves a place in all medical care.

Wise physicians know that they should use new drugs while they are still effective [43]. Many new treatments work for a while, that is, as long as they have positive expectations associated with them. However, as failures are reported and as the drugs or treatment procedures become commonplace, their efficacy often fades. Fortunately, positive expectations need not depend on the existence of new treatments.

In a review of various work on placebo effects, Henry Beecher found that about one-third of all patients are helped by placebo effects [2]. This is a significant percentage, and it means that *any* given treatment will help a substantial number of patients. Even "miraculous" cures such as shrinking cancer tumors have been reported, but they are very difficult to document systematically.

The mechanisms underlying placebo effects are not well understood, but two basic processes are probably at work. First, behavioral changes result from expectations. Patients who become optimistic may try harder; for example, they may drink more fluids and sleep and walk more, and these behaviors may lead to improved health. Second, a person's thoughts and feelings can produce physiological changes through the actions of the nerves and hormones. For example, a person's psychological state can affect heartrate, muscle tension, breathing, sweating, and many complicated endocrine processes [9].

Of course, placebos can also produce severe negative physiological effects, resulting from negative expectations. One example is the American soldiers studied by Frank, which was mentioned earlier. Negative placebo effects include fainting, vomiting, diarrhea, changes in blood flow, and detrimental respiratory effects.

Since placebo effects are probably closely related not only to the patient's expectations but also to the *doctor's* expectations, valid research on all new therapies demands the use of *double-blind* experimental procedures [40]. In this procedure, neither the doctor nor the patient knows whether the patient is receiving the new treatment being tested, the old treatment, or a placebo control. For example, a new pain reliever might be compared to aspirin, codeine, or a sugar pill, but neither the medical personnel nor the patients would know which treatment was which. Only the researcher would know.

It is sometimes difficult for medical personnel to believe that their expectations, which they try to keep to themselves, can influence a patient's recovery. They may assume that either a new treatment will or will not work, no matter what they do. However, such an approach is a serious mistake, and also very unscientific. Without strict controls in a double-blind procedure, the results of a study of a new treatment are scientifically worthless (see also Box 4-1).

SOMATOPSYCHOLOGY

In studying the relationship of the mind and the body, we must also look at the influence of disease processes on psychological reactions. The study of the influence of so-called physical states on

Box 4-1
The Ethics of Placebo Control Groups

To determine their effectiveness, new drugs must be tested against old drugs or inert substances. In this way any improvement caused by the specific activity of the new drug can be distinguished from any improvement resulting from placebo effects. However, if the new drug is truly effective, some patients would have been deprived of a potentially lifesaving drug during the period of the test.

Interestingly, the results of a two-year study of stroke prevention showed the importance of careful experimental tests. A new drug, contrary to expectation, was not effective when compared with a placebo and aspirin. However, there was some evidence that the aspirin itself was effective in preventing stroke. If this study had not been conducted, patients might have gone on receiving the new useless drug, while the discovery that aspirin was better would not have been made. In research any treatment has certain risks and costs, and these must be weighed against the likelihood of any benefit.

Ethics cannot be decided on the basis of the *results* of a study. New treatments must be compared against old treatments in an experimental design that also assesses placebo effects. Indeed, it is unethical if medical researchers do not conduct methodologically sound research to insure that every new treatment that is used is effective.

For further reading: S. Bok, The ethics of giving placebos, in R. Hunt and J. Arras (eds.), *Ethical Issues in Modern Medicine* (Palo Alto, Calif.: Mayfield, 1977), pp. 278–290.

---

so-called mental states is called somatopsychology. It should be remembered, however, that this perspective is only one of emphasis; in an overall sense physical and mental states cannot be separated.

One way in which the body affects a person's psychological state is through the reactions of others. For example, a disabled or a disfigured person may receive negative reactions from others and may incorporate these reactions into his or her own self-image. Another source of influence of the bodily state on a person's psychology involves sensory impairments. For example, people who cannot see or who cannot walk may learn to approach the world and understand it in different ways from people who are not handicapped. Health providers should be alert to the psychological adjustments that are made by people with various physical handicaps. The problems of chronic illness and disability are examined in Chapter 8.

The temporary impairment caused by hospitalization or illness can also affect psychological reactions. Bedrest imposed on a normally active person, or the lack of control over the environment that is so much a part of hospitalization, may produce anxiety or depression in a patient. Many of these reactions are mediated by the individual's explanations for and means of coping with illness. For example, some patients may explain their illness in terms of punishment for past sexual escapades or other wrong doings and may become especially upset as a result of illness and treatment. The meaning of illness is important, and it is discussed in detail in Chapter 6.

A final area of somatopsychology concerns the body's level of comfort and activity. Tense muscles, lack of sleep, excessive sleep, pain, sunburn, muscle fatigue, and similar "physical" ailments can affect a person's psychological state and produce a state far beyond simple discomfort. On the other hand, exercises, sexual fulfillment, muscle relaxation, and other such "physical" influences can also serve to produce a marked improvement in general psychological functioning. Such inseparable ties between the mind and the body are well illustrated in a key area of medicine—that of pain.

PAIN

When we touch a hot stove or a sharp needle we feel pain. At a young age we learn to associate the feeling of pain with the destruction of our body (as through burning or cutting). This is adaptive learning. Since the relationship is strong, many people assume that pain means that the body is sensing tissue destruction. People generally think that pain is a natural, fixed reaction to an intrusive stimulus, for example, if we are pricked by a pin, our nerves carry the message to our brain and we feel pain. This assumed sequence of pain perception is actually inadequate and misleading. There is no necessary and direct link between tissue damage and pain [33].

Soldiers who are injured on the battlefield often do not feel as much pain as they would if they received an identical injury at home in their kitchen. Athletes frequently report not feeling the pain of injury until they are off the playing field and in the clubhouse. People under hypnosis often have a greatly increased tolerance for pain. Two patients with the same degree of physical degeneration as the result of a disease may experience very different degrees of pain. Such phenomena are partly the result of social influences on pain.

In the early nineteenth century, before anesthetics had been discovered, mesmerism (hypnotism) was used successfully to control pain. It has been reported that the French surgeon Cloquet performed an extensive operation to remove a malignant tumor from a woman's breast. During the surgery the woman talked quietly to her doctor and showed no signs of pain. Pain-free surgery procedures done under hypnosis (and related techniques) still occur today [7, 48]. Thus even the enormous pain of surgery can be significantly decreased or eliminated with a process based essentially on interpersonal influence.

Why are pain and social factors related? Szasz and others have pointed out that the sensation of pain partly serves a function of communication [45, 53]. Expression generally brings compassion and help from others; the expression of pain may be a request for comfort. The rewards and punishments received from others may affect reactions to pain. Furthermore, interpretation of feelings is an element of pain.

There are many examples of the social benefits of pain. A child who reports a minor sensation of pain and is excused from school may soon begin to feel the pain more severely. Patients who report pain may receive significant attention from various medical practitioners, and it is also very difficult to rule out serious organic influences on pain; therefore a patient who seeks attention will be constantly rewarded for feeling pain.

For Sigmund Freud and his followers, pain may be symbolic of a psychological problem in interpersonal relations. For example, a patient may feel a pain in his or her derrière when in the presence of the boss. More commonly, people may feel headaches in various unpleasant situations. Furthermore, pain may be associated with emotional disturbances [44]. For example, people often feel pain when they are depressed. It is not necessarily true that such people have absolutely no organic disturbance (although it is possible, of course), but rather that *various sensations become painful when the psychological environment is right.*

Since the expression of pain is partly a communication to others that has been rewarded by others, the expression and even the feeling of pain can sometimes be eliminated through extinction or punishment. For example, if a child's minor pain is minimized and the child is sent to school despite it, the pain is likely to disappear. Similarly, if an employee loses pay for missing work because of headaches, the headaches may be minimized or disappear. Some suggest that successful pain management can be attained by medical practitioners if they ignore pain as a symptom when no organic causes can be found over a long period of time. On the other hand, if emotional disturbances seem prominent, psychological intervention (such as psychotherapy) may be necessary. However, given the complex nature of pain, it is likely that more active methods of treating pain such as those described below may be more useful than ignoring pain.

The discouragement of pain expression is valuable in pain management for another set of reasons. There is evidence that the suppression of pain responses and expressions may actually lessen pain. Examples of this process from common folk wisdom are "whistle while you work" and "let a smile be your umbrella." Behavioral changes are expected to produce psychological changes such that a person's body feels good and the person feels happy when working productively and smiling. In psychology this idea can be traced to Charles Darwin and William James [11, 22]. Darwin noted that the expression of an emotion intensifies it, while the repression of an emotion softens it. Expressing rage may increase a person's rage, while keeping it in may reduce the intensity of the experience. William James hypothesized that *all* emotion develops *following* bodily changes. According to this theory, the act of crying makes someone feel sad and the act of trembling makes someone feel fearful. Although more complex theories of emotion have since evolved, it is true that inner feelings can sometimes be affected by outer expressions.

Under what conditions can a smile or a whistle alleviate pain? It is obvious that the process is complex, for we cannot deal with the pain of a deep bleeding cut by whistling a happy tune. Two main factors are relevant: the feedback the brain is receiving from the body and what the person is thinking about. For example, a crying child with a scraped knee may have the pain reduced through distraction, entertainment, laughter, or through tickling, bouncing, massaging, and so on. In adults the influence of both bodily sensations and thoughts on pain perception was demonstrated in an experimental study by Sonia Blackman [5]. Since people receive detailed internal feedback from their facial expressions, Blackman manipulated whether people held a facial expression of pain or tried to hide pain (or smile) while experiencing pain from a tourniquet. Consistent with the "facial feedback" hypothesis, hiding pain expressions led to lower pain than a facial expression that showed exaggerated pain; cues from the body affected pain perception. However, Blackman also found that after five minutes, people's *thoughts* about their pain and their current situation became an increasingly more important influence on felt pain. In short, hiding (or covering) pain expressions can be a helpful technique of pain control so long as this process is consistent with what the person is thinking about the degree and appropriateness of pain.

Of course, if patients do not express pain, medical personnel do not receive valuable information about the progress of a disease or the course of recovery. Such information should not be suppressed. The suppression of pain expressions may be a valuable means of controlling pain *after* the disease is well diagnosed and charted. Patients should be encouraged to report difficulty but discouraged from excessive complaining.

Low Back Pain

"No amount of knowledge about the physiologic, anatomic and biochemical substrates of pain perception will suffice to fully explain the common clinical syndrome of low back pain" [30]. This striking statement from a pain researcher reaffirms the key role of social psychological factors in medicine. Low back pain is a common and important medical problem. In addition to chronic suffering for the individual, it may lead to early retirement and to disability benefits. Hundreds of thousands of Americans each year undergo surgery or are given dependency-producing medications for back pain. Yet significant bone or nerve dysfunction is generally not found in these patients. In many cases, low back pain will disappear in response to a variety of placebo treatments ranging from hot (or cold) compresses to doctors' orders to remain active (or inactive). The specific communication skills that medical practitioners can use to create positive expectations are discussed in Chapter 5. First, however, we discuss some of the physiological evidence for mind–body ties and some promising pain management techniques.

The Gate Control Theory of Pain

A promising physiological theory of Ronald Melzack and P. D. Wall, which is called the gate control theory, attempts to explain how psychological factors can influence pain perception [34]. Simply, this theory proposes that there are special nerves that carry intense sensation (such as from extreme heat like a stovetop) to the spinal column. But these signals do not necessarily go directly to the brain because there is a "gate" in the spinal column that can be closed by signals coming down from the brain. Thus thoughts and feelings can provide these gate-closing signals and influence whether the sensation of pain reaches the brain and is perceived as pain. Although the actual gate control mechanisms are not yet clear, this model in which psychological factors influence the processing of sensation does seem likely to be able to account for much of the existing data about pain (see Figure 4-1).

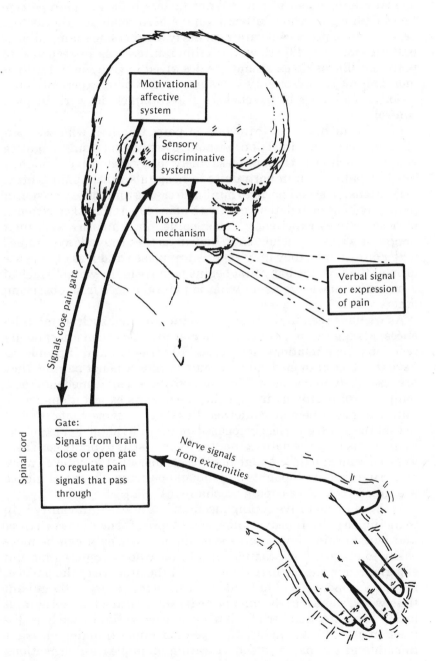

Figure 4-1. The gate control theory of pain.

What implications does this model have for the social psychological management of pain? What factors influence pain perception? Although various attempts have been made to describe the personality of people who are most likely to experience pain, no clear pattern emerges [49]. However, ethnic differences in response to pain and illness do exist and are described in Chapter 6. Furthermore, although personality variables predict pain experience only weakly, a number of psychological *techniques* do work in pain control.

First, modeling is an influence on pain. Children who see their mother receive an injection without overtly expressing negative emotion, such as crying, are less likely to cry themselves and may feel less pain. Even in burn units in hospitals, where pain is often very intense, a social norm to minimize crying and the expression of pain may help each patient deal with pain [49]. At the other extreme, men sometimes experience "labor pains" in sympathy with their pregnant wives, a phenomenon known as the "couvade syndrome" [38]. For example, they may experience nausea and loss of appetite around the time the baby first begins to move in the womb. Much of a person's knowledge about what is painful comes from observing others.

As we have seen in the first part of this chapter, such social influences as suggestion, hypnosis, and placebo effects can affect bodily reactions. This relationship is especially true of pain. If people believe that a certain medical procedure or illness is not painful, they are less likely to feel pain. These processes resemble modeling as a pain control technique in that they depend on expectations transmitted from one person to another. But they are somewhat different in that the process is clearly focused on the individual. For example, in hypnosis only the patient (not the hypnotist) is hypnotized. There are also related pain management techniques that focus even more on the individual's thoughts and thought patterns. These techniques are called "cognitive coping mechanisms" [32].

Practice in cognitive coping mechanisms may significantly help to minimize pain. If people know what types of sensations to expect and how to think about these sensations, their pain can be more easily managed. For example, an athlete who is prepared for and experienced in the feelings that occur in the practice of the particular sport is more likely to be able to continue activity without pain than would someone who unexpectedly suffered an identical painful bodily injury. A number of related cognitive variables such as distraction also affect pain [23, 27, 48]. For example, thinking pleasant thoughts as compared to concentrating on unpleasant sensations may minimize pain. Similarly, studies in attribution theory in social psychology have demonstrated that the explanations people have for their bodily feelings (e.g., "I am bench pressing" versus "I'm having a heart attack") affect their subsequent reactions to such feelings.

Biofeedback

The technique of *classical conditioning* is well known to social scientists. In this type of learning the body's autonomic responses become conditioned to a previously neutral stimulus in the environment. For example, when Pavlov paired the ringing of a bell with the presentation of food, his dogs learned to salivate to the bell ringing. The new behavior is known as a conditioned response. This type of learning differs from *operant conditioning* in which an organism learns those behaviors for which it is rewarded. For example, rats may learn to turn right in a maze if that is where the food is usually presented, or children may learn to brush their teeth if they are often praised by their parents for so doing. Learning in response to rewards is usually voluntary behavior.

In recent years research has indicated that autonomic responses such as heartrate and intestinal contractions may be subject to operant (reward) conditioning. That is, people can gain some control over their "involuntary" responses [4]. *Biofeedback* is a self-regulatory technique by which a person can learn to control some autonomic bodily processes and can gain increased control over some voluntary processes. For example, if patients hear a tone that changes from unpleasant to pleasant as their blood pressure drops, some patients can evidently learn to lower their blood pressure. Biofeedback holds promise in treating headaches by influencing bloodflow and in treating neuromuscular problems through control over muscle tension. However, much more research is needed to define the boundaries of biofeedback's effectiveness. This aspect of the mind–body link is not yet well understood. At the very least, however, people can learn muscle relaxation, which may be useful in combating anxiety, for anxiety is known to increase pain perceptions.

Acupuncture

Medical personnel are familiar with the phenomenon of referred pain; that is, stimulation to one part of the body is felt somewhere else. For example, the pain of a heart attack may be felt in the left arm or in the jaw. It is also known by most people that stimulation to one part of the body can reduce pain in another part. For example, a hot water bottle applied to the neck may reduce back pain for some people. We have also seen that pain is affected by expectations. These two phenomena function together in the Chinese technique of acupuncture [6].

In acupuncture, which is designed to minimize or eliminate pain, a patient may undergo major surgery such as removal of a lung or the stomach while fully conscious. The only analgesic (pain-killing) mechanisms are acupuncture needles inserted at certain critical points in the body *and* the patient's faith in the effectiveness of the technique. The precise mechanisms underlying successful use of acupuncture are not well understood because pain itself is not well understood. However, consistent with the gate control theory of pain, it seems clear that stimulation of one part of the nervous system can interfere with the sensation of pain produced by stimulation of another part of the nervous system.

Pain Clinics

Because of the complexity and prevalence of pain and because of the problems of addiction and drug abuse brought about by pain-reducing drugs like morphine and Darvon, some hospitals have developed pain control clinics. Such clinics create a comprehensive pain management program that begins with a detailed assessment of the patient's social situation and psychological state [12]. Training in relaxation, the proper way of thinking about pain, a monitoring of situational influences on pain, and perhaps biofeedback are all used in conjunction with such psychophysiological techniques as drugs, surgery, and transcutaneous nerve stimulation. The so-called special techniques of pain clinics take a truly holistic view of pain, an approach to pain that should be adopted in everyday medical care.

SUMMARY

In sum, there is substantial scientific evidence documenting the influence of psychological and emotional states on so-called physical health. Similarly, there is a link between the condition of a person's body and the resulting mental state. Thus a mind–body dualism is an inappropriate model for medicine. Health involves both the physical and psychological factors at the same time; they are inseparable. This link is most clearly seen in pain perception and control, where instances of the phenomenon of "mind over body" are readily observed.

Yet psychological and emotional factors are relevant, to a greater or lesser extent, in every illness. The "will to live" and related phenomena of placebo effects are a basic element of health care. We have seen that belief and faith can be understood in terms of expectations, most of which arise in interactions with other people. Even though the precise physiological mechanisms through which social psychological factors influence disease processes have not yet been identified, "faith" healing is not necessarily unscientific. It is up to health professionals to incorporate the proper social environment into the treatment regimen in order to provide the most effective, scientific health care.

5
Communication with Patients: Verbal and Nonverbal

Physician: "Well Mr. Johnson, the results of your tests are back," said Dr. Welton, with a slight frown at the fact that he was running behind schedule. "It looks like what we are dealing with here is a simple case of hypertension. There seems to be no kidney involvement at this stage, and your blood chemistries look pretty good." Dr. Welton continued looking at the chart, not at Mr. Johnson. "Since the hypertension is most likely being exacerbated by your obesity and excessive stress, I'd like you to follow this diet, which is designed both for weight loss and for decreased sodium, in order to reduce fluid retention. In addition, I want you to relax and take these pills three times a day—hydrochlorthiazide or water pills for diuresis. You should talk to my receptionist and make an appointment to come in again in three weeks. Do you have any questions you would like to ask me?"

Mr. Johnson: "No thanks, Doc," he smiled graciously. "See you in a few weeks."

Later in the Johnson home:

Mrs. Johnson: "What did the doctor say today?"

Mr. Johnson: "He said I have a chemical problem in my blood and that is what makes me a little overweight and nervous. He wants me to go back and see him in a while, and then after I see him again I should start taking some pills if I want to lose weight. I think he's worried about my health. I wonder if there's something he's scared to tell me."

The gross misunderstanding of the physician's explanations and instructions by this patient, Mr. Johnson, may seem a little farfetched. You may be thinking that such confused communication between the physician and the patient is unlikely to happen. Yet if we look at the research studies that have addressed this question of physician–patient communication, we find that such misunderstanding is actually common.

The Problem of Practitioner–Patient Communication

Research on the communication of medical information from health care professionals to patients suggests that faulty communication, and resulting errors in diagnosis and treatment, may be the rule rather than the exception. In one study, for example, researchers tape recorded twenty-five physician–patient interactions in which the physicians conveyed important information to the hospitalized patients [36]. These communications, for example, were about the need for surgery or the results of important diagnostic tests. The patients were questioned immediately after the physician left them. They were asked to tell the researcher what they had discussed with the physician. Ten of the twenty-five patients showed definite distortions of what they had been told. Analyses of the tape recordings showed most distortions to result from inadequate explanation by the physician. Furthermore, in all cases except one, the physician left the room before checking to see whether the patient had understood what was said.

In a related study patients were interviewed after a visit to an outpatient clinic [54]. A comparison was made between what the patient reported was told him or her and what the practitioner had actually said, according to a verbatim record. It was found that only 63 percent of the medical statements made by physicians were recalled accurately by patients. Furthermore, 56 percent of the instructions were reported erroneously, although this was true of only 27 percent of other statements such as diagnoses. While it is not possible to determine whether patients forgot quickly or never understood in the first place, the discrepancy between the physician recommendation and the patient perception may have seriously jeopardized treatment.

Work by Barbara Korsch and her colleagues documents significant problems in physician–patient communication [28, 29, 49]. In her studies at a children's hospital, Dr. Korsch tape recorded 800 patient visits to a pediatric walk-in clinic and then conducted follow-up interviews with the mothers of the children. Significant problems in communication were found in the physician–mother interviews. The primary problems involved the physician's failure to take account of the patient's concerns and expectations from the medical visit, and the lack of a clear-cut explanation concerning diagnosis, the cause of the illness, and treatment. In 800 visits, 19 percent of the mothers reported that they had not been told by the physician what was wrong with their child, and 26 percent said that they had not mentioned their greatest concern to the physician because either they did not have a chance to or because they were not encouraged by the physician to do so. The major finding of Korsch's research was that there was significant misunderstanding by patients of what their physicians had communicated to them. While the length of the session that the mother and child had with the physician had *no* relationship to patient satisfaction or to subsequent cooperation with treatment, characteristics of the communication strongly influenced these results.

The communication problems had little to do with language barriers. The most severe as well as the most common complaint of the dissatisfied mothers was that the physicians did not show enough interest to relieve their worries about the children and acknowledge their concern. The mothers believed that doctors were more involved with "technical" matters. The most successful outcomes in terms of patient cooperation and patient satisfaction occurred when the mother and physician each had active roles in communication about the illness of the child. It was concluded that attention to communication skills could make a valuable contribution to health care delivery. What specifically can be done?

Barriers to Effective Communication

Patient: "I don't understand why doctors can't tell their patients what to expect, or explain things in terms the patient can understand. Why do I feel frustrated and confused when I leave my doctor's office? He talks to me in gobbledygook and he thinks I understand. Then if I don't get everything exactly right—like if my blood pressure doesn't go down enough to satisfy him—he seems to get angry at me.... I think he just likes to keep me in the dark so I think I can't do without him."

Physician: "What do my patients want from me anyway? I tell them what I think their symptomatology means and I tell them what the results of the diagnostic examinations were. I explain to them carefully what they should do to effect a treatment regimen. I tell them all the implications of each of the treatment regimens. Still, so many of them come back having not followed directions, or having done few of the things I told them to do, or remembering a small proportion of the things I told them. I guess I assumed too much about what patients are capable of comprehending. They probably should not be given very much information."

Here we see some of the issues in the miscommunication between health care professionals and their patients, which is pervasively common. Incorrect assumptions about what the other can understand, and about what the other's motives are, tend to be significant obstructions in the flow of communication between the health care consumer and provider. Let us look at some of the reasons for these problems, so that we can better understand how communication can be enhanced.

In 1963 Samuel Bloom, a medical sociologist, proposed that the two functions of the health care professional involved the provision of "instrumental care" and the provision of "socioemotional care" [12]. The former involves the purely technical aspects of the treatment of the patient (e.g., surgery or the administration of a specific drug for a specific condition). The latter involves the emotional and interpersonal dimension of care—the communication of caring to the patient and the understanding of the patient's feelings [6, 7]. As we have noted in the preceding chapters, total care of the patient involves both of these dimensions, requiring both technical and interpersonal expertise by the health care provider. Interpersonal expertise involves two basic skills. First, the practitioner must have the proper orientation to and understanding of the role of the health practitioner in health care. This matter was discussed at length in Chapters 2 and 3. Second, the practitioner must be skilled in interviewing and must engage in effective *communication* with patients. The main barriers to effective communication generally fall into two categories: issues of *medical jargon* and issues of *nonverbal communication*.

MEDICAL JARGON

In a study by Julian Samora, Lyle Saunder, and Richard Larson [72], certain patients defined various medical terms as follows:

1. Abdomen: sides; buttocks; heart; bladder; entire area below the waist.
2. Appendectomy: a cut rectum; taking off an arm or leg; something to do with the bowels.
3. Digestion: a sick feeling; belching; what you eat.

4. Intern: same as an orderly; boys that help in the hospital; drugstore man; a man nurse; a doctor with no degree.
5. Pulse: a bad hurt or sickness; a nerve; temperature.
6. Respiratory: in the arms or legs; venereal; tiredness; a sickness in which you sweat and have hot and cold flashes.

In this study, randomly selected common medical words, which physicians and health care professionals had reported they would readily use with their patients, were repeated to 125 hospitalized patients and scored immediately by an interviewer according to whether or not the patients understood what the word meant. No respondent gave an adequate definition for all of the words, and no single word was known or understood by all respondents. While there was some relationship between education and knowledge of medical terms, there was no overwhelming tendency for patients

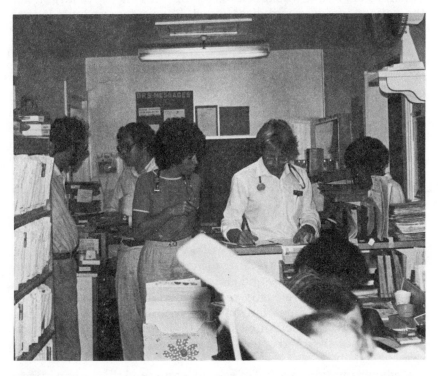

Figure 5-1. Communication problems in pediatric clinics have been well documented. In the clinic setting pictured here, psychosocial issues in child care are given special emphasis. (Photo by Howard S. Friedman, © 1982)

of higher educational levels to know many of the words. Thus, this study suggests that the vocabulary used by physicians creates significant problems in medical communication with patients. It is important to remember that these medical terms were terms that physicians and other health care professionals had indicated they would readily use in discussing a medical case with a patient.

Because it is medical jargon and very familiar to the practitioner, the practitioner may believe that the patient understands what has been said when in fact this is not so. Barbara Korsch has also documented the significant degree to which physicians speak to their patients in medical jargon and the detrimental impact that jargon has on a patient's understanding of what is wrong [28, 29, 49]. In this research it was found that physicians were much too technical in the language they used in communicating with their patients. In fact, in more than half the 800 physician–patient (mother) interactions that were recorded in the pediatrics clinic, the physician used language that was much too technical. This use of jargon left the patient confused and dissatisfied. Physicians used words that were totally misinterpreted by the mothers. For example, when one mother was told that the physician would have to "explore," she had no idea that her child would have to undergo surgery. Another mother thought that "incubation period" meant the length of time the child would have to say in bed [28, 29, 49].

In the totalitarian world of George Orwell's novel *1984*, there is a new language called Newspeak [66]. The purpose of Newspeak was to make it difficult or even impossible to think "unacceptable" thoughts. For example, words like *honor, justice,* and *morality* did not exist any longer, and words having to do with freedom were combined into the word *crimethink.*

The idea that our thought is influenced and controlled by our language comes from the psychologist and philosopher Benjamin Lee Whorf [84]. It is called *linguistic relativity.* For example, in English there is only one word for frozen water vapor—*snow.* But in Eskimo there are three words, describing different types of snow. Although we can all recognize snow and distinguish wet snow from dry snow, the Eskimo may more easily recognize and remember the type of snow that fell last winter and may be more sophisticated in thinking about snow. Words facilitate thought, and sometimes our thoughts and memories are interrupted because we cannot think of the right word.

Medical situations are full of special words, and this jargon affects patients. First, health practitioners who have facility with medical terms can think faster about medical topics than the patients with whom they are talking. In a discussion the practitioner may have gone on to a new topic while the patient is still trying to remember precisely what "abdomen" means. Second, practitioners may be better able to remember past discussions and problems than patients because of their greater knowledge of medical language. The patient may have forgotten the explanation received at the last visit because all the terms were new to the patient.

Third, medical jargon may lead practitioners to *think* about certain medical problems in very different ways from how their patients think about them. For example, "coronary thrombosis" may recall the image of a blocked artery to a nurse while the term "heart attack" may lead the patient to imagine a deadly substance attacking the heart. Consequently, the patient may not understand the treatment. Finally, medical jargon may create obvious problems of miscommunication, as in the following examples:

Doctor: "Have you ever had a history of cardiac arrest in your family?"

Patient: "No, we never had any trouble with the police."

Doctor: "Do you have varicose veins?"

Patient: "Well, I have veins, but I don't know if they're close or not."

Various surveys of randomly selected patients in the waiting rooms of clinics and private medical practices have found that a large percentage of the patients feel their doctors do not understand their problems, and that doctors and nurses use words that are too difficult for them to understand. Patients said that they would like doctors to simplify their language [4, 5, 48, 58].

Physicians and other health care professionals also use many abbreviations when talking to each other. For example, *DOA* means the patient was dead on arrival; *zero delta* means that there is no change in the patient's condition; *oids* are steroids—that is, corticosteroids. Physicians use this kind of jargon in talking to each other about patient's conditions. What is distressing for health care professional–patient communication is that health care professionals tend to use precisely this language when speaking to each other about the patient *in front of the patient,* and also sometimes when speaking to the patient.

Of course, medical jargon can be tremendously beneficial to practitioners in communicating with each other concisely and precisely. Everyone understands the necessity for scientific precision, but there may also be a more insidious use of medical jargon. It has been suggested by at least one observer of medical communications that health care profesionals do indeed talk a secret gobbledygook. Nicholas Christy, in the *New England Journal of Medicine,* has defined a language called *Medspeak* that health care professionals (particularly physicians) use to facilitate the sharing of information [14]. Medspeak often clouds scientific communication between the health care professionals themselves and is especially problematic when used in communications between health care professionals and their patients. An example of Medspeak is to use "symptomatology" synonymously with "symptoms." Actually, symptomatology is not a gramatically accurate substitute for symptoms, for it is defined in the dictionary as a field in which symptoms are studied. It confuses those not speaking Medspeak. "Armamentarium" is another Medspeak word. It is usually used by physicians to describe the collection of therapies they have available to treat a certain condition. It is a high-sounding, formal, frightening word—and while it has much to do with armies, arsenals, and baggage trains in wartime, it has virtually nothing to do with medical treatment.

Some writers have suggested that health professionals use their expectations that patients cannot understand medical issues as excuses for avoiding the time and trouble required to communicate with patients [60, 68]. Limited communication with patients also serves to protect the nurse or physician from encountering emotional reactions from patients [79]. It also may prevent a patient

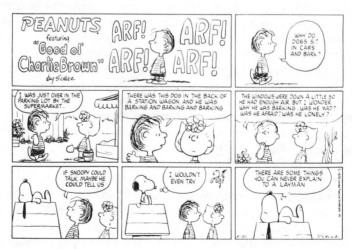

Figure 5-2. The use of professional jargon. (Copyright © 1978 United Features Syndicate)

from discovering neglect or error, and it may even prevent health care professionals from having to face their own emotional reactions.

Finally, it has been suggested that the control and withholding of information in the health care professional–patient relationship— the careful control of what is said to the patient about the patient's condition and how much is explained—represent an explicit attempt by the health professional to exert a measure of power over the patient [16, 30, 56, 57, 81, 82]. Obviously, most of the (power-oriented) reasons for the use of jargon benefit only the practitioner and only in the short run. In the long run, however, excessive jargon will destroy the interpersonal aspects of health care, with detrimental consequences for the patient's health, and as a result the entire medical care system will suffer. (See also Box 5-1.)

There is no way of knowing whether medical practitioners who allow jargon to interfere with the proper care of patients are doing so in a conscious effort to insure personal gain. The use of jargon may be so natural in certain medical settings that practitioners are not aware of the problems it creates. Special vigilance is needed to avoid this state of affairs. In fact, the use of jargon is so rarely necessary in communicating with patients that a good rule for practitioners is to always endeavor to explain any medical condition to a patient without using a single technical term. Medical names for conditions, drugs, and so on, can be provided later as needed in treatment.

The fact that most patients do not know medical jargon does not mean that they cannot understand medical explanations. Most patients can understand explanations of their medical condition, the cause of the illness, the prognosis, the choices involved in designing therapy, and the requirements for carrying out the therapy and cooperating with the treatment. In an interesting study by Lois Pratt, Arthur Seligman, and George Reader, clinic patients were questioned about the etiology, symptoms, and treatment of ten common diseases [68]. The questions were then given to physicians to see how well they thought their patients would answer. It was found that 81 percent of the physicians underestimated their patients' capabilities of understanding conceptual explanations. Patients actually had a surprisingly good understanding of medical problems when discussed in ordinary language. However, it was found in the analyses of physician–patient relationships that physicians rarely educated their patients. Patients seldom requested information from their physicians, and they seldom directed their physicians' attention to anything. Physicians tended to keep their patients at a very low level of information about their illnesses precisely because they believed that the patients were not capable of

Box 5-1
Ethical Issues in Deceiving Patients

The law of the courtroom insists that witnesses not only tell the truth but also that they tell "the whole truth and nothing but the truth." This demand protects against the case in which a statement is true but misleading. For example, if a doctor tells a leukemic youngster that he has a serious chronic disease but does not mention cancer, the doctor has told the truth but not the whole truth. Many people believe that adults are entitled to hear "the whole truth" from their doctors.

The medical setting is quite different from the legal setting, however, and there are various significant factors that complicate the issue of deception in medicine. The most troubling factor concerns placebos, which were discussed in Chapter 4. As we have seen, psychological factors can have a tremendous influence on health. Patients who expect to get better will often do much better than patients without hope. Indeed, the creation of positive expectations is a critical aspect of medical care. Thus if a patient believes that cancer is always painful and fatal, and the doctor consequently tells the patient that he or she has cancer, the communication itself may have a detrimental effect on the patient's health. Further complicating the matter is the fact that the doctor often is not sure of the patient's prognosis. Giving a patient unnecessarily bad news may thus be seen as a serious mistake in treatment. The patient's right to

know the diagnosis must be somehow balanced against the ambiguity in the diagnosis and the implications of knowing.

Another problem in telling the whole truth is the fact that medical knowledge can be very technical. Most people can understand the question "Were you in the victim's house on the night of the murder?" But many people cannot fully understand the meaning and implications of certain diseases. Thus it is almost impossible to communicate "the whole truth" to them.

Patient anger at physicians who did not tell them the whole truth is usually the result of the *reasons* why the doctor did not tell the truth. Patients may understandably be upset if they were deceived because the doctor did not take the time to talk to them, the doctor was protecting his or her own reputation, or the doctor did not want to face the emotional reaction of the patient. In such cases the doctor is simply another dishonest person.

The issue of the ethics of deceiving patients does not have to be decided in the abstract. If the doctor and patient are communicating well for the most part and if the doctor–patient relationship is generally positive (according to the criteria described in this book), deception is usually not a problem. Such patients in some situations want to and need to know more of the truth than other patients in other situations, and this matter can usually be dealt with directly in a healthy doctor–patient relationship.

For further reading: R. Hunt and J. Arras (eds.), *Ethical Issues in Modern Medicine* (Palo Alto, Calif.: Mayfield Co., 1977).

understanding the etiology (causes) of their illness, as well as its progress and treatment [74].

This unfortunate state of affairs suggests that medical care would be greatly improved and the patients' help enlisted if there were better interpersonal understanding. Techniques for obtaining accurate information from patients are considered in this chapter in the section, "Interviewing in the Health Care Context." First, however, we examine the subtle emotional communication that occurs between health practitioners and patients.

NONVERBAL COMMUNICATION BETWEEN PATIENTS AND PRACTITIONERS

Since ancient times healers have relied upon careful observation of patients as an aid in diagnosing illness. They have also developed certain bedside manners to promote recovery. Medical lore offers numerous suggestions for proper comforting of patients and for correct demeanor. In other words, experienced practitioners rely heavily on the subtle, unspoken messages of practitioner-patient interaction [65]. However, although scientific procedures have replaced art in much of medical practice, subtle interpersonal communication has not generally been studied scientifically. Such vague notions as intuition, empathy, sensitivity, caring, and similar suggestive but imprecise terms are often used in discussions of face-to-face patient care, and sometimes these terms are appropriate. But there have been many scientific studies about the meaning of these notions in terms of *nonverbal communication*. We can also apply this information to medical interactions [26, 32, 33].

Nonverbal communication involves facial expressions, voice tones, gestures, touches, and related cues that complement and illustrate aspects of the spoken word. They often express feelings that are not subject to direct conscious analysis by the practitioner or the patient. For example, a patient's grimace or shudder as well as a nurse's comforting touch or facial expression of sadness are messages that may be even more important than the words that are spoken [15, 46].

Many factors make it likely that patients will be especially watchful of providers' nonverbal cues. First, illness generally provokes anxiety and emotional uncertainty [52]. The patient must deal with such matters as the possibility of death, reactions to drugs, the presence of imposing equipment, new environments, and being separated from loved ones. In such circumstances, patients are likely to have a strong need for what psychologists call *social comparison*. That is, they want to reduce their emotional uncertainty and tend to look to those around them—often medical personnel—for subtle clues to help them understand what they are feeling and how they should respond [25, 73]. Second, patients are likely to be searching for factual information about their disease and its prognosis. Some of this information is provided by the verbal diagnosis, but we have already seen the many problems connected with verbal communication in the health care setting. Much of this information is not understood by patients, and more importantly it may not be fully believed. Practitioners may withhold or distort the whole truth for a variety of legitimate and not-so-legitimate reasons and patients know this fact. Since it is commonly believed that cues about deception are expressed through nonverbal channels, such cues may be given special attention by patients [47]. For example, patients may look for false smiles or a hurried manner.

Third, patients are especially likely to watch for nonverbal cues because of their position of weakness. Research indicates that inferiors may closely examine the nonverbal cues of their superiors; people with less power need to assess the mood of their superiors and ascertain which of their actions are creating a positive versus a negative effect [27, 41]. Patients are often completely at the mercy of the practitioner and want to please him or her. Furthermore, they may be hesitant to question a busy, high-status professional in detail and prefer to rely on messages left "unsaid" for clues about their medical condition. Finally, certain medical matters interfere with normal verbal communication and therefore require that more attention be paid to nonverbal communication. For example, orders to remain still, being attached to a respirator, and even holding a thermometer in the mouth all limit the patient's ability to question the practitioner and thus increase the importance of nonverbal communication.

In addition to patient sensitivity to nonverbal communication, it is also true that patients tend to be especially nonverbally *expressive*. That is, important information about the patient's condition is emitted solely through nonverbal channels. First, patients are likely to experience emotions such as fear, sadness, surprise, and anger. Research shows that emotions are often clearly revealed nonverbally, particularly through facial expressions [3, 23]. Practitioners can become experienced at recognizing these emotions. Second, patients are unlikely to have had much experience in hiding or controlling emotions in medical settings, and their usual social graces may disappear. For example, people may know how to control anger when provoked in a department store, but fear of hospitalization or pain caused by a doctor's probing may be directly revealed. Thus the attentive practitioner can detect valuable information. Third, some patients may prefer to communicate their feelings about certain difficult matters—their attitude toward death, embarrassing disabilities, a desire for additional services, and so on—through channels that are not too explicit, that is, through nonverbal communication. For example, a proud man may ask for pain medication with his eyes, but refuse to ask with words. Finally, various medical medical conditions may disrupt verbal communication and thus leave the patient with no choice but to communicate nonverbally. For example, weakness may make conversation too difficult for the patient but still allow the possibility of nonverbal messages such as a glance or gesture [11].

Probably patients will both be especially sensitive to the nonverbal cues emitted by health practitioners and be communicating a significant amount of important information through their own nonverbal cues. The likely meanings of specific nonverbal cues are described next.

The Face and Facial Expression

Hippocrates urged the physician to study the patient's face first. A face with "the nose sharp, the eyes sunken, the temples fallen in, the ears cold and drawn in and their lobes distorted, the skin of the face hard, stretched and dry, and the color of the face pale or dusky" usually portends death [42]. In addition to its general sense organs, the face has many muscles and nerves. In modern times facial features have proved useful in diagnosing genetic disorders [38]. Beyond fixed features, however, facial *expressions* of emotion provide valuable and detailed information.

Facial expression is an important element in the communication of pain. There is little doubt that valuable information about the intensity of pain and related negative feelings (fear, distress, sadness) is communicated to the health practitioner through the face, even when the patient is not fully conscious. For example, facial expression has been used to assess the amount of distress of women in labor [53]. In fact, the concept of pain itself has a communicative component in that its expression generally brings help from others; the expression of pain is, in part, a request for comfort [78]. Facial expression of pain may thus be expected to vary somewhat as a function of the nature of interpersonal relationships. If the expression of pain brings rewards other than pain relief (such as sympathy or insurance payments), the patient may show increasingly more pain. If the expression of chronic pain is ignored or punished, on the other hand, it may decrease, although at the cost of avoiding the possibility of relief through treatment.

This communicative function of pain expression is especially important because theory and research suggest that facial expression plays a role in the perception and management of pain. As we saw in Chapter 4, controlling the facial expression of pain (hiding pain) may help to reduce the pain [9, 50]. If you smile, you may temporarily feel better. Thus in some situations it may be advantageous for health providers to reinforce patients' suppression of facial expressions of pain. However, since such suppression in turn affects the other responses of the providers, who may now think the pain is gone and so not treat its cause, the issue is complex. In situations where nothing more can be done to treat the disease, the patient should be reassured, but the expression of pain should be discouraged.

The practitioner's expectations and the patient's emotions are often clearly and forcefully communicated through facial expression. The human face is fantastically expressive and people can easily and quickly recognize distinct emotional states from facial expression [22, 23, 80]. The six basic and easily recognized facial expressions are happiness, anger, sadness, surprise, disgust, and fear. Such expressions can effectively communicate a nurse's disgust at a wound or deformity, a physician's anger at a patient's failure to follow treatment regimens, or a technician's fear of a patient's deterioration. On the other hand, facial expressions can with practice be effectively controlled by most people [21, 22]. With proper training and motivation, practitioners' expressions might just as effectively communicate a nurse's sympathy and understanding or a physician's positive outlook and expectations. This psychological power of facial expression was not lost on tribal medicine men who wore elaborate masks during healing. In fact, in Ceylon different masks were worn for each disease [55]. Patients, paying special attention to nonverbal cues and especially influenced by the emotional nature of the social interaction, are usually strongly influenced by the provider's facial expression [6, 7].

Touch

Touch is one of the oldest and most widespread forms of traditional medical treatment. For hundreds of years during the Middle Ages, Europeans sought relief from the disease of scrofula (tuberculosis of the lymph gland) with the "King's touch" or the "royal touch" [10]. Many English and French kings treated thousands of people who came to them to receive divine healing. Despite a very low "cure" rate, the practice persisted, and many people obtained temporary relief. The power of this technique illustrates the tremendous symbolic value of touch in healing. Not surprisingly, the healing power of this royal touch tended to wane with the disappearing divinity of kings. However, some of this power may have been transferred to physicians. Patients may feel much better after a routine physical exam but may complain if the doctor "never even touched" them. In many situations touch has retained its symbolic value as a kind of blessing involving the transfer of special powers.

The tremendous symbolic value of medical touching can be easily seen in folk medicine. Faith healers have long used the technique of "laying on of the hands," and this "therapy" is still quite popular in American society. Since its efficacy is supposedly derived from the transfer of a healing spirit, just as the king transferred the divine spirit, this technique is of course generally viewed as quackery by modern medicine. We have seen the importance of expectation (Chapter 4), however, and at the least, touching may be fruitfully seen as a special sort of placebo effect. Imbued with a special symbolic value, the practitioner's touch may indeed promote healing. In modern American society, the concept of touching as basic to the process of healing has been enthusiastically adopted by the "human potential movement." Many popular encounter groups praise the healing value of touching. In short, touching has a significant psychological effect on many patients. Since positive expectations may result, even brief touches can be beneficial [69].

A recent study investigated the effects of being touched by female nurses during presurgical instruction [83]. In the hospital some patients were touched on the arm by female nurses while receiving information about upcoming surgery whereas other patients were not touched. Patients who had been touched reacted more positively to a variety of measures than patients who had not been touched, but this beneficial effect was confined to female patients. This study provides evidence that touch is important to medicine, but it also indicates that reactions to touch may depend on other aspects of the situation.

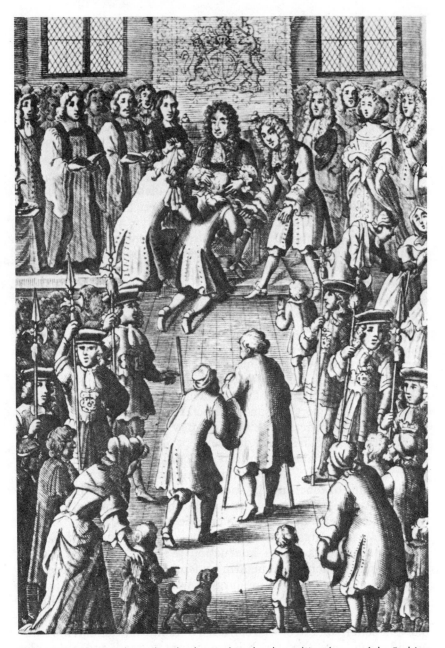

Figure 5-3. The royal touch: Charles II of England touching for scrofula. Etching by Robert White, the frontispiece to J. Browne, *Charisma Basilikon* (Part 3 of *Adenochoiradelogia*), 1684.

Touching for therapeutic purposes is not standardized and has been left as a relatively unresearched medical "art." However, medical practitioners palpate, poke, and otherwise touch their patients for purposes of diagnosis. Furthermore, diagnostic procedures such as temperature taking and throat and stethoscopic examination all involve touching the patient. Often, as in examinations of the breasts, vagina, prostate, and groin, the touch is in intimate areas not usually invaded by relative strangers. This kind of touching often produces important emotional and interpersonal reactions from patients.

There is little doubt that being touched is sometimes comforting and also sometimes emotionally arousing. Some medical touching may even be sexually arousing. However, a certain type of touch at a certain part of the body cannot be shown to have a general, predictable effect. First, there are tremendous individual differences in responses to being touched. Second, many differences arise from the fact that touch has social meaning. Two prominent interpersonal meanings of touch concern *intimacy* and *power*. In normal social interaction, the part of the body touched is generally clearly related to the intimacy of the relationship [44]. For example, the genitals are generally only touched by a close friend of the opposite sex or by a spouse. Violation of such norms in the medical setting may produce confusion. Nurses report incidents in which patients begin disclosing very personal information or become flirtatious during or after a backrub, a bath, or other usually "intimate" forms of touching, even though such behavior violates the role constraints of being a patient [43]. There are often technical reasons for providers to touch patients, but providers are also people and thus some patients may react to the *social* meaning of the touch.

Touching also communicates power [41]. If one man is touching another in a doctor's office, which man is the doctor? Practitioners touch patients routinely, but there is usually very little occasion for the patient to touch the practitioner. The practitioner is of higher status. Of course, most of this one-sided touching is for instrumental means in the technical side of medical care. Doctors do not touch patients for the purpose of asserting their power, although the implication of power differences remains. Thus on a social psychological level, touching can have an important effect on the overall relationship between the patient and practitioner.

Not all benefits of touching come from positive expectations. Classic studies of monkeys raised with wire and cloth surrogate mothers showed the importance of touch to healthy social development. Harry Harlow found that infant monkeys were very attracted to the contact comfort of a terrycloth surrogate "mother" [40]. This terrycloth mother aided the adjustment of the monkeys and was even preferred to a wire surrogate mother who had a nipple and provided food.

The comfort of contact is physiologically based. Indeed, the lack of touch retards development and has even been implicated in skin disease [64]. Certainly backscratching, patting, gentle massaging, and other touches are tension reducing. The successful use of water-beds in hospitals, to reduce the incidence of bedsores, may in fact partly result from an increased need for tactual stimulation in a tense atmosphere in which the patient is removed from usual family touching. In fact, nursing instructors acknowledge that "in nursing, touch may be the most important of all nonverbal behaviors" [11, p. 6]. An ill, anxious patient who is surrounded by cold equipment may be especially reassured by a warm touch. A similar conclusion was reached by the anthropologist Ashley Montagu, who wrote that "in every branch of the practice of medicine touching should be con-sidered an indispensable part of the doctor's art.... Touch always enhances the doctor's therapeutic abilities" [64, p. 223].

In sum, touch has significant functions in medical settings. Touch has symbolic value in healing, and it may create positive expecta-tions. Furthermore, even when it is used for strictly diagnostic pur-poses, touch may affect the interpersonal nature of the practitioner–patient interaction. Finally, touching has important physiological effects. Certainly this topic is deserving of a good deal of attention in medical practice.

Gaze

People generally are aware of and respond when they are being stared at [24]. Gaze is an influential nonverbal cue. Eye behavior is similar to touching in that its total meaning may depend upon other factors in the situation. A stare may be comforting if it inten-sifies a pleasant situation or opens communication in an uncertain situation; on the other hand, a stare may be arousing or threatening if it is excessive or if the context is negative [24, 25]. For example, glances from a sympathetic nurse or an unhurried doctor may en-courage a patient to cope with a difficult time or help a patient bring up a sensitive subject. Relatedly, the doctor described at the begin-ning of this chapter should have looked at the patient while giving good news. The practitioner's refusal to look a patient in the eye may produce negative reactions and be part of the process of dehumani-zation, common in medical settings, in which the patient is seen as (and comes to feel like) a body rather than a person (see Chapter 11).

A doctor who looks only at medical records while avoiding the gaze of the patient will have difficulty establishing rapport with a patient.

Excessive staring at a patient, with no apparent cause or in a troubling situation, is likely to have a negative effect, perhaps making the patient feel like a freak or a bad person. Presumably health providers will generally not stare at a patient's physical deformity, but constant eye contact to avoid doing so is also likely to be recognized by a patient. For example, interaction with a handicapped person (including eye contact) may be less variable, that is, more rigid and unchanging [45]. This difference in behavior is obvious to the handicapped patient. Refusal to look at or constantly staring at the chest of a mastectomy patient or avoidance of or excessive eye contact with a dying patient may have similar effects. It is a signal that something is awry, and it will intensify the emotions being communicated in other ways, through other channels. Fortunately, as with facial expression, people can learn to be more aware of where their gaze is directed.

Tone of Voice

As with facial expressions, the specific emotional and motivational states of patients and practitioners may be revealed through their tone of voice [17]. The tone of voice refers to sounds, primarily pitch variations, that accompany the spoken word. Emotions like fear, anger, sadness, interest, and joy and motivational states like pain are readily transmitted through vocal cues. Another message expressed through tone of voice concerns the nature of the interpersonal relationship. For example, some dependent elderly patients may be addressed in high-pitched "baby talk"—the tone parents use when talking to infants.

Although tone of voice is probably an important element in the overall "tone" the practitioner sets for an interaction, not enough research has been conducted in this area. Tone of voice does, however, seem important to the transmission of expectancies; it is probably an aspect of placebo effects [20]. For example, one study found a negative correlation (relationship) between the amount of "anger" judged to be present in a doctor's voice and his success in referring alcoholic patients for treatment [63]. Another study has shown a relationship between a physician's ability to express emotions through voice tone (and face and voice) and the way the physician is evaluated by his or her patients; physicians with better voice control were better liked [34]. Thus providers' voice tones are likely to affect the expectations and emotional reactions of their patients.

Smells

Communication through odors is sometimes important in the medical field. Some drugs and treatments may produce unpleasant odors in the patient. Various illnesses affect patient odor through actions on the gastrointestinal tract. On the other hand, medical practitioners may also be associated with particular odors. The use of anesthesia, alcohol, and other chemicals may give practitioners and their surroundings certain smells. Furthermore, the lingering odors of other patients may transmit an olfactory message to the patient.

Social psychological research on "person perception" has shown that negative personal attributes are often associated with malodor. A bad person may be labeled a "stinker" or "stinkpot." In fact, perceiving the outgroup as smelly is a prime characteristic of prejudice [1, 51]. The diseased person suffering from malodor is likely to be reacted to with negative feelings. Even some health care providers may unknowingly come to regard foul-smelling patients as less good or moral, especially if the patient has at least some control over the odor. Such reactions of distaste may then be transmitted to patients through facial expressions.

The particular and uncommon smells of practitioners' medical settings may affect the health care process through associations. For unknown reasons, odors often have tremendous power to evoke memories of forgotten times and places [1, 61]. People often associate certain smells with particular events in their past. Hence a doctor's office or a hospital may evoke vivid memories of the previous negative experiences of an ill relative or a childhood trauma. These memories may create, even unconsciously, significant negative expectations in the patient.

A final point about smells is that they have strict norms associated with them in American society. People who have a bad smell may feel embarrassed or unworthy, and they may avoid needed treatment and needed friends in order to avoid social contact. However, since most people do not like to talk about smells, the practitioner may be unaware of this problem. Therefore the practitioners themselves must take the initiative in dealing with the possible medical implications of odors.

Distance

Bad odors, disfigurement, fear of contagion, and other factors may all affect the distance that health practitioners keep between themselves and patients. Extra distance can have a significant psychological impact on patients since there are firm expectations about the distances that should be used in normal social interaction.

The anthropologist Edward Hall has written extensively about the effects of interpersonal distance [39]. He distinguishes four spatial zones: intimate distance, personal distance, social distance, and public distance. The intimate distance is of course the distance at which very intimate interactions usually occur. We have already seen that closeness and touching by practitioners may produce psychological reactions in patients that are out of place. Analogous problems can occur at other distances. For example, if a doctor on rounds in a hospital with a group of medical students stands back across the room and addresses the patient so that everyone can hear (public distance), the patient may become upset if intimate matters are being discussed. Intimate matters are supposed to be discussed at the intimate distance; the public distance results in a lack of privacy, a loud voice, more emphatic gesturing, and other incongruent cues that may produce psychological distress. Similarly, interpersonal problems can result if practitioners and visitors stand too far away from patients, maybe because of fear or poor habits, or stand too close, perhaps out of curiosity or a desire to comfort the patient. If the type of social interaction does not match the usual distance at which such interactions occur, the patient may be distressed by such deviations, perhaps without even realizing why.

Cue Discrepancy

One of the most important aspects of effective communication involves not what is said nor how it is said but rather the degree of *consistency* between verbal and nonverbal cues. People with medical problems and other stigmas are very vigilant in watching for clues as to how they will "really" be treated [35] (see also Chapter 8). Even the slightest inconsistency is likely to be noticed. A positive verbal communication, for example, "You're looking better today," accompanied by a negative nonverbal cue like a scowl is likely to be perceived as very *insincere* even if the negative facial expression results from the fact that the practitioner has just realized that he or she is running behind schedule [3, 31]. If the practitioner is angry, sarcasm and nastiness may be perceived. On the other hand, a relatively submissive, negative verbal message, such as "I hope you won't mind if I tell you that you need additional tests," will probably be perceived as sincere and sympathetic despite its negative verbal content if it is accompanied by a sad face [31]. This sentence may be

Box 5–2
Interpersonal Process Recall

In 1962 visitors to Michigan State University were videotaped as they lectured to students and other faculty. Videotaping of lecturers was relatively rare at this time, since the technology had just been developed. Many of the visiting lecturers asked to view their videotape recording right after the lecture. Norman Kagan, clinician and psychological researcher, was surprised to find that the videotape stimulated the visitors' detailed recall of the feelings they had during the lecture. Many recalled points in the lecture during which they were panic stricken, having forgotten passages in their prepared address, although the videotape showed only slight hesitation in their behavior. The visitors often commented on their own behavior, as they saw themselves as others saw them.

Kagan's observations led to the development of a multifaceted project aimed at understanding and influencing human interaction based on videotape replay as a stimulator of recall of feelings. The project and subsequently developed human relations training program are called Interpersonal Process Recall (IPR). It has been used in the training of psychiatric and family practice residents, medical students, nurses, social workers, psychologists, and psychotherapists. The IPR program includes materials such as film series, with illustrations, exercises, and color film recordings of actual sessions in teaching, psychotherapy, and medicine.

Participants in the IPR program watch films of actual therapeutic interactions. They are asked to label the affective states (or feelings) of the interactants. Students receive feedback based on the actual affective states labeled by the persons in the films. Another aspect of the training consists of the videotape recording of the student's interview of a trained actor or actress (or patient who has a prepared repertoire) portraying a particular character type or problem. The interaction is observed by other students in another room. The interaction centers around psychosocial problems of the simulated patient. The interaction is later discussed by the videotaped student along with the faculty facilitator and the other students in the small group.

Research on health professionals' training has pointed to techniques like IPR as a successful way to teach interviewing skills to health professionals, both improving their ability to gain psychosocial information from patients and increasing their empathy. It also helps to identify health professionals whose natural interaction skills are so deficient that they need remedial work to improve their relations with their patients. Similar techniques have been adopted at various medical schools.

For further reading: N. Kagan, Can technology help us toward reliability in influencing human interaction? *Education Technology,* 1973, *13,* 44–51; and A. Werner and J. M. Schneider, Teaching medical students interactional skills: A research-based course in the doctor–patient relationship, *New England Journal of Medicine,* 1974, *290,* 1232–1237.

seen as patronizing by some patients, however, if it is accompanied by a happy face [31]. The degree and type of verbal–nonverbal cue consistency creates the "innuendo" that can either be very distressing or very comforting to an ill person. The development of proper demeanor requires some time.

A related matter concerns the intimacy of the relationship. It seems likely that complex nonverbal communication increases in efficiency and becomes more specialized as a relationship between two people develops [2]. For example, spouses are probably better at quickly communicating and detecting distress or encouragement from each other than are strangers. However, illness brings practitioners and patients into an intimate relationship (especially from the patient's perspective) in which communication channels have *not* been fully developed. The relationship is intimate but its development has been forced. Hence confusions and omissions may result as patients emit special cues that practitioners miss or misunderstand. Practitioners should be aware that such mistakes in nonverbal communication are likely to occur (see also Box 5-2).

Deception

It is sometimes very important for the health practitioner to know that a patient is hiding some discomfort or is not telling the whole truth. Patients may try to deceive practitioners for a variety of reasons, including a desire to appear healthy to please the practitioner, a wish not to "bother" the practitioner, anxiety or fear about new symptoms, embarrassment about certain intimate matters, and so on. Fortunately, clues as to possible deception can often be detected through attention to certain aspects of nonverbal communication.

A major category of nonverbal communication involves body positions and gestures. Posture, hand movements, how a person is leaning, self-touching, foot tapping, and so on, fall in this category. These behaviors generally receive little conscious attention from people. However, such behaviors have important effects on the "immediacy" or mutual stimulation of an interaction [62]. For example, leaning forward indicates an interest in the interaction. These behaviors are also relevant to deception.

Many people believe that you can tell if someone is lying by carefully watching the face. However, there is theoretical and empirical reason to think that cues of deception are often emitted through *body* behavior rather than through facial expression [21, 22]. For example, skillful nurses recognize a patient's squirming, gesturing, pacing, and similar body signs of general restlessness [11]. They should also watch for these cues of anxiety when questioning a patient. The basic idea underlying this phenomenon is that through feedback from others and detailed internal feedback, many people learn to *control* their facial expressions, but they do not normally monitor their body postures and movements. Thus it seems that many people express or "leak" their true feelings through body rather than facial cues.

If body cues are important subtle indicators of distress, therapeutic success should be related to the skill of the practitioner in reading body nonverbal cues. In one research project, six studies of psychotherapy measured the nonverbal sensitivity of counselors with a test called the Profile of Nonverbal Sensitivity (PONS) [71]. The PONS test is a film test that provides a quantitative index of an individual's accuracy at decoding (understanding) facial, body, and voice tone cues of emotion. In these studies the counselors were also rated by their supervisors on clinical effectiveness. The studies found that counselors who were sensitive to body communication were more likely to be seen as clinically effective. Two additional studies were done in medical settings. These studies again measured physicians' nonverbal sensitivity with the PONS test. However, they also obtained actual patients' ratings of the interpersonal effectiveness of their physicians. It was found that physicians who were most sensitive to *body* nonverbal communication received the highest ratings of patient satisfaction with treatment [18, 19]. It is impossible to assign a particular meaning to each body movement. However, any changes in normal behavior are probably important, including such things as clenched fists, hand, foot, or body shaking, tapping—drumming—smoking, and tightly closed arms or legs (see Figure 5-4).

In sum, nonverbal communication is especially important in medical settings. Fortunately, it is no longer necessary for medical practitioners to rely solely on concepts like intuition and empathy in dealing with subtle interpersonal aspects of health care. We can

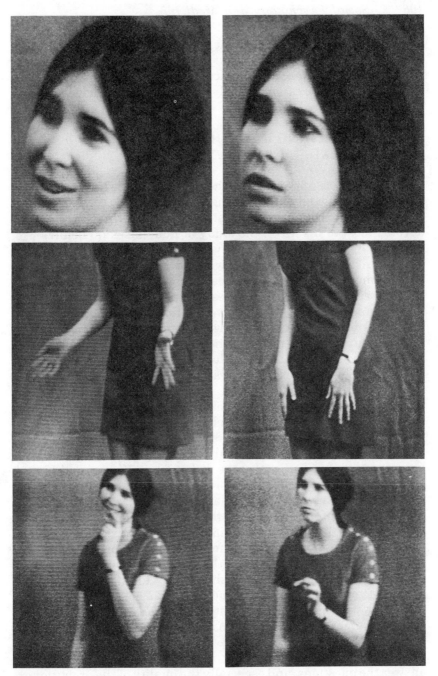

Figure 5–4. Nonverbal communication. These still photographs illustrate the visual channels in the PONS film—face, body, and figure. (Reprinted from Robert Rosenthal et al., *Sensitivity to Nonverbal Communication*, by permission of the publisher, The Johns Hopkins University Press.)

become more specific about what we mean by the "tone," "atmosphere," or "rapport" of practitioner–patient interactions.

Keeping in mind issues of medical jargon and issues of nonverbal communication, we can now analyze the medical interview in detail.

INTERVIEWING IN THE HEALTH CARE CONTEXT

As a professor and researcher at the Institute for Sex Research at Indiana University at Bloomington, Dr. Alfred C. Kinsey was one of the most widely known scientists of the twentieth century. Kinsey devoted most of his life to the study of human sexual behavior (of adults and children) by taking over 18,000 sexual histories of individuals from every walk of life. Overall, these people had engaged in an enormous range of sexual behaviors. Kinsey's research was ground breaking, and his analyses of sexual behavior were astoundingly complete. Kinsey interviewed various people in the country ranging from prostitutes and Bowery bums to powerful members of the community and members of the clergy. It is fascinating that this work was conducted primarily during the 1940s and 1950s, times when the subject of sexuality was taboo [67].

In these interviews Kinsey was able to elicit an extraordinary amount of detailed, sensitive information about respondents' most private behaviors. Kinsey was able to elicit, even from his most inhibited subjects, detailed accounts of their masturbation habits, of their pre- and extramarital sexual behavior, and of their sexual behavior with animals. People revealed much to Kinsey and his colleagues that they had never before told anyone.

The personal interview is a major tool of health care professionals for gathering information about the patient's medical history. It is also useful in discovering a comprehensive picture of the present problems the patient is experiencing. The widespread use of this technique is based, however, on the *incorrect* assumption that the interview is a straightforward, simple way to collect health information. It is a mistake to assume that, as usually conducted, the interview yields correct information. Actually, interviewing persons about medical facts is not in any way similar to retrieving information from a computer bank or from written files. Aspects of human memory, understanding of the questions, motivation to answer the questions, and especially the quality of the practitioner–patient relationship are crucial aspects of the process of interviewing and strongly affect the kind of information retrieved.

Charles Cannell and his colleagues at the University of Michigan have conducted a number of relevant studies, funded by the National Center for Health Services Research [13]. The studies involved thousands of individuals responding to questions about their present and past health; the responses were then compared with the information in their written medical records. Overall, this research found serious problems with the medical interview. For example, the studies showed a very high level of underreporting of illness incidents. Between 12 and 17 percent of recorded hospital episodes were not reported by people in their health interviews, and 23 to 26 percent of recent physician visits were not reported. Furthermore, it was found that at least 50 percent of the medical conditions that appeared in the medical records were not reported by the respondents in the interviews. Reliance on interviewing can thus be quite hazardous. Fortunately, the research also indicated that problems such as underreporting can be remedied [13].

Interestingly, inaccuracies in interview results are not strongly related to characteristics of the respondents (patients). Rather the characteristics of the interview itself were more important. Of course, people differ in the extent to which they provide accurate information about their condition, but the respondents' social characteristics and even level of medical sophistication are not so important as factors in the interview situation itself. How can accurate answers be obtained? What makes an interview bad or good? The following factors are especially relevant.

Interviewer Bias

Kinsey never asked *whether* a subject had ever engaged in a particular sexual activity, such as sex with an animal. Instead, he asked *when* was the first time that the respondent engaged in the activity. For example: "When did you first have sexual intercourse with an animal?" Kinsey thus communicated the acceptability of the activity. The burden was then on the respondent to disavow the behavior; the response, "I never did that," could be taken as probably true. In an analogous situation, a doctor might ask, "How many times have you had venereal disease?" rather than "You never had VD did you?"

The phenomenon in which a respondent's answer is influenced by the interviewer is known as *interviewer bias*. Careful phrasing of the question (such as asking "when" instead of "whether") is one way of making various answers socially acceptable and thus minimizing bias. The reporting of an event is more likely to be distorted in a socially desirable direction. People tend to underreport embarrassing conditions such as disorders of the reproductive system and diseases of the nervous system. Reporting is higher and more accurate for such diseases as gall bladder problems. This underreporting of threatening events can be partly reduced by creating an atmosphere in which the individual is not made to feel unusual because of having the diseases or condition. Relatedly, avoidance of medical jargon lessens the chance that a patient will fabricate a response so as not to have to admit a lack of understanding of the question. Incidentally, it turns out (according to Kinsey's long-time associate, Wardell Pomeroy) that of all the issues considered in the interview, the most embarrassing question, particularly for women, turned out to be "How much do you weigh?" [67]. It is important to remember that matters that seem routine to the practitioner may be very embarrassing to the patient unless proper expectations are created.

Bias can sometimes be minimized by suggesting a wide range of possible answers to the patient. Kinsey would sometimes encounter a respondent who found it hard to estimate the frequency with which he or she had engaged in a particular sexual practice. Kinsey was on guard against respondents who were highly suggestible. Thus a range of possible frequencies such as "once a week, four times a week, more than twenty times a week, or once a year" were suggested. In this way Kinsey did not communicate to the respondent an idea of what would be considered an appropriate answer.

Sometimes interviewer bias is the result of characteristics of the interviewer [37]. For example, it has been shown that white people are less willing to make prejudiced comments about blacks to black interviewers, and non-Jews are less willing to make negative comments about Jews to Jewish interviewers. Therefore, we might expect male patients to be less willing to discuss marital problems with female doctors than with male doctors. Or medical problems related to poverty might go unmentioned to an obviously wealthy physician. Such matters can be difficult to deal with since a health provider obviously cannot change his or her sex or status. However, the provider can do certain things to insure an open, supportive atmosphere in which personal characteristics of the provider become less salient.

Positive Regard and Patient Motivation

Cannell found in his research that the interpersonal dynamics of the interaction between the interviewer and the respondent strongly influence the accuracy of reporting. The behavior of many health interviewers was observed by the researchers and their behaviors subjected to intense scrutiny. An important set of interviewer errors emerged. One of the most striking findings of the research was that the interviewer delivered positive feedback (yes, um hum, nods, etc.) for both good and poor respondent behavior. Unfortunately, adequate responses received proportionately *fewer* positive feedback responses than did less desirable answers. In fact the worst possible response on the part of the patient, that is, a refusal to answer the question, received the most positive feedback. When the patients were uncooperative, the interviewers acted warmly, thus rewarding and encouraging patients for being uncooperative.

Feedback, if *properly* used, is an effective means of influencing the behavior of respondents in desired directions. Laboratory studies in social and learning psychology have shown that an experimenter can reinforce specified classes of respondent verbal behavior. For example, some studies have shown that nodding used as a reinforcement can increase in respondents the production of plural nouns. Expressed attitudes toward various topics have also been shown to be reinforceable—that is, the listener can subtly reward a speaker for expressing some attitudes and not reward him or her for others, thereby increasing the expression of the first attitudes.

Research by Kent Marquis was designed to test the hypothesis that the number of health events reported would be greater in an interview with proper reinforcement [57]. The interview that produced the most information in a total of 429 interviews was one in which for every report of morbidity (health symptom, condition, illness, or residual impairment), the interviewer used a programmed reinforcing statement. These statements were used in a natural tone with the interviewer looking directly at the respondent. They included such statements as:

"Yes that is the kind of information we need."

"This is all valuable information."

"Yes, we need to know about things like that."

"I see, you had . . . (repeat what respondent said)."

"Yes that is the kind of information I need to know."

The interviewer also smiled, leaned forward, and used appropriate hand gestures.

In the control condition the interviewer did not look at the respondent, did not lean forward, smile, or use hand gestures. In effect, the interviewer eliminated what some practitioners would consider superfluous activity and the interview was conducted in a very businesslike manner, as are most medical interviews. This interview was very poor and ineffective.

Kinsey took great pains to describe to his respondents how the confidentiality of their responses would be carefully guarded. Confidentiality is very important, but it is not enough. A warm, positive interpersonal atmosphere must be created through the use of what is called "unconditional positive regard." The provider should not reward a close-mouthed, nondisclosing patient. But once the patient is talking about his or her condition, the provider should give positive responses no matter what the nature of the medical problem. An effective practitioner is generally nonjudgmental.

The social psychologists Judith Rodin and Irving Janis [70] suggest that the first step toward an effective practitioner–patient relationship involves encouraging the patient to disclose his or her troubles and feelings while offering unconditional positive regard. In this way the provider comes to be seen as an understanding person who can be confided in. For example, the practitioner should encourage the patient to describe problems with alcohol, overeating, and so on, and should *not* make any critical statements or express any negative nonverbal cues during the interview process.

Precision of Questioning

The questions chosen by Kinsey were always simple as well as single-barreled; that is, only one concept was dealt with in each question. For example, if a respondent was asked about becoming aroused after seeing nude pictures, the effect of male and female pictures were asked about separately. If questioned about male *and* female pictures most males would say, "Yes, I am aroused by female pictures." Unfortunately, in this way arousal from seeing male nudes could be kept secret, and it would not have to be admitted to answer the question fully. Health professionals often ask double-barrel questions and as a result receive little information of any value from their patients. If a physician were to ask, for example, "Are your allergies better and does your back hurt less now?" a "yes" response would be confusing. The health professional does not know whether the allergies, the back, or both, are better. Questions should be unambiguous. If the meaning of the patient's response is not obvious immediately, the question is not good [37].

The careful sequencing of questions is very important. In Kinsey's research, impersonal, nonthreatening questions were asked first, with the interviewer working slowly to the more sensitive topics. The first question asked was usually "How old are you?" Common questions about the subject's childhood (where he or she lived, etc.) were also asked. Religion and early sex education followed. Then questions about current sexual practices were asked. What was considered sensitive for the individual depended upon the meaning of that particular issue for the person. The questions became quite detailed (e.g., fantasies during masturbation). Any leads into rare or unusual sexual activity were followed up by the researchers with additional questions that were reserved for these situations. Throughout the interview Kinsey was careful to use the patient's own language in describing a particular sexual practice. Progressing from less personal to more personal questions is necessary because of patients' natural aversions to the invasion of their privacy. However, if the physician or nurse proceeds in a considerate manner, the patient will probably become progressively more relaxed and cooperative [8].

In eliciting relevant information from patients, it is also useful to begin with general questions and gradually become more specific, although never becoming too limiting. The process of starting the interview with the most broad questions and then moving to more specific detailed questions is called *narrowing*. This method is particularly useful for eliciting spontaneous patient attitudes. A patient will tend to lead the interview toward the specific issue that he or she is interested in and that is relevant to his or her life. Nevertheless, it is also important to help the patient to continue talking freely. Thus questions should be worded in such a way as to elicit complex answers in many cases—particularly when the health care professional wishes to explore a number of related issues. While the closed-ended question can be answered very quickly, the open-ended question gives the patient a chance to elaborate and to provide valuable information.

Example: Closed-ended: Was the pain sharp or dull?

Open-ended: Tell me about the pain—what was it like?

It is usually best not to limit the patient's responses.

When combined with interviewer bias, the wording of a closed-ended question can lead a patient to a particular response that might in fact be inaccurate. For example, questions like "You've been taking your medication haven't you?" or "You aren't having any more pain are you?" lead the patient directly to a response that might not be completely true. In both cases the patient's response is drastically limited by the expectations of the health professional.

If deception is suspected, it is important to pay very close attention to the patient's responses and behaviors, especially nonverbal cues. To minimize deception in Kinsey's research, simple questions were asked in rapid succession in an attempt to insure that patients would answer spontaneously without too much time to think and to fabricate responses. Kinsey also maintained eye contact with his subjects. If he thought that the respondent was not telling the truth, he would pay close attention to the nonverbal clues given by the respondent, and he would *repeat* the question. If the suspicion still remained Kinsey would confront the interviewee, asking "Now will you please give the story to me straight?"

In Kinsey's research, guarding against respondents' covering up information was done by cross-checking histories of husband and wife where possible. Furthermore, a number of retakes were done two to four years after the first interview. Health practitioners should similarly be on the lookout for information that confirms or disconfirms information gathered in the initial interview. Conversations with relatives, the results of medical tests and exams, and the overall cohesiveness of a medical condition or story are valuable checks on interview information. Even the most skilled interviewer can be deceived from time to time.

Finally, it should be noted that many cognitive factors can affect interview responses [13]. As one might guess, as the time between an event and its recall (the interview) increases, there is increased underreporting of the event. What is surprising is the *rapidity* with which the failure to report information increases with time. In one study of visits to physicians, for example, the failure to report the visit increased from 15 percent one week after the visit to 30 percent two weeks after the visit.

A related factor concerns *salience*. Events that are more important to the individual are more completely and accurately remembered than events of less importance. Note, however, that this is *subjective* importance. An event may be very useful to know about for the doctor, but the patient will not report it unless it had an important impact on the patient's life. While there is no single way directly to improve the patient's cognitive functioning in an interview, proper use of the techniques described above will tend to have a beneficial effect.

The Computer–Patient Relationship

We have seen that communication between practitioners and patients is a complex process, susceptible to dangerous errors. Perhaps machines can help; at least, computers may be valuable supplements in the part of the communication process that is most mechanical.

Computers are now being used in both diagnosis and treatment. In diagnosis a patient interacts with a computer terminal that asks questions about background, history, and symptoms. This information is then either summarized and stored for the physician or compared to existing knowledge in an attempt to provide a diagnosis [75, 76, 77]. In treatment the computer provides relevant information about the matter in question, especially in such areas as venereal disease, where factual knowledge is very important but frequently lacking to patients. Not surprisingly, the computer excels at collecting and providing neat, detailed, accurate, and complete information of a factual nature. Perhaps more interesting is the fact that reactions from both patients and health professionals seem to be quite positive.

The medical histories of patients have traditionally been recorded by using the longhand method (the health professional asking the patient a series of detailed questions, such as "Is there any diabetes in your family?", "Do you have any allergies?", etc.). This method, however, can take so much of the health care professional's time that shortcuts often must be taken; the resulting histories are then unstandardized, illegible, and often incomplete. Such an interview may also limit the time available for discussing social and emotional matters. The overload of a medical care system can also affect the amount of time that is available for carefully developed and executed patient education. Thus developers of computer-based patient interviewing and education are primarily oriented to producing complete, legible, consistent clinical histories and effective, efficient education of patients with various conditions (such as diabetes) that require self-care.

In most computerized interviews, the patient and computer communicate by means of a typewriter-style keyboard, called a teletype, and a cathode ray tube (TV) screen. Messages from the computer to the patient and from the patient to the computer appear in words on the screen. The program can be operated very easily by someone who has no training at all in computer techniques. The computer begins the interview program with a welcome message and explains the purpose of the interview, asking the patient to forgive the inadequacies in the program. In response to the many questions that are asked, the patient presses terminal (teletype) keys indicating "YES," "NO," "I DON'T KNOW," or "I DON'T UNDERSTAND." When the patient does not understand a question, the patient can ask that it be reworded or explained further. Depending on responses to the various patient history questions, the computer program can branch off into further detailed questions about symptoms. During the interview the computer offers words of encouragement and some humor. When the program is finished the computer thanks the patient, and then a summary of the patient's responses are printed out for the health care professional and stored on magnetic tape in the computer. Studies have shown that there is good agreement between computer-acquired data and physicians' medical records, but the computer-recorded data are more legible and at times more complete.

Computer programs can also be used to obtain psychosocial data from patients. General questions concerning personal, family, social, marital, or financial conditions can be explored. Psychological screening instruments can be included in the programs, and scoring can actually be done by the program to begin to evaluate the psychological condition of the patient. Patients are afforded privacy in their responses, and they may feel better answering personal questions when given a considerable amount of time to think about them. The computer can also be used to evaluate the life changes that the patient has gone through (life changes and illness are discussed in Chapter 7).

Computer programs have also been used successfully in educating patients about preventive health measures that are applicable to them, and they have helped to evaluate patients' usual dietary behaviors, teach them insights into their eating patterns, and plan meals for them. The programs are versatile and allow the patient a considerable amount of time to think. They serve as tireless instructors in educating patients. Evidence suggests that many patients actually might learn more from computers than from human instructors [77].

It should be obvious that there are two major problems that arise when a computer takes the place of a person in this health setting. First, there is a computer's limited flexibility. An experienced physician or nurse may want to follow up certain symptoms or complaints or may be more adept at recognizing certain conditions without going through a laborious series of questions. (Note that computers are not limited in this way in principle but only by the near impossibility of programming all the information available to an experienced clinician.) Second, there is the matter of nonverbal communication, both from the patient to the practitioner and from the practitioner to the patient. A computer cannot easily deal with facial expressions, voice tone, and other nonverbal cues. (Actually, providing for nonverbal communication by computers is difficult, but perhaps not impossible given sufficient knowledge of interpersonal relations and programming skill [76]. For example, attempts have been made to assess the patient's heartrate and latency of response by computer; that is, a computerized medical interview records the patient's heartbeat and the time it takes him or her to answer a question [76]. This information can be very useful in determining a patient's emotional reaction to a particular set of questions in order to see what is upsetting to the particular patient. However, such approaches may destroy the human element of the medical interview and provoke resistance by patients.)

Is computer interviewing and education more or less empathic in the medical setting than interviewing and education by the health care professional? Have we moved, with computer interviewing and education, totally into the clutches of modern technology with machines taking care of patients instead of people? These questions are as yet unanswered. Enlightened progress will come only if sufficient attention is paid to the complex, important issue of communication between practitioners and their patients.

SUMMARY

Communication between practitioners and patients, both verbal and nonverbal communication, is a key element in effective medical care. Sensitivity to nonverbal communication and good interviewing skills are essential to proper diagnoses. Avoidance of jargon, coupled with an understanding of the patient's frame of reference, is crucial to the transfer of information necessary in treatment. Perhaps most importantly, the process of communication is the central component in the creation of the rapport and positive expectations that we have seen are so important to health care. Social psychology provides knowledge of specific verbal and nonverbal skills that can be learned and practiced by health professionals as part of their medical training.

6

The Nature of Illness

Between 50 and 70 percent of patients who experience an acute myocardial infarction (heart attack) die before receiving any type of medical treatment. The deaths are most often the result of ventricular fibrillation (uncoordinated quivering of the heart chamber), which occurs in the earlier phases of the infarction. With medical help this condition is potentially reversible. However, many patients get to the hospital too late. Why?

One might expect that a person who is experiencing the symptoms of a myocardial infarction—chest pain, perspiration, shortness of breath, and dizziness—would seek immediate medical attention. Despite the serious consequences, however, help is often not immediately sought [8]. The typical response of the patient is to delay seeking medical advice or treatment beyond the critical period of one hour after the onset of acute symptoms. In fact, while about 56 percent of coronary patients arrive at the hospital within four hours of the onset of symptoms, 28 percent take from four to fourteen hours, and 16 percent arrive after more than fourteen hours. The median time from onset of symptoms to arrival at the hospital is between two and one half and four hours [8, 9].

The delay in seeking treatment is *not* primarily because of transportation problems. Transport takes only about 10 percent of the time from the onset of symptoms to the arrival at the hospital. Rather, most of the delay is caused by patient *decision time*. Deci-

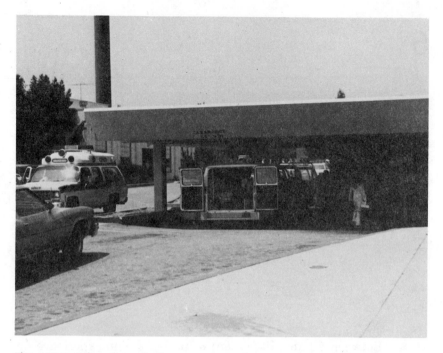

Figure 6–1. When the ambulance gets many heart attack victims to the hospital, it is too late. The problem is not one of transportation but rather the patient's delay in seeking treatment. (Photo by Brian Gordon)

sion time is the interval between the onset of symptoms and the patient's decision that medical help must be sought. Decision time depends upon the person's coming to the conclusion that something is wrong and that it requires medical attention. This time is precious, as it may be the most important determinant of the patient's survival.

The length of the delay before a person seeks medical attention is influenced by three basic factors. Together, these factors help to answer the important question, "What is illness?" These factors are the subject of this chapter.

The first factor involves the background of the patient. Reactions to physical symptoms vary as a function of cultural and demographic differences such as social class, age, sex, and ethnicity. For example, studies have shown that older or female patients take longer to seek help than younger or male patients. As another example, persons of British descent tend to be stoical and therefore may be reluctant to express the pain of a heart attack [4, 33, 36, 39, 46, 47].

The second factor that influences reactions and delay time is the psychological process involving the patient's perception of illness. The decision to seek help requires that the patient perceive the symptoms (the chest pain, perspiration, etc.), recognize their meaning and seriousness, and realize that medical care is necessary. Some patients fail to attribute their initial symptoms to a cardiac problem. They attribute their pain to such things as gall bladder problems or a cold. In two studies fully 70 percent of the coronary patients misinterpreted the causes of their symptoms. Other studies have found that many patients use denial to deal with the anxiety aroused by the symptoms; they avoid defining their sensations as symptoms of serious illness [8, 9, 28, 44]. While denial may have a useful purpose in momentarily reducing the feelings of overwhelming anxiety in the coronary patient, it may also reduce the patient's chances of survival by preventing the patient from seeking the emergency medical care that could save his or her life.

The third and final factor involves the social situation. The social context in which the symptoms first appear has a significant effect upon how long it takes the patient to seek medical treatment at the hospital [25, 44]. The day of the week and the time of day when the symptoms begins is one of the best predictors of delay in seeking care. For example, it has been found that the greatest delay occurs when the symptoms appear during the day on weekends. Patients are most likely to seek help right away if the symptoms occur at work. There is less delay if patients are in the presence of other persons, particularly spouses, when the symptoms begin [25, 44]. Social rewards and punishments also influence illness behavior, and these effects are described in this chapter.

The earlier the heart attack patient arrives at the hospital, the more likely is recovery. There is a significant difference in survival between "early" and "late" arrivals at the hospital (10 percent mortality compared with 27 percent mortality). This situation itself justifies a detailed social psychological study of the meaning of "illness." Yet the same three sets of factors also influence the decision to seek medical treatment in cases where life is not immediately threatened. Will a child with a runny nose stay home from school? Will a woman with a breast lump tell her doctor? Will a man with back pain ignore it, complain to his friends, quit his job, or travel from hospital to hospital?

WHAT IS ILLNESS?

The Sick Role. Starting with some insights from the work of the sociologist Talcott Parsons, we can explore and try to understand illness and illness behavior. People with symptoms can adopt a role in society known as the *sick role* [3, 31]. A person can enter the sick role if a doctor confirms that the person is ill, or if the family or friends of the individual define this person as ill. An individual enjoys certain advantages as a result of adopting the sick role. For instance, the ill person is not considered responsible for the illness—it is beyond the patient's control. As a result, the sick individual has a legitimate basis for exemption from normal activities and obligations. That is, the patient does not have to go to work or fulfill other normal expectations. If a mother of many children is hospitalized, she is not labeled a bad mother if she cannot take care of her children. Illness (the sick role) is a legitimate basis for seeking assistance from others. Thus illness is a social phenomenon; it is usually distinguishable from "disease," which is an organic problem with the body.*

However, certain responsibilities also apply to those who adopt the sick role. The patient cannot stay in the sick role forever. In fact, one of the obligations of the sick role is that the individual see the role as undesirable. The patient is expected to feel uncomfortable in the role and try to cooperate with others to get well. The person must also seek help from health care professionals when such care is seen as available and beneficial [3].

How do we understand and deal with an individual who, after exhibiting various symptoms, is defined as being ill, but then does not profess any desire to get well, or to cooperate with the treatment prescribed by health professionals? Suppose that Mrs. Carter, a 40-year-old woman, complains of headaches, is defined as ill, and is exempted from her role as part-time school librarian and as caretaker of her two children. Further suppose, however, that after a visit with the family physician who prescribes a certain drug, Mrs. Carter forgets to take the drug. What do we conclude? Is she ill? Is she refusing to properly play the sick role and simply using it to loaf? Is she perhaps refusing to cooperate with treatment for some hidden reasons stemming from her background or social relations?

There are many factors that affect patients' decisions that they have become ill and must seek health care. Similarly, many factors influence decisions to exempt people from their usual roles in society and to define them as ill. And, finally, various factors influence both patients' desires to care for themselves and the manner in which they deal with distressing symptoms. Let us examine some of these influences.

*Some authors make further distinctions among related terms, but this simple dichotomy is sufficient for our purposes here [13].

Becoming Ill. A number of conditions that cause people to interpret their symptoms as illness (and to exhibit illness behaviors) have been identified by the sociologists David Mechanic and Irving Zola. These factors are listed below, and in considering them, it is important to note that illness is relative, not absolute. *Illness depends upon interpretation.* It is defined by people and hence can only be fully understood by taking social psychology into account.

Mechanic has suggested seven groups of variables that are important to someone in deciding if he or she is ill [19, 20, 21]:

1. The number of symptoms and their persistence.
2. The individual's ability to recognize the symptoms.
3. The perceived seriousness of the symptoms.
4. The extent of social and physical disability resulting from the symptoms.
5. The cultural background of the person and of the defining group in terms of emphasis on stoicism.
6. The amount of information or medical knowledge available to the person.
7. The availability of sources of help—this includes not only the availability of clinic and hospital care but also the patient's physical distance from it and its cost in money, time, and effort. This factor includes the fear, stigma, and feelings of humiliation associated with treatment, and the patient's relationship with the health care professionals.

Irving Zola identified five triggers affecting the *timing* of a patient's decision to seek medical care. They are as follows [49]:

1. An interpersonal crisis that serves to call attention to the symptoms, causing the patient to dwell on them.
2. Social interference that occurs as the symptoms begin to threaten a valued social activity, such as work.
3. The individual receives sanctioning for seeking care; that is, others encourage the patient to seek care.
4. The patient perceives the symptoms as threatening in nature.
5. The symptoms are seen as similar to previous symptoms, or to those with which the person is familiar because relatives or friends have had them.

These various factors are now discussed in terms of the three categories noted above: cultural and demographic influences on illness (background); social perception, attribution, and illness (the psychological processes of perception); and the social context of illness (the social situation) (see also Box 6-1).

Box 6-1
FUO and the Rewards of the Sick Role

The sick role is made up of expectations about what it means to be sick. One set of expectations is that the patient wants to get better, that is, recover from the illness. Sometimes these expectations are not confirmed, however, and the patient may be a fraud. One such instance involves patient-induced fever of unknown origin, or FUO.

Fever is a symptom that attracts serious attention since it may be a sign of a significant medical problem. However, it is often difficult to isolate the cause of some fevers. Thus a patient with a fever of unknown origin may receive intense and prolonged attention from medical personnel, including hospitalization. Unfortunately, fevers can be self-induced by patients, either by artificially heating thermometers or by injecting themselves with noxious substances. Thus it is possible for some

people to turn to "phony" fevers in order to acquire the benefits of the sick role. By contracting this form of "illness," the patient may be excused from work or family life and given lots of attention. Insurance may even pay the bills for the "vacation."

Faked illness may be difficult to detect if health personnel do not recognize that there are many social aspects to illness, and medical testing could continue indefinitely. However, if the health provider carefully studies the patient's background and becomes familiar with the patient's current lifestyle and beliefs, the problem is much more likely to be resolved.

For further reading: D. Mechanic, Social psychological factors affecting the presentation of bodily complaints, *New England Journal of Medicine*, 1972, *286*, 1132–1139.

CULTURAL AND DEMOGRAPHIC INFLUENCES ON ILLNESS

The ways in which patients perceive, evaluate, and act upon their symptoms depend to a great extent upon their cultural and social backgrounds and early experiences. Some people make light of their symptoms, avoid seeking medical care, and refuse to enter the sick role. Others respond to a slight amount of pain and discomfort by avoiding work and other obligations and by developing a dependency upon other people.

Throughout the following discussion, it should be remembered that the type of symptoms may influence whether a person adopts the sick role. If someone has a raging fever of 105 degrees and a bright red rash, for example, this person is very likely to define him or herself as ill. Social psychological factors, however, always influence the rapidity with which the individual seeks medical care, and the response the individual has to the (organic) disease.

Social Class Determinants of Illness Behavior

In 1954 sociologist Earl Koos conducted a door-to-door household survey in order to examine the manner in which people from different social classes interpreted the seriousness of various medical symptoms [16]. He gave the respondents descriptions of various symptoms (some as nebulous as lower back pain, others as serious as vomiting blood) and asked them whether they would seek help from the medical system (go to a doctor) if they had these symptoms. He found large differences in the willingness of respondents to seek medical help as a function of their socioeconomic status (defined by their economic status and their level of education) [16].

Koos reported that less than one-fifth of the lower-class patients in his sample thought chronic fatigue or persistent backache was worth mentioning to a doctor. Loss of appetite would be ignored by about 80 percent of the lower-class, fainting spells by 67 percent, and continued coughing by 77 percent. Overall, Koos concluded that upper-class persons were more likely than lower-class persons to view themselves as ill when they had particular symptoms, and they were more likely than lower-class persons to say that specific symptoms would lead them to seek the advice of a physician or other health care professionals.

It is important to understand that such differences among people in various socioeconomic groups probably have little to do with their interest in keeping themselves healthy or with the extent to which they value health. Instead, the reasons for the differences in interpretations of symptoms as serious or not serious (whether or not they require medical attention) stem in large part from the ability of the various individuals to spend family or personal resources for health care. A worker whose monthly earnings barely cover the expenses required for basic necessities is unlikely to readily define a symptom as needing medical attention or warranting a day off from work—with the resultant loss of a day's pay. A decision about the seriousness of the symptom is made in the context of the resources of the individual or the entire family, and the importance of the symptoms is considered relative to other potential drains on the family's limited financial resources. In addition, among patients of the lower class good medical care is not always accessible [40].

One of the major problems facing patients from lower socioeconomic classes is that state health (e.g., MediCal, Medicaid) payments to physicians are usually lower than payments made to physicians by private insurance companies for the same services. Therefore many physicians refuse to take patients whose only source of insurance is state or federal assistance programs. The few physicians in a given area who do take MediCal or Medicaid patients are usually quite busy. If the accessibility of care is low, patients tend to avoid seeking care. It can also be troublesome to receive MediCal/Medicaid—filling out forms can be confusing, tedious, and embarrassing. Patients become frustrated, and thus may deny or minimize symptoms to avoid care. The special health care problems of the poor are discussed later in this chapter.

Culture and Medical Care

Cultural factors have an enormous influence upon patients' interpretations of symptoms and their responses to these symptoms [5]. Anthropological work has shown that conceptions of illness in any culture are part of a learned cultural complex and that responses to symptoms are culturally conditioned as are responses to other environmental threats. In comparing Anglo- and Spanish-speaking cultures, for example, we find that Anglos tend to prefer medical science and hospitalization to deal with illness, while many Mexican-American patients tend to prefer to rely more heavily upon folk medicine and family care as an important aspect of treatment [4, 26, 36].

Some of these cultural differences are very important. An obvious example of cultural differences involves symptoms that are usually indicative of mental health problems. Mexican-American (Chicano) patients may have different perceptions of reality from Black and Anglo patients. In one study only 16 percent of Mexican-American teenagers interpreted "hearing voices" as evidence of insanity or hallucination as compared to 90 percent of the Anglos [29]. The Mexican-American children tended instead to regard hearing voices as evidence of a religious experience.

The Mexican-American population in the United States is rapidly increasing, and frequently the communication difficulties encountered between Anglo health care professionals and Mexican-American patients are significant [34]. They illustrate the profound influence of culture on perception of illness: To many Anglo physicians illness means disease—an organic condition brought about by a natural agent, and as such it should be dealt with unemotionally. To Mexican-American patients, however, illness relates to their life, to their community, and to their family and interpersonal relationships [15]. Furthermore, Mexican-Americans traditionally believe that illness exists only when there is pain or visible symptoms. Thus preventive care is difficult [4, 15].

Folk beliefs may also be important in the understanding of disease by Mexican-Americans. These beliefs are sometimes thought to stem from factors such as magic, dislocation of internal organs, or a hot-cold imbalance. Anglo physicians and other health care practitioners often view these beliefs as superstitious and expect the Mexican-American patient simply to accept modern medical practice. However, it may be extremely difficult for the Mexican-American patient to accept diagnostic tools in place of beliefs indigenous to the culture since these beliefs are reinforced by the culture [4, 17, 35].

The folk curer or *curandero* tends to be an important source of medical care for the Mexican-American patient. The folk curer is a member of the community, makes house calls, and deals with the entire family of the patient. The efficiency of the Anglo physician's office may be distressing to the Mexican-American patient, who prefers a friendly, calm, courteous physician. Patients expect and get sympathy and warmth from the curandero, and Anglo medical efficiency may be regarded as rudeness. Because the curandero provides so many of these interpersonal aspects of healing, the patient may prefer the curandero. Considering the other issues discussed in this book concerning the body and mind, we might reasonably conclude that the curandero has a greater chance of effectively treating conditions that have a strong emotional component [4].

Traditionally oriented Mexican-Americans may also feel that in-depth discussions of their illness must involve their families, and only after family consideration of the components of treatment can the patient be assigned a treatment regimen. The patient may agree to a treatment plan, but the family makes the final decision. Any infringement on the family rights by the health care professional may result in noncooperation on the part of the patient [4].

Other cultural factors are also relevant to health care. The role of culture in influencing patients' illness behaviors was shown in a classic work by Mark Zborowski in 1952. Zborowski conducted research in New York City on the reactions of patients from various ethnic groups to pain. He noted that Jewish and Italian patients tended to exaggerate pain experiences, responding in a very emotional manner, while patients of English ("Yankee") or Irish descent were inclined to be more stoical and to deny pain. While the outward expressions of the Jewish and Italian patients were usually similarly emotional, there was a difference in the meaning of pain to the patients in these two ethnic groups. The Jewish patients were concerned with the cause of the pain and its future significance, whereas the Italian patients tended to seek relief from the pain and were satisfied when they felt better regardless of the future consequences [46, 47].

Zborowski's basic findings have been supported by other researchers [20, 42, 48]. For example, it has been found that Italians and Jews are more likely than other groups to report a great number of illness symptoms when questioned in surveys. What is important to recognize is that certain aspects of *cultural and social conditioning* bring about differences in illness behavior. These illness behavior patterns can have either healthy or unhealthy consequences.

Most illness behaviors are learned in childhood. For example, Italian and Jewish parents are often extremely protective about their children's health, and crying in response to illness or pain is usually responded to by the parent with sympathy and attention. The children learn to pay attention to painful experiences and distressing symptoms, and also to seek assistance. Zborowski believes that familial responses to illness behavior of the child set the pattern for the child's life.

Patients' illness behaviors can sometimes have a profound impact on the attributions that are made about these patients in the health care setting. Although some illness behaviors stem from cultural differences in expressiveness about symptoms and discomfort, these illness behaviors can influence how the health care professional evaluates the medical condition of the patient. Research that illustrates this point was conducted by Dr. Irving K. Zola at Massachusetts General Hospital [50]. The subjects in the study were patients who voluntarily went to the ear, nose, and throat clinics with symptoms for which no medical disease could be found. Zola found that patients' modes of cultural expression strongly influenced the way in which they expressed the symptoms, which, in turn, influenced strongly the physicians' decisions about their care. It was found that psychogenesis (psychiatric origin) was implied in the records of eleven of the twelve Italian patients but in few of the remaining cases. Patients were, according to Zola, very similar on other dimensions, including present life stresses. Patients' usual methods of expressing symptoms (primarily culturally based) affect how they are viewed and evaluated by the physician.

Age and sex roles—what is expected of people because of their age and sex—also partially explain illness behavior. Chest pain in a teenager is unlikely to be interpreted as a heart attack by the teenager or by others. Failure to take medication may be seen as rebelliousness in a 30-year-old but may be excused as forgetfulness in a 7-year-old or a 70-year-old. Differences in expectations also apply to males and females. Traditionally, females have been seen as weak, and sometimes as very frail. In fact, weakness has sometimes been viewed as attractively "feminine." Hence the same symptom—weakness or fainting—may be interpreted very differently depending on the sex of the patient.

A final but striking example of the influence of culture and background on reactions to bodily functions concerns menstruation [30]. Since biblical times and throughout history, the same biological process has been given many different and often strange interpretations. Menstruating women have been subjected to many rituals, often involving isolation and even including special menstrual huts. Even the word itself is often avoided, and euphemisms such as "the curse" are used. Depending on the culture, women will not cook, pray, exercise, have sexual relations, go out in public, and so on, when menstruating. The tremendous variety of reactions illustrates that the "illness" is not solely biological; reactions depend instead on social factors. Even in modern American society, relationships between menstrual distress and social factors have been found to be related to religion [30]. For example, Catholics who are very traditional in their views (e.g., believing that a woman's place is in the home) are more likely to experience menstrual distress than are more liberal women. Among Jewish women menstrual distress tends to occur among women especially concerned with social rituals and personal hygiene during menstruation. The way in which people are reared affects their illness behaviors.

Thus various factors in culture and upbringing may affect whether a person senses certain symptoms, whether the person defines the symptoms as illness, and whether the person thinks it necessary to seek medical attention for the symptoms.

SOCIAL PERCEPTION, ATTRIBUTION, AND ILLNESS

Consider the following interview with a first-year medical student:

Questioner: How do you know that a person is ill?

Med. Student: He says that something hurts, or that he doesn't feel well, or cannot manage to work as before or fulfill other responsibilities. Of course once the person comes to the hospital or doctor's office, we look for a specific organic cause of the symptoms.

Questioner: So it is the *report of symptoms* to the health professional that defines illness?

Med. Student: Well, of course a person can be ill and not seek health care. He or she could simply stay home from work, or simply act sick. Then again, the doctor could find something wrong even if the patient feels okay.

Questioner: How do you know how ill a person is?

Med. Student: That is a tough one. There are objective indices such as fever and tissue damage. Also with regard to a specific pathogen, we have measures of the extent to which the disease is life threatening. The more life threatening the disease, the sicker the person is I guess. However, with most conditions, since they are not life threatening, we often go by how much the condition tends to impair the functioning of the individual. For example, I just met a lady the other day who went back to work five days after a radical mastectomy. She said that it was psychologically healthier for her to do that. She reported a little pain but did not let it interfere with her work. Another lady had the same operation and took months to go back to work and really take on her family responsibilities again. The two women had the same amount of tissue damage and the same cancer prognosis. They had the same surgeon and a very similar course of surgery. I still don't completely understand the difference between the two.

Questioner: How do you know someone has gotten better?

Med. Student: He or she acts healthy.

This interview with a health care professional-in-training demonstrates two important issues: The first is that illness may not be discovered until a person begins to exhibit "illness behaviors"—behaviors such as complaining of discomfort, missing work, minimizing social responsibilities, and seeking health care from professionals. Thus to understand the onset of illness, as well as its course and its cure, we need to understand the illness behavior associated with the particular illness. The second important point is that we tend to confer upon an individual the label of "ill" if this person exhibits these behaviors. Of the two women who had had radical mastectomy surgery, the woman who continued to exhibit illness behavior was defined as ill. The woman who went back to work was considered recovered (although perhaps not completely healthy).

The process of interpreting a symptom or behavior is one of *attribution* [11]; that is, we search for a causal explanation for an event. Consider the case of a co-worker who calls in sick and does not show up for work on a fine spring day. We are not only concerned about this person's behavior, that is, the fact that the person failed to come to work, but we are also very interested in the reason for the absence. We make attributions of responsibility for behavior, attributions that are influenced by many factors. First, we might recall the past behavior of the co-worker. If this person always calls in sick when there is something interesting to do away from work, we may become suspicious of his or her present motives. Or we might examine this person's past medical history, assuming that he or she is justified in staying away from work if we know that this person recently underwent a series of operations. We might also discuss the matter with other co-workers, asking them how this person looked yesterday and why they think he or she is absent from work. If we find that our absent co-worker is often absent from the job, likes to have a good time, does not spend much time visiting doctors, and loves to go to baseball games on nice spring days, we may then conclude that the co-worker is not really ill. That is, there are systematic influences on our attributions. Note that the behavior or action—the fact that this person is not at work—remains the same; only our explanations change. And of course there may be severe consequences for abusing sick leave. Although we constantly make attributions about behavior in our daily lives, attributions about illness are especially important because of the importance of the sick role. Illness is in part a function of a psychological inference process. An element of *interpretation* must enter into play before we are willing to speak of *illness* [45].

Sometimes the attributions we make are about ourselves. As we saw in Chapter 1, aspects of our identity come from other people. We are not born knowing what a headache or a stomachache is. A young boy who looks pale, is holding his stomach, and has just eaten a bowl full of chocolate, may be asked by his mother, "Do you have a stomachache?" It is in such ways that we learn to interpret symptoms and behaviors of illness. Understanding the attribution process is important because our decisions are not always rational but are often biased, that is, distorted by the social situation. Fortunately, there are regularities in these biases that help make them predictable.

An interesting insight into how people interpret internal body events is provided by research on the self-labeling of emotion, which was pioneered by the social psychologist Stanley Schachter [38].

Schachter noticed two interesting phenomena. First, he noted that sometimes people feel that their body is physiologically aroused, although they are not sure about the cause of the arousal. For example, something may be affecting their hormonal balance, or they may have received a drug or treatment that (unknown to them) produces sympathetic nervous system arousal (e.g., the drug ephedrine, which is an over-the-counter drug given to relieve bronchial asthma symptoms and nasal congestion caused by an allergy).* Second, Schachter noticed that people sometimes gather information about their own feelings and reactions from other people. For example, in times of fear people seem to gather together and look to each other to decide how to deal with their fear. In fact, experiments have shown that people who have had fear aroused in them are more likely to want to be with other fearful people than are people who have not been made fearful [37]. Using these two observations about arousal and social comparison, Schachter concluded that emotion involves a process of providing a cognitive label for a physiologically aroused body condition. That is, there is no simple one-to-one relationship between bodily states and feelings and reactions. Instead, each body sensation must be interpreted before it has meaning. If we are surrounded by people who tell us that our symptoms are typical of a heart attack, we are much more likely to think that we are ill and to seek medical attention. Thus a man experiencing chest pain in the presence of his worried wife is more likely to seek medical assistance [8].

As we have seen in Chapter 4, our thoughts can have significant effects on our bodily reactions. Specifically, the attributions we make for our symptoms can in turn affect the symptoms. An interesting case concerns insomnia. While there are many factors that can interfere with a person's sleep, a prominent factor in chronic insomnia seems to be a person's anxiety about being an insomniac. That is, insomniacs worry that they are insomniacs, and this worry helps keep them awake even more. Hence an important means of treating sleeplessness involves breaking this vicious circle of insomnia leading to anxiety leading to insomnia. One way is to convince the patient that the insomnia is caused by a common problem such as noise, which can be solved. The anxiety then disappears as the attributions change from "I'm an insomniac" to "I can't sleep because of a problem in the environment." It may be relatively easy

---

*Ephedrine causes bodily changes similar to (although slightly weaker than) the amphetamines, including insomnia, restlessness, tremor, alertness, and feelings of anxiety, tension, and agitation.

to modify the environment and reduce the insomnia. In an interesting related study researchers gave insomniacs a placebo pill but told them that the pill would produce the symptoms of insomnia [43]. Since the patients now had an external explanation for their insomnia, their anxiety was reduced, and they were indeed able to go to sleep more quickly. By the same token, a patient who cannot fall asleep after taking a sleeping pill may become even more anxious about the problem and have even more difficulties. Thus the use of pills must be considered in light of the attributions that the patients will make about them.

An important factor that influences the interpretation of symptoms as illness and produces the desire to seek medical care is the *salience* or prominence of the symptoms. The salience of symptoms is dependent on the disruptive effect of the symptoms. For example, if we are at work and feel so weak that we cannot continue working, we may see ourselves as ill; however, if we are at home and do not feel well enough to continue watching the late show on television, we might simply decide that we are tired and go to bed. Social interference is usually the most important component of salience, but other matters can also be very significant. These variables are the visibility of the symptoms, the extent to which they are life threatening, and their frequency of appearance.

A related factor influencing reactions to illness is the *availability* of relevant information. Can the patient match the symptoms to previous illnesses or to illnesses others have? For example, when there is a flu epidemic it is easy for both doctors and patients to diagnose the flu. But if a patient has an exotic parasitic infection while there is a flu epidemic, definition of the illness may be much more difficult.

The attribution process also operates in relations with other people. We often try to understand and interpret another person's actions, given the information available to us. That is, we infer causes of behavior using certain general principles. For example, we generally give special weight to actions that seem unpopular or that go against our expectations. If a surgical patient refuses postoperative pain medication, cooperates with and compliments the health care personnel, and is able to leave the hospital early, we are more likely to make inferences about this patient than we are about the patient who proceeds in the usual normal manner [14]. Other attribution principles indicate that the consistency of information affects the inferences we draw. Suppose a friend catches the flu and responds distinctively by going to bed with the illness. If this is something this person has not done during past illnesses, you may conclude that your friend is now very ill. If it is also true that almost everyone else who has this type of flu is very ill and also must stay in bed, you then become very confident that your friend is really quite ill and it is legitimate for your friend to stay home in bed. In other circumstances, for example, if everyone else says this flu is like a minor cold, you might conclude that your friend is not really very ill. It is important to note that the interpretation of a friend's ill behavior does not depend to a great extent on biological symptoms. Our interpretations are instead a function of the patient's behavior in the context of what we know about the patient, the circumstances of the illness, and a comparison with other people. Interpretations occur in the minds of observers; in this sense illness is *socially* defined.

Differences in Point of View

A patient's perspective on illness differs from that of health care personnel. For example, consider a patient with a nonspecific virus that causes this person to be very weak, fevered, nauseous, and depressed. The person may be aware of having an aching body, being unable to stand up, feeling dizzy when lifting his or her head up, being unable to eat, and being better off resting than trying to carry on normal conversation with people. However, to health personnel, such as nurses, this patient may appear in a very different light. The virus may produce no obvious physical symptoms except perhaps the fever; there are only behavioral symptoms. Furthermore, the nurses probably had never seen this patient as a well person leading an active life. These differences in information and perspective between the patient and the practitioner may produce an *actor-observer difference* in attributions [12]. The patient or "actor" will interpret his or her behavior (such as the refusal to talk or eat) as caused by the illness. This interpretation is a *situational* explanation ("I don't usually behave this way"). However, the nurses or "observers" may attribute the same behaviors to something characteristic of the patient, such as seeing the patient as uncooperative or as a "crock." That is, the nurses will tend to make a dispositional attribution (explanation), and they will blame the behavior on the personality of the patient. This difference in interpreting identical behavior can thus lead to unfortunate conflicts between patients and practitioners. It is therefore important for the health provider to look at the patient's perspective and try to learn more about the patient's point of view. The proper type of interviewing is helpful in this attempt (see Chapter 5). Practitioners should also try to imagine themselves in the patient's position.

With all these factors to be kept in mind, it becomes clear that there can be a vast difference between what the patient considers an important symptom and what the health care professional considers important. Patients' judgments of saliency do not necessarily coincide with those of the medical professional. Certain symptoms that are disruptive to the patient may be medically trivial and not require attention. Other symptoms, such as initial signs of cancer, might be very serious but have no disruptive effects. Illness behavior usually represents the patient's rational attempt to make sense of the symptoms and to cope with the problem given the limits of the patient's knowledge, social situation, and culture. But this behavior may not be at all rational from the point of view of the medical professional.

The competing interpretations of symptoms affect the decision of patients to seek care. If patients can place the symptoms in a normal frame of reference, they are unlikely to seek medical care or define themselves as ill. An example of this phenomenon is the symptom of "fatigue." People who are accustomed to pushing their body (e.g., a working mother with two children and a house to take care of, who is also taking night classes) may try for a while to interpret extreme fatigue in a normal frame of reference and thus delay as long as possible the conclusion that they are ill.

THE SOCIAL CONTEXT OF ILLNESS

In addition to the cultural and background factors and the attributional processes that affect definitions of and reactions to illness, the presence and actions of other people are important in the definition of illness. Social factors that affect many everyday reactions may have a special meaning for illness.

Different people respond to what seems to be the same physical condition in a variety of ways. One person might have a severe form of a condition and respond in such a way as to minimize its effects on his or her life, while another person with a more mild form of the same illness will become disabled psychologically and socially. In the next chapter we examine the considerable research that has been done in an attempt to understand the role of stressful life events in the etiology of illness. We discuss a possible explanation for the connection between stress and illness, which is that *life difficulties influence illness behavior.* It has been suggested that somatic (body) complaints might often be signs of underlying emotional problems [2, 21, 22, 23]. The emotional problems might be motivating the expression of physical distress. In fact, emotional distress may be more influential in the patient's decision to express illness and to seek help than is the actual occurrence of any organic condition [18]. Complaining of a physical symptom (however trivial the symptom) is one way for a person who is emotionally distressed to seek reassurance and support.

The ill individual might not recognize the existence of underlying emotional problems. Even if they are recognized, emotional problems are often difficult for a patient to reveal (disclose) in an undisguised form. A socially acceptable source of help—the physician—is consulted instead of a psychologist, clergyman, or social worker [32]. Illness behavior may be part of a coping repertoire—an attempt by the patient to make a challenging situation (e.g., losing a job) more manageable by imposing a familiar explanation on it ("I am upset because I am sick"), especially if this person can deal better with being ill than with losing a job. Under conditions of manageable difficulties, people may ignore the same symptoms.

Not everyone acts ill when upset. People vary in the extent to which their reactions to serious life stress are translated into the expression of symptoms to a health care professional. One study suggests that emotional stress leads to an attempt to cope on the part of the patient [23]. Someone who has successfully used the sick role in the past (i.e., has been a high utilizer of medical services) will use this particular coping strategy more frequently than someone who has not often utilized health care services. A person who reports being lonely and anxious is more likely to use medical services (reporting some somatic complaint) if this person has been a patient before [23].

Illness is recognized by society as an acceptable reason for withdrawing from certain social obligations. We have noted, for example, that if a woman is ill, she is not expected to continue to go to work, and she is also relieved of the social obligations tied to her role as mother and wife. The Jones's can be excused from attending a boring social event if Mr. Jones is ill.

The sick role may actually draw some people into it who desire to obtain advantages or rewards that go along with the role. The sick role gives the individual an acceptable excuse for making claims on others for care and provides a reason for failure. Hence the individual may be motivated to adopt the sick role, and others may be motivated to grant the individual entrance into the sick role in order to avoid social difficulties. If a student is doing poorly in school, for example, and exhibits a vague symptom like a persistent nonproductive cough, this child might use the cough as a vehicle to gain entrance into the sick role and avoid school altogether. The parents might be motivated to grant the sick role to this child (define the child as ill and let

Box 6-2
The Munchausen Syndrome

Baron von Karl Friedrich Hieronymus Munchausen was an eighteenth century German soldier and adventurer who told unbelievable tales. In medicine the Munchausen syndrome refers to patients who tell wild tales, often to gain admission to hospitals. A recent case concerned an impressive sounding man who claimed to be an oceanographic physicist working with Jacques Cousteau. He complained of chest pains and claimed to have sustained many injuries in the Vietnam war that had necessitated extensive surgery. Later investigation showed that this same man had been hospitalized in other medical centers around the country, sometimes as a major in the Strategic Air Command and other times as a counter-intelligence agent. This "patient" seemed to be attracted to medical centers because of the narcotics and other drugs he would receive. This treatment, which rewarded his behavior, evidently continued for many years. Other patients with this syndrome are reinforced by more "social" rewards from medical settings, and they may derive great satisfaction from the attention they receive from medical professionals. They are also likely to become litigious (bring malpractice suits) in an effort to retaliate against health professionals who try to end their treatment.

For further reading: Chronic factitious disorder with physical symptoms, in *Taskforce on Nomenclature and Statistics, Diagnostic and Statistical Manual of Mental Disorders* (DSMIII) (Washington, D.C.: American Psychiatric Association, 1980), pp. 288–290.

the child stay home from school) partially to explain or provide an excuse for the poor performance of their child. Such a situation further illustrates the point that illness is socially defined. In fact, it may be very difficult for a person to see him or herself as ill if no one else will define this person as ill. Others around the individual must *legitimize* this person's adoption of the sick role and support (reward) the exhibition of illness behaviors (see Box 6–2).

Ultimately, people's use of the illness label (the ability to define themselves as ill) depends on legitimization by a health care professional. People cannot continue calling themselves ill for long if no physician agrees. Other people will say, "Why haven't you been to the doctor?" or "What did your doctor say?"

The ability of the health care professional to assign the illness label to the patient depends in part upon societal values and the restrictions placed upon health care professionals. In present-day American society, the medical system is not heavily controlled by external manipulation (e.g., by the government). The physician's behavior is determined by the profession's standards and by personal values. In some countries, for example, the Soviet Union, government influence makes it very difficult for a physician to assign a person to the sick role [7]. Each individual who is defined as ill is lost to the production pool in society. Illness is seen as a threat to the society's well-being. Therefore it is difficult and nonrewarding for a person to adopt the sick role. In American society, in contrast, an individual only has to say that he or she is ill or in pain and this person is given at least a preliminary (or partial) excuse for social failure, being allowed to neglect his or her social responsibilities. The individual may even receive monetary compensation for the illness— such as sick pay or workman's compensation. Receiving money for being ill might actually encourage the individual to exaggerate the inability to perform the routine tasks of daily life, and discourage attempts to cope with the disability. Problems like this make the social principles of medical care a major political question in the modern world.

In most social situations people want to present themselves in a favorable light; that is, they want to look good. The sociologist Erving Goffman has described the many ways in which people try to present a certain "face" to the world and hide potentially embarrassing information behind the scenes [10]. For example, persons with a stigmatizing condition such as epilepsy or a colostomy may try to present themselves as perfectly "normal." This desire may directly affect how they define illness and their reactions to it. People who suspect that they have syphilis may try to ignore the symptoms and not immediately seek medical help. Similarly, people who have symptoms of a heart attack may refrain from calling the doctor in the middle of the night in order to avoid bothering health personnel and appearing stupid if it turns out to be a false alarm.

If you think about it, you can probably list certain symptoms that are socially undesirable, some that seem neutral, and perhaps others that are desirable. Consider the different *social* meanings of such diseases as lung cancer, flu, breast cancer, tennis elbow, hemorrhoids, runner's knee, stroke, indigestion, gonorrhea, muscle strain, cirrhosis of the liver, myopia, sunburn, and leprosy. An important element influencing the reactions to these problems involves their social desirability.

Conformity to group pressure is very relevant to people's reactions to illness [1]. It is well known that people often conform to the be-

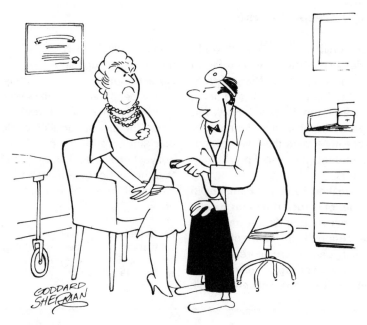

"I don't care if you are listed in 'Who's Who'. . . . You still have just plain old fashioned hay fever."

Figure 6–2. The sick role. (Reprinted by permission of Goddard Sherman)

haviors of others, both to gain rewards from others and to establish a sense of their own proper identity. People look to relevant others—that is, to members of their *reference groups*—to determine what behaviors are appropriate. For example, American teenagers often dress alike and appreciate similar music; lawyers may have similar-looking offices and similar automobiles; and so on. Such conformity pressures also apply to the definition of and reaction to illness. Little boys soon learn that it is not "proper" for them to cry when they scrape their knees. This "manliness" may be carried into adult life, causing some men to avoid complaining about serious symptoms so that they will not appear "soft." Reactions to flulike symptoms may vary among people as a function of how their friends have responded; if their friends recently stayed home in bed when they had the flu, so probably will these people (see Box 6–3).

Box 6–3
When Do People Cough?

A traditional medical model would consider a cough as an innate reflex in which air is rapidly discharged from the lungs. Complex muscle and nerve actions are seen as central. However, the psychologist James Pennebaker has recently shown that even coughing is influenced by social psychological factors.

Pennebaker monitored coughing in a number of natural situations such as classrooms. He found three important influences on the incidence of coughing. First, people are more likely to cough in large groups than when they are in small groups. Second, people are more likely to cough when they hear others cough and when they are close to someone who is coughing. Finally, people are more likely to cough in boring rather than interesting situations. The precise social psychological mechanisms affecting coughing have not yet been isolated, but it seems likely that the subtle suggestions and expectations of others have a pronounced effect.

For further reading: J. W. Pennebaker, Perceptual and environmental determinants of coughing. *Basic and Applied Social Psychology*, 1980, *1*, 83–91.

A more dramatic but relatively rare instance of the group's influence on definitions of illness involves collective behavior. The term *collective behavior* refers to actions that seem to arise spontaneously, are guided by a general rationale, and spread rapidly from one member to another in a group [41]. Fads are an example. Most interesting is "mass psychogenic illness" or "assembly line hysteria." A typical case involves the "blue mist" that someone in a midwestern furniture assembly plant thought she saw. One by one, the women workers began to feel dizzy, lightheaded, and weak, supposedly from the blue mist. Actually, analysis of air samples showed that the air was fine. A similar incident occurred recently in West Virginia. Workers in a shoe factory began fainting, felt weak, and had headaches and nausea. Government tests found no toxins, which makes it seem likely that the workers were victims of mass psychogenic illness.

This phenomenon is well known to social psychologists. In one case in a textile factory in which an imagined insect caused nervousness, nausea, and weakness, psychologists found that the spread of the "disease" affected persons who were nervous, isolated, and knew others they thought were bitten. This process is a special form of suggestion in which illness is created purely from the social psychology of the group. It is important to recognize that the individuals involved do indeed feel ill and may even vomit or faint; however, the cause of these symptoms is the *belief* that one is sick. This suggests that the social situation may strongly affect the collective illness behaviors of a group of people [20, 51].

Thus the same physical symptoms may be interpreted and reacted to in different ways depending on the social situation. In fact, illness is especially likely to be subject to the influence of other people since it usually has important implications for a person's friends and associates. If a man is defined as ill and stays home in bed, there are often important consequences for his wife and children, his employer and co-workers, his bowling partners, and so on. Hence it is difficult to overestimate the importance of social influence in deciding "What is illness?"

MEDICAL CARE AND THE POOR

We have seen that social factors strongly affect definitions of illness. An important application of this analysis concerns medical care for the poor. In the United States today, complete access to good health care is not the right of every individual, for the socioeconomic status (SES) of the patient affects the kind of care received. Although maintenance of health and success of treatment depend upon early recognition of symptoms, accurate diagnosis, and application of appropriate treatment, failures at various steps occur all the time for patients of low economic status. These failures are responsible for the higher mortality rates of the low-income population.

One of the failures of medical treatment for the poor involves the health care professional–patient relationship. Persons of low socioeconomic status in this country often do not have a personal physician, and consequently they enter the medical care system through the emergency room of the hospital. Persons who enter the medical care system in this way are usually more seriously ill than patients who enter the system via their private physician.

Patients of low SES are more likely than those of higher SES to delay treatment. First, they have *less information* about disease than do patients of higher SES and higher education. They are not exposed to health information as much as higher-income groups are, and they are also less likely to have a long-term relationship with a physician who can provide health education. Second, patients of low SES delay treatment longer because they simply do not have the resources to obtain the care they need. Life is, for the poor, often a constant battle to make ends meet; sociologist Lee Rainwater calls it the "crisis life of the poor." Care of their body may have a high priority for upper-income people, but the poor have many other problems to address with their limited resources. A poor person may compare their body that is not functioning correctly with a poorly working car and other aspects of their lives that do not run well. Only when their health difficulties interfere with the rest of their lives (their ability to go to work, to take care of their children, etc.) do they feel it is necessary to attend to them. Earl Koos reports interviews with survey respondents who are poor who answered questions about their health in ways such as: "I plan to get this hernia fixed, but it really does not bother me that much right now. My car is a wreck and I need the money to get a new one. There really are other things more important to me right now." Another respondent remarked on the difficulty of taking time out to acknowledge illness: "Sometimes I feel so bad I could curl up and die, but I have to go on because the children need me to take care of them, and besides I have to go to work and cannot spend the money on doctors" [16].

Third, patients of low SES delay treatment because they are commonly treated in public hospitals where they may undergo procedures done in part for the education of physicians in medical training. Poor patients who receive public assistance in the form of free medical care are sometimes teaching material for the residents and medical students at public institutions. Patients of high SES are less likely to be "practiced on" in private hospitals. Therefore many poor people who realize this consider even a top-notch medical center a "butchershop" [27]. Patients' fears are confirmed if they find that physicians-in-training are interested in their diseases, not in them as a person.

In a classic study of patients in a large urban teaching hospital, Raymond Duff and August Hollingshead documented the distressing treatment of patients of low SES by health care professionals in the hospital [6]. This treatment was compared with the treatment of more well-to-do patients. The researchers found that in this elite academic medical center, attached to a famous medical school, patients became acutely aware of their social status in the hospital by the way in which they were treated. The health care professional–patient relationship was influenced tremendously by the social class of the patient. Poor patients received impersonal treatment in the medical center, and poor patients also endured unnecessary procedures so that the house staff could practice medicine on them, even though the patients knew that they were teaching material for the young physicians. In addition, poor patients tended to be grossly uninformed about the details of what was happening to them, mostly because the health care professionals viewed them as uneducated and incapable of understanding what was happening to them. Finally, because of differences in social class and education, none of the health care professionals could easily identify with poor patients. The physicians and other health professionals preferred to communicate with patients of their own social class.

Thus the factors of background, psychological inference, and social situation, all of which affect the definitions and reactions of everyone to illness, have a special influence on poor people [24]. Together these factors may seriously increase the time that elapses before a poor person seeks treatment and therefore produce more serious disease states.

ILLNESS AND WELLNESS

Consider the following two patients:

Mr. Johnson complains of being tired, lethargic, generally uneasy, uncomfortable, and has a sore back and headache. He is grumpy with his family and misses a number of days of work, calling in sick. Mr. Johnson's wife finally convinces him to go to see his family physician. Many tests are done and a detailed history is taken. Still the family physician, even in consultation with others in his group practice, can find no definable organic condition to explain Mr. Johnson's symptomns. The physician explains to Mr. Johnson that a specialist can be called in if it turns out to be necessary, but that the family physician would first like to explore some other issues, like Mr. Johnson's relationship with his boss at work, how many heavy things he has been lifting lately, and his feelings about approaching his fiftieth birthday. While no specific pathogen or tissue damage has been found, Mr. Johnson is obviously not "healthy."

Mrs. Smith is medically normal in every way—all of her blood chemistries are in the normal range, she feels okay, and there are no unusual results from a complete physical exam. However, Mrs. Smith does not exercise at all—she has virtually no muscle tone and she has little stamina. Physical stressors are potentially devastating. It would be hard to recover from surgery because she has little strength. Her diet is adequate but not very well balanced. She smokes filtered cigarettes. Is Mrs. Smith healthy?

Box 6–4
Exercise and the Concept of Wellness

Each year millions of Americans visit their family doctor for an annual physical checkup and are pronounced "healthy" or are given a "clean bill of health." Yet, according to Dr. George Sheehan, heart specialist, author, and expert on running and exercise, only 2 percent of Americans get enough exercise to be considered physically fit. True, Dr. Sheehan's definition of "normal" and "healthy" and "fit" is very stringent. It involves a well-trained body at its maximum efficiency. This state is difficult for most people to attain, for few can spend most of their time in the pursuit of physical conditioning. But he points to the limited concept of wellness that is used by most physicians—the absence of detectable disease. The traditional definition ignores fitness, physical adaptability, strength, speed, and quality of daily living.

While not everyone need be an athlete, moderate regular exercise reduces the risk of many health problems. A sedentary lifestyle is one of the factors contributing to heart disease, yet most individuals receive relatively little or no physical exercise at their work. Even in sports, people have become spectators instead of partici-pants. A Gallup Poll in 1977 found that only about half of all American adults engage in some form of exercise to stay fit. Most participate in activities that are not nearly strenuous enough, or which provide only intermittent demands on the body.

Physical fitness helps people feel better, have more energy, and require less sleep, as well as develop greater muscle strength and flexibility and lose excess weight. Psychological benefits reported by exercisers include decreased anxiety and depression.

Health professionals, according to a U.S. government report, largely *ignore* promotion of exercise for their patients. This is probably because they do not engage in exercise themselves or do not know how to motivate people to seek out healthy behaviors. More interest and concern on the part of health professionals are necessary if a broader conception of wellness is to be achieved.

For further reading: G. Sheehan, *Dr. Sheehan on Running* (Mountain View, Calif.: World Publications, 1975); and The Surgeon General's report on health promotion and disease prevention, *Healthy People* (Washington, D.C.: USDHEW, PHS Pub. #79-55071, 1979).

There is a wide range of fitness among people who are free of disease; people may be more or less healthy. For this reason some medical practitioners have adopted the concept of *wellness*. People who are well are not only free of disease but are also taking positive action to improve their health. For example, they may exercise regularly, eat nutritious and well-balanced meals, avoid tobacco, and carefully monitor physical signs such as their blood pressure. In addition, wellness-seekers pay attention to the special, individual needs that are unique to their own bodies, rather than merely following general medical advice. From this perspective, wellness-seekers are actively responsible for all matters relating to their health, with a special emphasis on prevention of illness. This view is quite different from the traditional view in which medicine is seen as a curing or repair system needed only when medical problems strike.

Wellness can be viewed as an ideal state of self-realization toward which a person strives but never reaches. Prevention of disease is an important part of wellness, but an active striving is central. We have seen that a large part of illness involves the inability to engage in normal kinds of behavior. The wellness-seeker builds stamina and fitness, thus expanding the range of what is to be considered "normal," and perhaps may also develop added flexibility in dealing with life (see Box 6-4).

Because it is a new concept in medicine, wellness has been misunderstood by many traditional medical practitioners and even some of its most vociferous proponents. Unfortunately, wellness is sometimes viewed as a crazy new fad or as some kind of mystical road to truth and self-fulfillment. Actually, the concept is a sensible antidote to the narrow but well-established view that achieving health involves the "fixing" of a passive, diseased body. Wellness concepts, on the other hand, tend to emphasize that there are many aspects of a person's lifestyle that affect well-being. By focusing attention on healthy ways of living, concepts of wellness can have a beneficial effect on resources people bring to the challenges of their daily life.

SUMMARY

Although physical symptoms are associated with disease, these symptoms do not in themselves define illness; illness instead involves a process of interpretation. People have certain expectations about illness that create the sick role, and people make certain attributions about their own sensations and about the illness behaviors of others. Hence symptoms ranging from a headache to acute chest pain may or may not be seen as illness depending on the background of the individual, the particular attribution processes at work, and the social context in which the symptoms appear.

In this chapter we have mostly ignored the biological aspects of illness because our emphasis has been on the social psychological aspects of illness. It goes without saying, of course, that biological processes (organic diseases) are a significant part of illness. The social psychological aspects, however, are too often ignored even though they are an equally important part of illness. A complete understanding of illness can come only with an understanding of *both* the biological and the social psychological answers to the question of "What is illness?"

7
Psychological Factors in the Etiology of Illness

Art Jennings is a 52-year-old hardworking executive for a large New York City firm that manufacturers computers, line printers, and teletype machines. Art has a college degree and has been working for the company for about sixteen years. He is married and has three children who are headed for college. Art's company recently informed him that he will be transferred to their midwestern office. Selling his suburban house and making plans for the move have been trying for Art because his wife and children do not want to move. However, Art feels he must make the move for financial reasons; a policy instituted by his company makes it impossible for Art to turn down the transfer.

Complicating Art's career problems at this point are some personal problems. Six months ago Art's best friend died suddenly of a heart attack; this friend was someone with whom Art could talk freely and openly. Art had never really developed any other close friendships, and he took relatively little interest in community affairs and belonged to no social organizations. Art and his wife, although together now, were separated for some months during the past year in an attempt to iron out some of their marital difficulties. Art's mother, an 80-year-old widow who was relatively independent until she broke her hip, is now confined to a nursing home on Long Island near Art's home, and as an only child, he is solely responsible for his mother's welfare. Finally, Art's youngest son has been getting into trouble in school.

Art is overwhelmed with a feeling of loss of control over his life. He feels that many constraints have been placed on him, and because of the demands of his job and family, his mother's needs, as well as the loss of his friend, he is becoming progressively more depressed. He wonders about the purpose of his life. He is afraid that because of his age he will not be able to find another job if he leaves the job that he already has. Art feels trapped in a very uncomfortable situation. To compound these problems, Art has an intermittent pain in his chest that is accompanied by shortness of breath.

Although the details may differ, many people are in situations similar to that of Art. Such people may be at high risk for health problems, for they and Art Jennings are facing many life stresses. Research suggests that the experience of life stress can play a role in the etiology (causes) of illness.

Earlier in this book we considered how various social psychological factors affect the course and outcome of illness. For example, we saw how the relationship between the health care professional and the patient can influence the patient's willingness to cooperate with medical treatment. We considered how the art of medicine can lower the anxiety level of the patient and bring about a more positive outcome. We also considered how communication can affect the patient's understanding of the health measures that should be followed and what is likely to occur in treatment. We discussed how this understanding may, in turn, have an important effect on the patient's well-being. In Chapter 6 we directly analyzed the social nature of illness and reactions to illness.

In this chapter we examine how life events can contribute to illness. We show how the social stresses facing Art Jennings—loss of his friend and his old job, for example, as well as agitated patterns of behavior and the inability to cope effectively—are critically important in the etiology of illness.

There are at least two major psychological factors that play a part in the precipitation of physical illness [10]. The first involves *personality and coping style*. Certain characteristic modes of responding to relatively usual and normal life events—that is, typical patterns of behavior—can predispose an individual to illness. These behaviors include such things as constant anxiety, giving up hope, overeating, not sleeping well, and chain smoking. The second major factor involves *stress stemming from difficult life situations*. A person may experience a great amount of physical disruption as a result of a major life change (such as the death of a spouse). In the research on the etiology of illness, these two psychological factors have typically been examined separately. That is, researchers studying social psychology and medicine have examined *either* the contribution of a patient's personality characteristics to illness *or* the role played by a multitude of stressful life situations in the development of illness. These two variables actually operate in concert, however; people respond differently to different life crises [10]. Some people become extremely upset, anxious, or depressed when faced with a slight change in their normal routine, whereas other people take certain major problems in stride with a minimum of emotional trauma. An individual's personality—the usual way of responding to life—thus tends to "interact with" the situational stresses.

There are many different ways in which psychological factors can precipitate or increase the likelihood of illness. Before we consider them, however, we should examine the notion of *stress*.

What Is Stress?

Stress is a concept that has been defined in many different ways by researchers. A satisfactory definition considers stress to be the *state of an organism when reacting to new circumstances*. Stress is produced by an unexpected event in the environment, and a stressful event is an event that induces stress by requiring the organism to readjust itself [1, 52, 72].

A great variety of environmental conditions (both positive and negative) can produce stress, but different individuals respond to the same conditions in different ways. Some experience stress easily, whereas others can barely tolerate the same event. Even the response of a given person to a stressful event may vary depending upon the physiological and psychological state of the person. This person may react differently to the same kind of environmental event, such as a term paper. The term paper deadline might be dealt with in a straightforward manner by the individual when feeling well, but the same person may experience severe stress when facing a deadline when tired or suffering from a virus. The degree of stress that the person experiences depends, too, upon the meaning attached to the environmental event and upon the resources the person has available for coping with the event. Thus reaction to environmental states varies considerably among individuals and within each individual as well.

Stress affects everyone, not just the harried executive. Stress is necessary for the psychological growth and change of each individual. An individual experiences stress when attempting a new endeavor. Increasing stress is usually associated with increasing opportunities and potential resources for the individual. Stress is an inevitable feature of modern life, and a certain amount of it can be beneficial, for it can help to keep a person alert and interested in life. However, sometimes (as in the case of Art Jennings) the amount of readjustment required at a given time in a person's life is so excessive that the person's level of stress is overwhelming [75].

A MODEL OF STRESS AND ILLNESS

There are many ways in which the relationship between stress and illness can be examined, and here we combine the important elements of the various explanatory models into one model. Figure 7-1 illustrates this comprehensive model of stress and illness.

One model linking stress and illness is described by the pathway *a-b-d-h* in Figure 7-1. This model suggests that certain people respond to certain stressful life events by entering the sick role [45, 47]. For example, Art Jennings might respond to the pressures of moving to a new job by avoiding his responsibilities—by losing his appetite, oversleeping, and being lethargic, by staying away from work and remaining home sick in bed, and by complaining of headaches and other pains, such as in his chest. He may exhibit enough illness behaviors to be defined as ill and excused from having to move away. Note that in this model no organic condition such as heart disease or brain tumor is involved. Rather what is evident is the person's behavior (including what the person says). People sometimes turn to unhealthy habits and exhibit illness behaviors in situations that are extremely stressful.

The attempt to cope with stress makes a person more likely to attend to physical symptoms. There is some evidence in the research literature that certain symptoms (e.g., headache or backache) are attended to (and medical help sought) by the person under stress [45]. If things are going well in someone's life, attention tends to be focused elsewhere. For example, it has been found that most apparently *healthy* people (those who are functioning normally in day-to-day life) report at least one or two symptoms of illness if they are asked whether they have any symptoms. As we saw in Chapter 4 in discussing pain, recognition of these symptoms is not directly related to the physiological state of the person. The reporting of symptoms is clearly affected by psychological processes [54, 77].

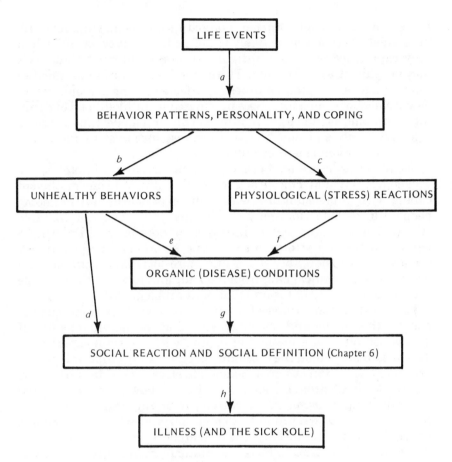

Figure 7-1. A general model of stress and illness.

The psychologist, James Pennebaker, has suggested that symptom reports are affected by three factors [53, 54]. First, a person's attention to bodily sensations increases the incidence of reported symptoms. For example, sports contestants are often unaware of sprains and muscle pulls and sometimes even broken bones when they are deeply involved in the competitive game. Medical students, on the other hand, constantly direct their attention toward bodily functions, and as a result, they often report experiencing a cornucopia of symptoms [46]. Second, symptom reporting is influenced by "interpretive set"; that is, symptoms are affected by what people *think* about their sensations—what meaning they attach to them.

For example, if people think prolonged fatigue is a symptom of illness, they are much more likely to define themselves as "ill" when they experience prolonged fatigue. Others might see fatigue as a normal part of everyday life. Third, the interpretation of a bodily sensation as a symptom of illness is affected by the person's mood. Negative moods such as depression increase the likelihood of defining symptoms as indicative of illness. This first model thus suggests that Art Jennings could become ill in response to stressful events without the involvement of an organic condition.

Social rewards are also crucial. As discussed in Chapter 6, the sociologist David Mechanic suggested that illness is one method of coping with unpleasant or unsatisfying experiences [45]. For some people illness behaviors may be an attempt to make an unstable situation more manageable. Illness behaviors provide the person with an opportunity to gain social and emotional support. In our society, it is considerably easier and more socially acceptable for a person to seek medical care from a doctor and to adopt the sick role than it is to seek help for an emotional problem [55].

The psychologist Frances Cohen has reviewed the research supporting this model and has suggested that an individual's use of illness behavior as a method of coping with stressful experiences depends, in part, upon the individual's personality [10]. Some people are more likely than others to respond to stress by exhibiting illness behaviors that, through social definitions, allow them to enter the sick role. Studies using standardized personality tests have shown that people who are prone to depression and who have low ego strength (people termed by the researchers as "psychologically vulnerable") also tend to have a somatic hypersensitivity. That is, they tend to be more sensitive than most people to normal fluctuations in physical states [8].

In sum, there is one pathway connecting the stress of life events to illness that involves no physiological mechanism. Stressful events can lead certain people to pay more attention to fluctuations in their bodily state and to interpret fluctuations as illness. The sick role may then provide relief from the changes in the environment.

Stress, Unhealthy Behaviors, and Organic Disease

We have seen that the first model linking stress and illness does not involve an organic condition (e.g., heart disease). Although the remaining two models *do* involve organic conditions, they differ significantly in the character of the link between stress and physical condition. The second model is described by the path *a-b-e-g-h* in

Figure 7-1. In this model, the person's psychological responses to stress lead the person to unhealthy behaviors such as cigarette smoking, alcoholism, poor diet, and lack of rest and exercise. These behaviors in turn lead to disease or trauma. There are many unhealthy behaviors that place people at high risk for various medical problems, and many of these behaviors are instigated by stress. A simple example involves traumatic injury: Stress leads to careless or fast driving, which then leads to injury in an automobile accident [35]. Another common example involves stress, alcoholism, and cirrhosis of the liver.

Physiological Stress and Illness

The third and final model of the link between stress and illness also involves organic conditions. However, in this model there is a *direct* link from stress reactions to organic conditions through physiological responses. This path is represented by *a-c-f-g-h* in Figure 7-1. This third model is provocative and is taken up in the next major section of this chapter, on loss, life change, and illness.

Other Models

Of course, it would be possible to draw in other links in Figure 7-1. For example, someone who is defined as ill would be likely to experience different life events from someone not defined as ill. In addition, organic conditions can affect personality and coping mechanisms. For example, the physical weakness resulting from a serious illness can induce depression. Personality might also affect the life events that people encounter and with which they must deal. For example, some people are naturally cautious and therefore remain content to take few risks in their lives. They might be less likely than others to put themselves in situations where they must deal with a new job or a new city in which to live [10]. The web of interlocking relationships that affects health actually constitutes the entire subject matter of this book. The purpose of Figure 7-1 is to focus attention on the processes that we examine in this chapter.

LOSS, LIFE CHANGE, AND ILLNESS

When a person becomes seriously ill soon after the death of a loved one, we might say that the person is suffering from a "broken heart," and we may not be surprised when we hear of such cases (see

Box 7-1). We also may find that some people become ill after a big change in their life occurs. For example, Richard Nixon became seriously ill with phlebitis soon after he resigned the presidency, and his wife Pat had a stroke. Many people respond to social psychological events such as loss and life change with a physiological reaction that leads to actual organic disease.

In 1932 Dr. Walter B. Cannon of the Harvard Medical School wrote that bodily alterations occur in conjunction with emotional strife and the experiencing of "violent" emotions such as anger or fear [6, 7]. He said that stress causes an increase in the blood sugar level, a large output of adrenalin, an increase in pulse rate, blood pressure, and respiration rate, and an increase in the amount of blood pumped to the skeletal muscles. Cannon called this the "fight-or-flight" response. When an animal perceives a threatening situation, its reflex response is an integrated physiological reaction that prepares it either for running away or for fighting [6, 7].

Scientists have demonstrated that the physiological characteristics of the fight-or-flight response exist in people as well. In some studies healthy young adults were put into resting positions. Then, while trying to solve arithmetic problems under time limits, they were verbally harrassed and pressured with statements from the researchers, such as "I did that better than you did—You're not doing very well." Measurements were taken of their pulse and respiration rates, blood pressure, and the amount of blood pumped to the skeletal muscles. A *physiological response* was found to occur in the person on whom an *emotional stress* was placed. This is the same response as the fight-or-flight response. Although this response may still be necessary in some cases for actual survival, the stresses of society today usually do not require such behavior (physical fight or flight). Yet the response remains. According to Cannon and others, stressful life events trigger continuous bodily arousal, and this continuous arousal can cause lasting changes in basic physiological processes.

A researcher-physician, Adolf Meyer, proposed in the 1930s that stressful life events may be important in the etiology of illness [49]. These events need not be negative or bizarre or catastrophic to be pathogenic. They must simply be interpreted by the individual as an important life change, requiring some degree of coping. Examples are changes such as moving from one city to another, changing jobs, the birth of a child, marriage, a death in the family, and other fundamentally important life events. Meyer noted the effects of these stresses on patients with respiratory, gastrointestinal, cardiovascular, and skin diseases. However, while Meyer noted the relationship between life change and illness clinically, he never documented his findings with systematic empirical research.

In time more illustrations of the relationship between stress and physical deterioration appeared. Cannon, for example, in 1942 wrote about a phenomenon that he called "voodoo death" [7]. Various examples are known in which a person received some kind of curse (e.g., from a witch doctor), became overcome with fear, and died within a few days. Cannon believed that the continuous stress on the body from severe emotional activation produced this effect. The precise physiological mechanisms are unknown, but there may be rapid breathing with a rapid pulse rate until the heart finally gives out. (Curt Richter called this phenomenon "sudden death," although he studied it only in rats [61].)

Related to this physiological response to emotional stress is another phenomenon proposed by Martin Seligman [71]. Seligman suggested that people (as well as animals) who are in highly stressful situations that they cannot control develop "learned helplessness." They can no longer cope, and therefore they may give up and die. A physiological response develops from a psychological stress. (Learned helplessness is considered in more detail in Chapter 11 when the effects of institutionalization are discussed.)

All the phenomena considered so far suggest that stress may lead to disease. Yet this does not always occur. Stress is inherent in life— it cannot be avoided, but many people remain healthy. A number of questions therefore arise concerning the relationship between stress and illness. What are the properties that distinguish more stressful life events from less stressful life events? Do specific kinds of stresses lead to specific kinds of illnesses? And, most importantly, why do some people become ill while others do not, given the same stressful life events?

These questions have occupied the attention of researchers who study the relationships among stressful life events, coping, and illness. These researchers have tried to determine the extent to which illness can be predicted from knowledge of stressful life events. They have also tried to delineate the determinants of succumbing versus not succumbing to illness, for if more is known about the specific effects of certain kinds of stress on health, health care professionals and their patients can then be better equipped to combat the ill effects of life stresses.

The General Adaptation Syndrome Model

One of the earliest theories that linked stress to illness was that of Hans Selye [72]. Selye proposed that any noxious stimulus (emotional or physical) results in a biological response that is character-

Box 7-1
The Broken Heart

Social support and the existence of strong, meaningful relationships are crucial coping mechanisms that weaken the link between stressful life changes and illness. Social support helps the individual to cope with a stressful situation and may reduce the severity of the physiological response to a life change. On the other hand, some people die from a "broken heart."

Lack of human companionship and love has been thought since antiquity to contribute to death and disease, but the effect of human contact on the health of a person's heart has not been carefully examined until recently. James Lynch, a researcher, studied the effects of human contact and of loneliness on the heart. He began with a qualitative analysis of "folklore"—of the many instances in human interaction in which the heart is implicated as a significant participant in the drama. For example, people use phrases such as "heartbroken," "heartsick," and "a broken heart." Lynch also observed that human contact had important effects on the hearts of patients in the coronary care and other intensive care units of hospitals. He examined systematically how cardiac rhythms are affected by human contact. He found that human contact with laboratory animals (especially dogs) could have marked effects on the animals' hearts.

Lynch then examined death statistics. In examining the *average annual death rate* per population of 100,000 between the ages of 15 and 64, he found that widowed, divorced, and single people have significantly higher death rates than married people. For all age groups (in 1959–1961), the rate of death from coronary heart disease was about twice as high among divorced people as among married people and about one and one-half times as high among among widowed and single people as among married people. Thus the loneliness of a broken heart may be a factor in heart disease.

It is interesting to examine how Lynch reconciles his theory of broken hearts with other explanations of heart disease. He considers, for example, the statistics showing a low incidence of coronary heart disease in Japan as compared to the United States. Experts have attributed this difference to the diet in Japan and have shown that when Japanese move to the United States, their risk of heart disease goes up. The conclusion has always been that when Japanese men change their diets, they become prone to heart disease. Lynch, however, noted that the family structure in Japan is very strong —there are almost no divorces. People live in extended families and there is a great deal of love and companionship. When people come from that environment to the United States, they often experience a great deal of loneliness and their family ties are weakened. Similarly, research on Type A versus Type B behavior patterns and coronary heart disease (considered in detail later in this chapter) might also be explainable with Lynch's hypothesis. Meyer Friedman and Ray Rosenman found that the Type A person is involved in a chronic, incessant struggle to "achieve more in less time." Type A individuals are often addicted to work to the point where they grossly neglect their families and friends. The link to disease might be that persons with love and security from their families, friends, and community can cope better with stressful psychological situations than individuals deprived of such support. When social psychological factors are considered, the "broken heart" becomes a legitimate medical concern.

For further reading: J. J. Lynch, *The Broken Heart: The Medical Consequences of Loneliness* (New York: Basic Books, 1977).

---

ized by an arousal in the body's system of defenses against the noxious stimulus. Simply stated, the general adaptation syndrome consists of three stages: the alarm reaction, a stage of resistance, and a stage of exhaustion. Selye proposed that there is a basic, specific physiological response developed for defense against noxious stimuli, and that it is possible that many different diseases could result from prolonged adaptive processes using this response. Different organs are affected, depending on the characteristics of the organism, and different diseases result. Often the "weakest link" gives out first. It is important to note, however, that in Selye's model, stress does not lead to disease unless the adaptive responses are required for a *prolonged* period of time; that is, unless the individual is constantly attempting to adapt.

While Selye's model does not propose a specific answer to how noxious stimuli produce physiological responses, there is an emphasis on the part played by the adrenal cortical hormones in response to stress. Selye caused stress in rats by pulling their tails, and after sacrificing them, he examined their adrenal glands and found the adrenal glands to be affected. He thus hypothesized that as a result of the activation of the adrenal system, bodily resistance to disease is lowered and other biological changes take place. The findings of other researchers fit into this framework as well [39, 43, 44]. The suggested link in this theory is that such physiological responses to life events can affect the person's general susceptibility to illness.

In Figure 7–1 this model is represented by path a-c-f-g-h, as noted earlier. Life events trigger responses by the individual that produce physiological reactions, and these reactions in turn may lead to an

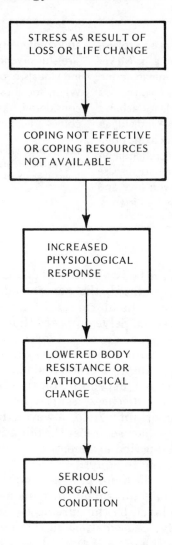

Figure 7-2. Adaptation syndrome and disease.

organic condition such as hypertension or heart disease. Part of this model is expanded and presented in Figure 7-2. There has been quite a bit of research attempting to identify the physiological changes that occur and their mechanisms of operation. Unfortunately, the precise physiological processes are poorly understood, although the body's nervous and hormonal systems are obviously very important

[10]. In any case such matters are outside the scope of this chapter. Our interest here is to understand the social and psychological factors that affect people through their reaction to life events. Our goal is to understand how people can learn to cope with these events.

Giving up or Relinquishing Control—Loss and Its Effects on Health

It has been suggested that the loss of a significant component of a person's life, particularly an interpersonal relationship, can bring about stress for a person because of a need to then reorder life. Furthermore, the loss may remove a significant source of emotional support for the person. Loss can influence the state of health of an individual [14, 15].

The response of "giving up" as a result of a severe loss has been linked with vulnerability to illness. While the biological mechanisms that underlie this phenomenon are still in dispute, an empirical relationship seems to have been demonstrated. Research on human beings has been done by George Engel and his colleagues that suggests that a "giving up" response in the face of situations of loss may precede the development of illnesses of all types in individuals who have predispositions to the particular illnesses. While Engel emphasizes the occurrence of loss, he also clearly specifies that the key component of the problem is the ability or inability to cope in the face of a negative environmental event [16, 66, 67]. The giving up behavior of the individual involves a sense of psychological impotence—a feeling that, at least for a while, the person is totally unable to cope with the changes in the environment. In the extreme, the person loses all interest in life and in other people (see Box 7-2).*

Before we discuss this research in detail, we examine the methodology used in these studies [10]. Research linking psychological factors and illness is often *retrospective*. The research is conducted by asking the patient (*after* diagnosis of the illness) to recall and report the pre-illness emotional state or stressful life events. The knowledge that someone is ill as well as the actual experience of illness (e.g., the debilitation and pain of a heart attack) can affect the recall of the events leading up to the illness. Illness can also affect how people recollect their personality characteristics before the ill-

---

*The inability to cope may actually be related to the loss. For example, if a person's spouse has always been a source of support in the face of stress, the loss of the spouse removes the usual coping mechanism in addition to being a change that must be adjusted to.

Box 7-2
Taunts and Death

A sad event can provide a dramatic reminder of the link between stress and illness. This case, recently in the news, concerns a seven-year-old black girl with sickle cell anemia.

This little girl was bussed to a new elementary school in a white neighborhood of Chicago. She and other black children were met with cries of angry whites to "go back where you belong." The little girl was quite upset by the incident. After some time at the school, she went to the principal's office crying and complaining of chest pains. She died later that day in the hospital, apparently from a sickle cell crisis brought on by stress. As she died, she kept repeating "go back where you belong."

---

ness (e.g., "I used to be very energetic—running around all the time" or "I was very nervous"). Hence retrospective reports are often biased.

Let us look at a specific example related to the research on stress and illness. A study of stress reactions contributing to a heart attack is *retrospective* if the researcher assesses precoronary life stress *after* the heart attack. This is done by asking the patient to recall the life events and stresses leading up to the time of the heart attack. Such an approach is biased because of the patient's knowledge of having had a heart attack, and also by the patient's physical and emotional state after the attack. Anxiety, hopelessness, helplessness, fear, and agitation resulting from hospitalization and the threat to life can affect the patient's recollections and reporting of the precoronary events. The patient might focus only on the stressful life events or exaggerate their intensity, thereby giving a distorted picture of the relationship between the stress and the subsequent heart attack. Thus retrospective analyses have inherent biases, and caution must be exercised in drawing conclusions.

Another example of how this retrospective methodology can lead researchers astray involves research on Down's syndrome (Mongolism). Researchers once believed that Down's syndrome was the result of emotional stress during pregnancy, because when asked about their pregnancy, mothers of Down's syndrome children recalled very stressful events. But after it was discovered that Down's syndrome was actually the result of a chromosomal abnormality, stressful events during pregnancy were no longer the focus of research and were no longer reported [5].

A more valid method is a *prospective* research study, which involves collecting predictive information *before* the event to be predicted. For example, we might examine life events and reactions to these events by interviewing a large number of people. After all the data are collected, the researchers simply wait to see which persons develop illness (e.g., who suffers a heart attack). If there is a correlation between how much stress a person reports and whether or not this person eventually has a heart attack, we have a good indication that the connection is not the result of biased reporting.

Unfortunately, much of the data that support the theory of "giving up" and its relationship to illness are retrospective in nature. There has been some prospective research, however [68, 69]. These studies were of patients who were asymptomatic for cervical disease, but who required a diagnostic biopsy because of suspicious cells in their PAP tests. The researchers interviewed the patients prior to the biopsy for evidence of loss and feelings of hopelessness. The researchers made predictions on the basis of the patients' psychological state about which patients would be found to have cancer. Predictions of cancer were based on the hopelessness expressed by patients in the face of loss. These predictions were confirmed statistically as better than chance occurrences. While all studies are limited by the special characteristics of the patients, we still can draw some conclusions from this kind of research, particularly when it is coupled with other research. Some studies have focused on illness and mortality after a loss, particularly the death of a spouse. These studies have supported the central importance of hopelessness as a factor in illness. Researchers reported significantly increased mortality among widows and widowers usually in the first six months after the death of their spouse [9, 28, 65].

Losses and even a temporary sense of hopelessness are quite common in most people's lives, and loss can be found in the history of most people. The research has shown, however, that how a person *copes* with the loss may be more important to health than the occurrence of the loss itself [10].

Life Change

All of us have heard of cases in which a person seems in worse health several months after changing jobs, or someone dies soon after retiring or even while on a long-anticipated vacation. In other words, illness follows an important change in a person's life. Working within Selye's adaptation model, researchers [24, 26, 57, 58, 60] investigated the relationship between stressful life events and the onset of illness. They looked at life stress in terms of events that required a significant amount of adaptation in the ongoing pattern of the individual's life, including life changes that were both positive and negative. It was hypothesized that exposure to life stresses does not cause disease but rather may alter the individual's susceptibility to illness.

As noted above, the role of stressful life events in the etiology of illness has been studied for many years. A half century ago, the physician Adolf Meyer organized medical data as a dynamic biography that contained information not only about a patient's medical history (specific illnesses) but also about the patient's psychosocial history. He began to recognize the importance of life events preceding patients' illnesses. Meyer called this method of organizing data the *Life Chart*. In the late 1940s other researchers [24, 26, 57, 58, 60] began to use the same method. In studies of more than 5000 U.S. Navy personnel patients, they showed that stressful life events tended to cluster within two years before the onset of disease. They noticed that social and personal transactions of significance in the social structure of American life affected people's health very strongly (see also Box 7-3).

Measuring Life Change. Research on "life events" attempted to demonstrate a connection between the onset of illness and the sheer *number* of life-change events that require adaptive responses. The effects of these events were assumed to be additive; that is, more events were expected to have a greater effect. Initially, the researchers counted the number of stressors, but then it became clear that some events are more stressful than others. They found a way to measure the general impact of these events by having a large number of people rate various events as to how much readjustment was required. The scale indicating these ratings is called the Social Readjustment Rating Scale (SRRS) [26] (see Table 7-1). For example, death of a spouse is rated 100, the highest point on the scale; marriage is rated 50; and a change in recreation is 19 and a vacation 12. Most investigators working in this field adopted either the original or a modified form of the 43-item checklist developed by Thomas Holmes, Richard Rahe, and colleagues. The items represent common situations that arise from family, occupational, personal, or financial aspects of an individual's life. They are events that require an adjustment in the individual's way of life.

The life events in the SRRS were used by Thomas Holmes and Minora Masuda to construct the Schedule of Recent Experience (SRE) [25]. This instrument, a self-administered questionnaire,

Box 7-3
Public Recognition of Stress

The idea that stress is often an important component of illness has made its way into the public consciousness. Stresses that used to be considered the personal problem of the individual are now being used in claims of illness and disability. For example, workers may take a sick day when they become very anxious on the job. A more striking example is claims for disability payments.

According to various news accounts, some public employees are claiming that the stresses of their work are so severe that they are ill and deserve full disability payments. In one case, a county assessor claimed that the nerve-racking pressures of his job incapacitated him. Instead of simply quitting his job, the official saw his problem as an illness and decided to fight for a retirement pension. In another case, a transportation officer claimed that certain problems on his job led to shot nerves and an aggravated case of gout. He too can no longer work and has filed a medical disability claim.

allows the respondent to document the occurrence of various life events over a 10-year period. Variations of the technique require the person filling out the SRE to cover only the past 6 to 24 months. Some modified forms of the scale are available for specific populations such as children, college students, and athletes.

The early studies by Richard Rahe and colleagues were retrospective. The researchers asked Navy personnel to report life changes and instances of illness during the ten years before the study. The number of illness episodes that occurred was found to be related to the amount of social readjustment that was required during that period. Scores on the SRRS are referred to as LCUs—that is, Life Change Units. The researchers claimed that subjects who reported fewer than 150 LCUs for a given year reported good health for the following year. However, among those with an annual LCU rate of between 150 and 300, about half reported serious illness in the next year. When the LCUs exceeded 300, as they did for a small portion of subjects in the research, illness followed in more than 70 percent of the cases. Furthermore, the higher the LCU rating, the more episodes of illness that occurred in a given period. Of course, there are dangers in drawing conclusions from retrospective studies, as we have seen.

Table 7-1. Social Readjustment Rating Scale

Rank	Life Event	Mean Value
1	Death of spouse	100
2	Divorce	73
3	Marital separation	65
4	Jail term	63
5	Death of close family member	63
6	Personal injury or illness	53
7	Marriage	50
8	Fired at work	47
9	Marital reconciliation	45
10	Retirement	45
11	Change in health of family member	44
12	Pregnancy	40
13	Sex difficulties	39
14	Gain of new family member	39
15	Business readjustment	39
16	Change in financial state	38
17	Death of close friend	37
18	Change to different line of work	36
19	Change in number of arguments with spouse	35
20	Mortgage over $10,000	31
21	Foreclosure of mortgage or loan	30
22	Change in responsibilities at work	29
23	Son or daughter leaving home	29
24	Trouble with in-laws	29
25	Outstanding personal achievement	28
26	Wife begin or stop work	26
27	Begin or end school	26
28	Change in living conditions	25
29	Revision of personal habits	24
30	Trouble with boss	23
31	Change in work hours or conditions	20
32	Change in residence	20
33	Change in schools	20
34	Change in recreation	19
35	Change in church activities	19
36	Change in social activities	18
37	Mortgage or loan less than $10,000	17
38	Change in sleeping habits	16
39	Change in number of family get-togethers	15
40	Change in eating habits	15
41	Vacation	13
42	Christmas	12
43	Minor violations of the law	11

Source: Reprinted with permission from *Journal of Psychosomatic Research, 11,* T. H. Holmes and R. H. Rahe, The social readjustment rating scale, p. 216. Copyright 1967 by Pergamon Press, Ltd.

In *prospective* studies of 2500 naval personnel between the ages of 17 and 30, shipboard medical records for an entire six-month cruise were examined. These medical records were compared to a record of life events that had occurred six months prior to shipboard duty, information that was collected before the start of the tour. A statistically significant difference was noted in the amount of illness found during the six months on board ship by individuals who had experienced *many* life changes versus those who had experienced *few* life changes before the tour of duty. Personnel who were in the lowest quartile of LCUs had an average of only 1.4 illnesses in six months, whereas personnel in the highest quartile of LCUs had an average of 2.1 illnesses [57, 59].

Various studies by other investigators have followed a similar format, and they have shown that the number and intensity of life events and the probability of future illness are related. The more severe the life change, the more serious is the ensuing illness. In most of these studies, the data about life events were gathered from very large homogeneous samples using questionnaires. Information about illness was gathered from medical records. The samples included military personnel, employees of large corporations, and clinic or hospital patients. In both retrospective and prospective investigations, there have been statistically significant relationships noted between a life change and the occurrence of sudden heart attacks, accidents, athletic injuries, leukemia, tuberculosis, diabetes, and many minor medical complaints. High scores on life change have also been associated with psychiatric symptoms and disorders. Finally, some researchers have noted that the number and magnitude of life change events experienced influence the course of recovery in some medical patients [56].

Do we know for sure that stressful life events cause the onset of illness? In reading the research literature, we are almost overwhelmed with the number of studies supporting this relationship. The variety of populations and the large sample sizes are impressive, although closer scrutiny of the methodological and theoretical aspects of the research leads to a host of problems. Since the alleged connection between stress and illness has received so much attention in the news media, it is important for us to consider the methodological issues very carefully in order to make a scientific evaluation.

Problems in Life Change Research.   There are several methodological problems in the stress and illness research, some of which we discussed earlier [59]. First, as already mentioned, many studies involved retrospective accounts of life changes and retrospective accounts of illness. Since people were asked to report both their recent life changes and their illnesses, the hypotheses of the study may have been obvious to the subjects. In addition, illness may make a person more aware of stresses. Furthermore, the researchers made no attempt to tell the subjects what types of illnesses to report. Therefore subjects made their own judgments about what to report, and they reported only the illnesses that were salient to them. Second, although the results were statistically significant because of the large sample sizes, the results were of small magnitude; that is, actual differences between the high LCU subjects and the low LCU subjects were often quite small. In some studies, characteristics of the occupational environment and demographic variables such as socioeconomic status, age, and sex were better predictors of illness than were the life events. Third, it has been pointed out that some of the life events in the Schedule of Recent Events (SRE) could be considered indicative of oncoming illness. For example, subjects are asked to report changes in eating or sleeping habits. These changes could either bring about illness or be indicative of developing disease. Thus life change may be a *result* rather than a *cause* of illness. In short, although life stress does seem to be associated with illness, its degree of importance is not yet known.

There are also some theoretical problems in the Holmes and Rahe approach. One criticism is that the researchers theorized that *all* life change, whether it is positive or negative, increases the probability that disease will develop. However, there is evidence that *undesirable* (negative) events are the events most strongly correlated with reports of illness [40]. More research is necessary in order to examine the theoretical questions concerning the impact of positive life events on illness frequency. Although Holmes and Rahe state that positive changes require adaptation and thus can also bring about illness, their data do not strongly support this contention. Their measures of life change are weighted in the direction of negative changes. Another question involves whether *no change* might have negative effects on an individual's health. It could be imagined that the absence of certain changes could have a negative impact on the individual, and might itself require adjustment [19, 23]. For example, if a person does not get a job promotion this person feels he or she deserves, or does not have an opportunity to move to a different location, a negative impact on the individual may result from frustration or understimulation. Some researchers have suggested that understimulation (as well as overstimulation) by the environment could lead to physiological activation, the *need* for adjustment, and the wearing down of the person's resistance to disease.

Finally, the life-change approach emphasizes the negative effects of life changes; it examines social events. It does not, however, focus on the substantial number of people who undergo a major life change and benefit from it without developing illness. It is important to study the characteristics of individuals who do not suffer illness as a result of life change. Research discussed later in this chapter further addresses the question of why some people experience a significant life change and yet do not develop illness as a result of it. Because of various mediating variables—personality, usual coping style, behavior patterns, the social support received from others, and specific coping strategies—there is no simple relationship between life change and illness.

The medical sociologist Aaron Antonovsky has proposed a theory of "salutogenesis"—a theory of how people stay healthy [2]. He points out that everyone is subject to environmental pressures, but some people can cope with them very well. Central to successful coping is what Antonovsky calls *coherence*—the person's confidence that the world is understandable. There are striking individual differences in the extent to which people can remain healthy despite life change, and these differences seem to be related to such social psychological factors as "a sense of coherence." We return to attributes of successful coping later in this chapter.

We begin our consideration of individual psychological and social differences in the effects of stress on illness with the study of a behavior pattern. This is the Type A behavior pattern and its relationship to heart disease. We then focus directly on behavioral and social factors in coping with stress.

TYPE A BEHAVIOR AND HEART DISEASE

The medical community has long suspected a link between emotional behavior and heart disease. Of course, it has been known for thousands of years that excitement increases pulse rate and that emotions like fear and love can make the heart beat faster. As early as the nineteenth century, the medical educator Sir William Osler proposed a link between high pressure activity and coronary heart disease [38]. In the 1930s Karl and William Menninger, brothers who were famous American physicians and psychiatrists, asserted that coronary heart disease is related to repressed aggression [48]. However, the dichotomy between body and mind, in which many physicians believed, delayed systematic study of the association between emotional behavior and heart disease until the 1950s.

The incidence of heart disease in the United States has increased dramatically during the past 75 years, with perhaps every reader of this book knowing (or having known) someone who suffers from angina pectoris (chest pain) or who has had a "heart attack." Heart disease is now the leading cause of death in this country [76]. Epidemiological studies have isolated differences in the incidence of heart disease in different cultures; however, cultures obviously differ in numerous variables (such as diet, exercise, and living habits) that may affect health. Thus it is difficult to ascertain which variables are critical. Nevertheless, research has focused on the high pressures and stresses of twentieth-century American life as causal factors in coronary heart disease.

Serum cholesterol, a substance found in the blood, is associated with coronary heart disease, in which the blood supply to the heart muscle deteriorates. Since some foods such as eggs are high in cholesterol, some scientists believe diet to be an important factor in heart disease. However, the human body processes the cholesterol in food and makes its own cholesterol through complex physiological mechanisms, and the level of cholesterol in the blood is affected by stress [20, 21]. Thus it may be that stress is actually an important factor leading directly to heart disease. Taking this argument a step further, there may be a causal link among behavior patterns, stress, and heart disease: Certain behavior patterns are stressful, and stress leads to heart disease.

In the 1950s, two cardiologists, Meyer Friedman and Ray Rosenman [18], noticed some interesting relationships between behavior and heart disease. When an upholsterer arrived to repair the chairs in their office waiting room, he asked them what kind of physicians they were. He wondered why only the front edges of the chairs were worn out. In other words, it seemed that heart patients were especially likely to sit on the edge of their seats! Of course, this incident is only illustrative, not scientific proof, but it does suggest a possible link between persistent agitated behavior and heart disease.

The Type A Behavior Pattern. Two decades of research on the possible links between personality and heart disease have identified the *Type A behavior pattern* or Type A personality. Type A people are involved in a constant struggle to do more and more things in less and less time, and they are sometimes quite hostile or aggressive in their efforts to achieve them. Type A people always seem to be under the pressure of time, constantly having a deadline to meet. They take life very seriously. Research has shown that such people seem especially likely to suffer heart disease. On the other hand, people who do not show these characteristics are called Type B; they are able to relax, do not worry about time, and are less concerned with accomplishment and more content with themselves. These people show a lower incidence of heart disease [12, 20, 30].

Extreme Type A individuals live a life characterized by competitiveness, and are always striving for achievement. They are hasty, impatient, impulsive, hyperalert, and very tense. People who exhibit this pattern tend, for the most part, to be deeply committed to their professional life to the exclusion of other aspects of their life, including their family and friends. When under pressure most people may exhibit some behaviors that are similar to this Type A pattern, but Type A individuals exhibit this behavior *very often,* for example, turning even the most potentially relaxing situation (recreational sports such as tennis) into a high-pressure event.

Type A behavior is assessed by means of a structured interview or a questionnaire [18, 33]. In the standardized, structured interview, the interviewer asks people a number of questions and observes their responses. The *manner* of the response is much more important than the answers themselves. The speed, volume, and tenseness of the individual's words are important, as are gestures, posture, and body movements. Voice analysis is sometimes used. Unfortunately, the precise characteristics of the Type A behavior pattern have not yet been completely defined, but it seems most Type A people walk and eat rapidly, hurry others along in conversation, speak with a very strong emphasis, clench their hands and teeth, try to do two things at once, and experience great time pressure [18]. The questionnaire measure of the Type A behavior pattern is called the Jenkins Activity Survey (JAS) [33]. The measure consists of 52 multiple choice items that inquire into a person's degree of impatience, job involvement, and competitiveness. A number of studies have found a relationship between high scores on the JAS and coronary heart disease [31, 32].

The issue of retrospective versus prospective data collection also appears in the study of the Type A personality. Until the mid-1970s all the research was retrospective. However, in a prospective study, the Western Collaborative Group Study (which lasted almost a decade), it was found that knowledge that someone was Type A as opposed to Type B could *predict* occurrence of coronary heart disease. Furthermore, the Type A pattern also predicted subsequent (second and third) heart attacks as well as hardening of the arteries [62, 63].

A panel of specialists recently assembled by the National Institutes of Health evaluated the evidence to date concerning the Type A pattern and heart disease. They concluded that Type A behavior is significantly related to heart disease and that this risk is independent of and comparable in importance to other risk factors such as smoking, high blood pressure, and genetic endowment. Thus, although this link between personality and illness may sometimes be mediated by unhealthy behaviors such as chain smoking, there is also a *direct* link between the Type A behavior pattern and heart disease [30].

COPING, STRESS, AND ILLNESS

The fact that negative life events such as divorce have a greater impact on health than positive events such as marriage indicates that the *meaning* of the change to the individual, rather than the change itself, is of significance. The meaning of interpretation of events is influenced by personal or social coping mechanisms. In Figure 7-1, for example, in the links between life events and illness all pathways included link *a*, which passes through "behavior patterns, personality, and coping." We now consider in more detail the use of coping mechanisms in the face of life change.

Successful Coping

There are many people who experience severely stressful life events and even a traumatic life change who do not become ill. This is probably because they engage in a variety of behaviors to reduce the ill effects of stress. They may even use the stress for a positive end. For example, an individual may be successful at channeling the physiological arousal that accompanies the experience of stress into positive outcomes such as accomplishment or opportunities to gain social support. It is interesting to note that the definition of the verb *to cope* in the *American Heritage Dictionary* is "to contend, to strive, especially on even terms or with success." This suggests that coping with stress involves not only *contending* with stress, but also *contending successfully* and using the stress to bring about a better outcome. Coping refers to behavior that people use to protect themselves from being harmed by new situations. Coping mediates the impact that stress has on a person's health.

At the heart of the concept of coping is the fundamental assumption that people are better off if they respond *actively* to the forces that impinge upon them. Coping is not passive, but involves an active response to stress. Leonard Pearlin and Carmi Schooler have suggested that coping mechanisms can take three forms: psychological resources, social resources, and specific coping responses [51]. *Psychological resources* are personality characteristics upon which people draw from within themselves to help them deal with threats imposed by the environment. Examples are self-esteem (the positive attitudes people have toward themselves), feelings of mastery and competence, and the feelings of control people have over their lives. Self-esteem and feelings of mastery can head off helplessness and hopelessness. On the other hand, self-denigration may lead to giving up and can interfere with successful coping. *Social resources* are aspects of people's interpersonal networks. They involve the social support available from family, friends, fellow workers, neighbors, and other associates. Although social support is usually equated with emotional support, it may also involve tangible resources such as information and cooperation. Finally, while psychological resources represent the characteristics that people have and social resources represent supports that they have, *specific coping responses* represent the things that people *do*—their concrete efforts to deal with specific strains of life. These specific coping responses may be influenced by both the psychological resources of the individual and social resources. Specific coping responses include techniques such as the relaxation response (see Box 7-4) and exercise, for example, running [37, 73]. In the next section we consider the empirical research on psychological resources, social supports, and specific coping responses.

Psychological Resources. Studies that examine the psychological resources of individuals concentrate on the effect of personality structure on coping with illness. These studies determine the personality structures that differentiate individuals who become ill under stress from those who do not. Overall, the personality differences are best characterized by what the psychologist Suzanne Kobasa [36] calls *hardiness*. Theoretical work in personality psychology suggests that hardiness involves living life to the fullest, a feeling of competence, and a productive orientation. Hardy persons possess three general characteristics: They believe that they can control or influence events; they are able to become deeply involved in and committed to activities in their lives; and they view change as an exciting challenge to their further development as people. In a study of executives under extreme stress, Kobasa examined personality differences between executives who became ill and those who did not. She compared 86 executives in the latter category and 75 in the former. In this study she found that personality characteristics did mediate the link between stressful life events and illness. First, the executives' feeling of control was important. Those who remained healthier did not feel powerless in the face of external forces but instead had an "internal locus of control"* [64]. The second characteristic of executives who did not become ill involved their commitment to something they felt was important as well as their sense of meaningfulness. Those who felt committed to their work, social institutions, interpersonal relationships, and their family were less likely to become ill. They also had a strong commitment to themselves and were able to recognize distinct values, goals, and priorities. By being committed to *other* aspects of life, executives who remained healthy were able to see that work was not the only thing that defined them as people. Third, individuals who did not become ill as a result of stress viewed life changes as challenges rather than as threats. Those who felt positive about life change tended to respond with excitement and energy. They were cognitively flexible— that is, they were able to integrate and to appraise new situations effectively. They were *not* engaged in irresponsible adventurousness. Rather, they were searching for novelty while remaining true to the fundamental life goals that they had already established.

It is important to note that Kobasa's study is essentially *retrospective*. There are indications from other research, however, that the psychological characteristics found in Kobasa's study are indeed important in mediating the stress–illness relationship. Many supporting ideas come from basic theories of psychology. *Growth psychology* and the work of Carl Rogers, for example, fit into this framework quite well. Rogers has suggested that the characteristics mentioned in the study of executives are also necessary for the development of the healthy personality and the fully functioning person. The "mentally" healthy personality is able to maintain a healthy physical condition as well [70].

Related to this research is work on coping mechanisms in facing the stress of surgery. This work was initiated during the 1950s by the psychologist Irving Janis [29]. His research showed that before surgery some patients were worried about their operation and felt very vulnerable; other patients were somewhat concerned and asked for information about their surgery; whereas still other patients were extremely cheerful and relaxed before their operation and did not want to know anything about it. Reactions also differed after surgery, and these differences were related in systematic ways to the presurgery behaviors. The highly fearful as well as the fearless patients experienced poor postoperative reactions while patients with a moderate amount of anticipatory fear recovered best. These pa-

*Internal locus of control refers to the generalized tendency of people to believe that whatever happens to them is under their own control; also see Chapter 11.

tients rehearsed ways of dealing with the stresses they faced—a phenomenon referred to by Janis as "the work of worrying." Mental rehearsal of solutions to realistic problems, a moderate level of anticipatory fear, and a preparatory "working through" of difficulties helped the patients deal with the stresses of medical procedures. This process has been proven effective by subsequent research in medical settings [34].

Social Resources. A second major source of coping is *social support*. When faced with life change and the stress experienced as a result of it, the support of family and friends can be a significant aid to coping [13, 42, 50]. Social support comes from the friendly ties an individual has with family, associates, neighbors, and the community (also see Chapter 8 for an expanded discussion of social support). A single person who moves to a new job in a new community may be isolated and have little or no social support, whereas a married person living and working in the town where this person grew up (who still has childhood friends and an extended family) probably has a great deal of support. Social support can influence an individual's coping by affecting how stressful events are appraised. For example, if many other people whom a person knows have gone through the same experience, a person may see the experience as less stressful. More importantly, social support may help the person deal with the emotional consequences of stress, thus minimizing the risk of illness. One study of unemployed men, for example, found less illness, lower cholesterol levels, and less depression among men with supportive marriages and friendships than among men without this kind of support [22].

Social support may also aid the individual in coping with life stresses in the following manner: Assume that a crisis event is experienced that creates anxiety in the individual. The usual coping mechanisms such as trying to relax are ineffective. If the individual has a social support network available, however, disclosure to the network is likely to initiate a series of interrelated behaviors directed toward dealing with the stressful life event. First, the social support network can help the individual to become aware of his or her feelings, to minimize the feeling of stress (but not deny it), and to accept the stressful life event. Second, the social support network can encourage a person to take control of the situation, and to take responsibility for action. This responsibility could head off any sense of hopelessness or helplessness that the individual might feel. Third, social support will help the stressed individual develop new coping strategies by providing *information* about how to deal with the

Box 7-4
The Relaxation Response

Dr. Herbert Benson, of the Harvard Medical School, has described an interesting technique that can be used by individuals who face stressful situations. Individuals who are pressured to the point of physical illness or emotional misery can engage in a meditative behavior that may cause them to feel better. This technique also has some specific physiological effects. There is evidence, in fact, that this procedure, called the *relaxation response*, can actually reduce an individual's blood pressure and respiration rate and other physiological indicators of stressful arousal [4].

The techniques of the relaxation response have been familiar to people in the Far East for many years and have been used in various religions. This method of relaxation is geared to reducing the physiological characteristics of the "fight-or-flight response" (an increase in activity of the sympathetic nervous system). According to Benson, the technique is very simple and requires only four basic elements: a quiet environment, a mental device, a passive attitude, and a comfortable position. First, Benson suggests that the person choose a convenient quiet room. Second, a mental device must be employed; this device is usually a syllable that is repeated silently or in low gentle tones. Although many different words or sounds have been used in traditional religious and other meditation practices, Benson suggests

the use of the syllable "one" because of its simplicity and neutrality. Third, a passive attitude is necessary. The person should not think about his or her own performance or try to force the relaxation response. Whenever a person becomes distracted—that is, whenever a thought enters the individual's mind—the distraction (the thought) should simply be disregarded. Finally, the "meditator" should sit in a comfortable position. The purpose is to reduce muscular effort to a minimum.

Benson suggests the following technique: In a quiet environment, sit in a comfortable position and close your eyes. Deeply relax all your muscles beginning with your feet and progressing up to your face. Allow them to remain deeply relaxed. Then, breathe through your nose, establishing an awareness of your breathing. Concentrate only on your breathing. As you breathe out, say the word "one" silently to yourself. Then breathe in. As you breathe out again, say "one" to yourself, and breathe in. Whenever a thought enters your mind disregard it. Continue this practice for 20 minutes, arranging a gentle reminder (not an alarm clock) that the time has passed. At the end of the 20 minutes, sit quietly for a few minutes at first with your eyes closed and later with your eyes open. It is important not to worry about whether success has been achieved in relaxing, and not to think about any kind of evaluation.

Benson found that the relaxation response helped hypertensive individuals reduce their blood pressure over a period of time. He also found that people who engaged in the relaxation response were better able to reduce their intake of hard liquor, their abuse of drugs, and their cigarette smoking.

stress. Finally, disclosure to others who are close, with their resulting support, can directly reduce the anxiety of the individual. This may happen partly because friends and family provide a sense of perspective on the problem; but friends and family may also provide comfort. For example, one study of stress and social support in Chinese-Americans measured social support in terms of feelings about the neighborhood, interactions with friends and neighbors, and involvement in community activities [41]. Illness was defined in terms of such symptoms as restless sleep, depression, overeating, drinking, anxiety, and lack of concentration (all self-reported). The researchers found that the greater the social support, the fewer the symptoms. (Social support and its effects on coping with the stress resulting from chronic illness are discussed in Chapter 8.)

There are studies indicating that married people are healthier on the average than divorced or widowed people (see Box 7-1). The difference is due partly to the stress of losing one's partner, but it also seems as if single people have a more difficult time dealing with environmental stresses. The loss of other social ties seems to have a similar effect. A striking example of the importance of the community to one's health is provided by the sociologist Kai Erikson [17]. Erikson studied the effects of a terrible flood in the mountain town of Buffalo Creek, West Virginia. Social ties and the sense of community were destroyed by the flood, and many people became ill. They felt drained, exhausted, and weak, and often these feelings were incapacitating. As Erikson put it, their emotional shelter was stripped away and the community could "no longer enlist its members in a conspiracy to make a perilous world seem safe" [17, p. 240].

Coping Techniques. The third class of coping mechanisms involves specific coping responses that help the individual to deal with specific stresses. There are two classes: the first involves cognitive mechanisms and the second concerns behavioral mechanisms. The former (cognitive mechanisms) involves efforts at controlling the effect of the stressful life event. The individual can learn to think in certain ways in order to make the stressful life event less important or less traumatizing. For example, the person who is experiencing a great deal of stress at work can learn to view work as only one part of life. The degree of stress experienced may be reduced simply because the critical importance of work, a large contributing factor to the stress, is minimized. In addition, a person may actually change the meaning of the event. For example, the individual can seek to reduce stress by interpreting the event as a challenge. Someone who is facing a job transfer, for example, might chose to interpret the transfer as a new opportunity. This person has thus changed the meaning of the situation to allow successful coping. Many "self-help" or "self-insight" groups and classes seek to facilitate coping by changing the person's view of life's challenges.

Coping responses may also be behavioral. Examples of these behaviors are running, meditation, biofeedback, and behavioral modification involving systematic desensitization. Such techniques are examined in Kenneth Pelletier's book *Mind as Healer, Mind as Slayer* [52]. These various behaviors attempt to encourage a different physiological reaction in the individual from the usual fight-or-flight response. An example is the relaxation response (see Box 7-2). Similarly, as noted in Chapter 4, various distraction and feedback techniques provide a chance to control the physiological arousal resulting from anxiety. Along these lines, the writer Norman Cousins has pointed out that *humor* can be very useful as both a mechanism for neutralizing the stress and as a method of actually changing the meaning of the situation so that it is no longer stressful [11].

A report by the U.S. Surgeon General suggests that running, as well as many other forms of vigorous physical exercise, can help a person cope effectively with stress [74]. The exact mechanisms by which this relaxation occurs are not clear [37]. Most simply, it is probable that going outdoors to run serves to remove the individual from the stimuli that cause stress—such as work pressures at the office or family pressures at home. In addition, focusing on one's body, breathing, and visceral sensations with repetitive movements may serve the same purpose as in the relaxation technique (see Box 7-2) [4]. Physiological responses are also implicated, such as the "runner's high," which is perhaps caused directly by physiological factors [37].

Self-Induced Stress

Throughout this chapter we have discussed stress in terms of external circumstances that require adaptation and introduce a strain on the individual. Sometimes, however, stress can occur even though no external conditions can account for it. This kind of stress is generated internally; it consists of the demands that people place on themselves, their own fears (which may be irrational), and their tendencies to reproach themselves. Unlike Mr. Jennings, some people have no obvious external problems to account for the stress they experience. The physician or other health care professional may try to tell the patient simply to stop worrying about benign situations. Such statements as "You worry too much" or "You take things too seriously," however, merely reinforce the person's own perception of him or herself as unstable, inferior, and unable to deal with stress. More complex solutions are needed.

In his book, *Cognitive Therapy and Emotional Disorders,* Aaron Beck has suggested that the stereotypic hard-driving business person may be likely to develop a peptic ulcer as a result of *internal stress* [3]. This person appears to be in a constant state of tension. Health care professionals often call such a patient "nervous," and they may even label the patient "neurotic." As a result of the health professional's label, it may not be long before patients like this begin to see themselves in those terms as well. The motivation behind this constant state of tension may be a fear of not reaching their goals. Because their self-worth and self-image are based on achievement, these people usually exaggerate the importance as well as the difficulty of what must be achieved. They underestimate their capacity to deal with the requirements to accomplish the task and exaggerate the ultimate consequences of failure. These people operate on the assumption that the only road to happiness is through total success. Because they regard each task as a major confrontation with major consequences, they are constantly racing to try to prevent some fantasized disaster. People whose stressors are internally originated may operate from what Beck has called "faulty cognitions." The health care professional can sometimes help these patients by logically and rationally sorting out the consequences of failure (pointing out their continued value as an individual) and also by helping them assess realistically their probability of achieving their goals. Social support and specific behavioral coping responses may also be helpful, although psychological counseling is sometimes necessary.

SUMMARY: WHAT CAN THE HEALTH PROFESSIONAL DO?

Among the coping techniques we have considered, it is not yet clear which techniques are most effective. A hardy, competent

Box 7-5
The Autonomous vs. Identified Person

Deviation from psychosocial norms—that is, going against the expectations of the cultural group—can be a source of stress for the individual. If someone is willing to go through life fitting in with the behavior that is expected by members of his or her religious group, community, family, and so on, this person may never have to experience the stress of thinking about how to behave. However, people differ in the extent to which stability, lack of change, and predictability are important to them. People differ in how much they rely on continuity in social and cultural structure to keep stress at a manageable level for them. These different orientations have different implications for the life course of the individual.

The sociologist Gordon E. Moss has called the individual who accepts psychosocial norms fully and merges his or her identity into that of the community an *identified person*. The *autonomous person*, on the other hand, resists psychosocial norms and tries to achieve a sense of identity outside of and apart from the community. There is of course a range of behaviors that falls between the two extremes. People who are identified attempt to reduce the amount of uncertainty in their lives and to maximize their security by associating themselves closely with organizations and other established social structures. They will abide by existing norms in order to fit in, and they will accept the beliefs and goals of the

group as their own. Autonomous people see uncertainty as an unavoidable aspect of life. They believe that security can be achieved only through complete self-sufficiency. Autonomous people develop their own moral codes in a variety of settings. Their expectations for their own behaviors and achievements are those they have formulated for themselves. They may be considerably more socially and geographically mobile than identified people. Autonomous people train themselves to deal adaptively with changes. They develop inner resources to deal with challenges without having them disrupt their lives or throw them off balance.

As you might guess, identified individuals experience less social change than autonomous individuals. In their insulated structure, identified persons will probably have fewer stress-related health problems. This is true, however, only if the structure remains completely intact. Because this is often not possible, these protected individuals might then begin to experience stress in reaction even to minor disruptions. Autonomous persons will experience more stress than identified persons as a matter of course in their attempts to develop independence and autonomy. They build up a tolerance for stress, however. If the group or social structure to which they belong is destroyed or if their place in the group is lost (e.g., because of the death of a spouse or loss of community), autonomous persons can better manage the change.

Which orientation is healthier? That of course is not an easy question to answer. It depends on what happens in the social structure of the individual. If it can be guaranteed that the group (community, family, religious or cultural structure) will continue, then the least stress and the best health are likely to be experienced by identified persons. But it is never certain that the social structure will be maintained. Thus autonomous people may be better off in the long run if they are prepared to deal with any situation using their own resources.

For further reading: G. E. Moss, *Illness, Immunity and Social Interaction: The Dynamics of Bio-social Resonation* (New York: John Wiley, 1973).

---

person with a sense of control, adequate social support, and healthy recreational activities will do well, but such a state is not always easy to achieve. A combination of techniques can often help a patient during a stressful time. It is also important for the health professional to recognize when the life stress is *related* to the social support system; for example, when through the death of a spouse, the individual loses his or her closest source of support in addition to experiencing a life change. Unless friends and family can be rallied to bolster the individual at such a time, the stress is not only in itself *life stress*, but also represents a significant reduction in the person's capacity for coping.

A health care professional must assess each patient's coping repertoire—that is, the usual behaviors in which the patient engages in order to cope with stress. Early recognition of maladaptive coping mechanisms (such as excessive drinking or excessive smoking) is important so that such behaviors can be changed by substitution of more healthful coping mechanisms. Understanding a patient's usual coping repertoire, supporting healthful coping behavior, and extinguishing unhealthy behaviors may constitute an important goal for preventive health care. While it may also help to assist the patient in avoiding stressful "life events," this kind of approach is usually unsuccessful. Stressful events may be closely tied to the patient's social and economic situation (e.g., the person is likely not to be willing to give up family and work responsibilities). In addition, the individual may desire new and exciting things in life. As mentioned in Chapter 6, health is not simply the absence of disease. It may, in fact, involve the resiliency to deal with potentially stress-

adapt to life change (see Box 7-5). Development of techniques for coping and for adaptation are part of health care.

Evaluation of a patient's social and emotional stressors and coping mechanisms has been systematized in the *Psychological Systems Review* [27]. This system is an interview guide developed to help the health professional understand the patient's psychosocial status. The Psychological Systems Review examines the patient's emotional state, life situation, and personality. Emotional state is assessed through questions about feelings, tensions, hopes, and expectations. Life situation is assessed through questions about family, work, friends, and recreation. Personality is assessed through questions about the individual's way of adapting, including self-esteem, independence, sociability, responsibility, and outlook on life. This information is entered on a medical chart in addition to details about the physical condition. Such systems are modern extensions of the "life chart" begun by Meyer more than a half century ago.

Let us return to Mr. Jennings. He is experiencing a great deal of life stress and is facing decisions that have serious consequences. An effort needs to be made to reduce Mr. Jennings's anxiety. One approach may be to help Mr. Jennings employ personality characteristics, attitudes, and styles of thinking that are adaptive for him. This can be done by reinforcing his personal efforts to cope as well as through empathic communication with him. Coordinated health care by physicians, social workers, nurses, marriage counselors, psychologists, school administrators, and community agencies can help relieve some of the pressures on Mr. Jennings and help his entire family function better as well. Health care professionals should also encourage Mr. Jennings to find other sources of social support such as friends and colleagues.

People are under stress each time they are in a situation that requires adjustment to personal, social, and environmental influences. There have been numerous changes in our culture in recent years that require a lot of adaptation and may thus be highly stress-inducing. On a social level, these changes include the status of women, equalization of the roles of minority members, and the enormous mobility of people. Other stress triggers are inflation and economic instability, growing old in a youth-oriented culture, and the removal of constraints preventing marital instability and breakup. In addition, technological advances may require adjustment on the part of the individual to situations that have never before been encountered [75]. The overwhelming impact of these changes makes the topic of psychosocial factors in the etiology of illness a major medical issue.

8
Chronic Illness: Psychosocial Aspects of Disability

When Orville Kelly was diagnosed as having cancer, he reacted as many patients do—with shock, disbelief, and despair. People, however, usually do not die on the day the illness is diagnosed, but rather they face a crisis of adjustment to their new condition. They may need to deal with a period of physical impairment that may last many years. While cancer is a well-known disabling disease, there are many illnesses that result in chronic physical impairment and limitations. Although it may seem hopeless to them at first, people do learn to cope with various physical handicaps. Physical impairment is, however, only one part of the problem of chronic illness. Social and emotional difficulties are of tremendous importance as well. Unfortunately, traditional medicine has not been well equipped to help patients cope with these socioemotional problems. Orville Kelly met the challenge of chronic illness by founding an organization of cancer patients called *Make Today Count** [26].

What is chronic illness? The term is usually applied to conditions that have one or more of the following characteristics: The condition is permanent (the person will never recover fully); the condition involves some disability; it is caused by nonreversible pathological

---

*Kelly died in 1980 of lymphocytic lymphoma, seven years after being diagnosed. He died just after winning a fight for veteran's disability benefits; he attributed his illness to exposure to nuclear radiation in the U.S. Army.

requires training and motivation on the part of the patient to care for him or herself. Chronic illness may involve all of the problems of acute illness, but it brings special problems as well. The onset of the illness can be sudden or gradual, but one characteristic common to all chronic illnesses is that the patient can never fully return to the pre-illness state of health [39].

In a survey by the U.S. Public Health Service (1965–1967), it was found that about 50 percent of the U.S. civilian population, excluding residents of institutions, had at least one chronic medical condition. Of these 95 million Americans, about 22 million experienced some degree of limitation in activity because of their chronic illness [39, 41]. About 4 million persons (i.e., about 2 percent of the total population) were unable to carry on major activities such as work, housework, school, or recreation. Another 12 million (6 percent) were somewhat limited in major activity. It was also found that the average number of chronic conditions per person was about 2.2; multiple chronic illnesses were very frequent.

Examples of chronic illness are heart conditions, impairments of the back or spine, and hypertension. Various forms of cancer cause many chronic conditions. Up to age 44 the most prominent chronic conditions involve paralysis (primarily from accidents) and impairments of the lower extemities and hips. After age 45 the most common chronic illnesses are arthritis, rheumatism, and heart conditions. Other chronic illnesses include diabetes, Parkinson's disease, multiple sclerosis, epilepsy, kidney disease, asthma, and emphysema.

While elderly people are more likely than younger people to have one or more chronic conditions, it is *not* true that chronic disease is merely a geriatric problem. It has been estimated that in the United States, 40 percent of those 65 years old or over have one or more chronic conditions that limit a major activity. Of those from age 45 to 64, 14 percent of the people have at least one chronic condition that limits a major activity [39, 41].

Chronic illness is becoming an increasingly important health problem in the United States. Many acute, infectious diseases can now be prevented or cured. Furthermore, better emergency treatments allow many patients to survive the initial critical stages of acute illnesses or trauma (e.g., stroke, accident, or heart attack). Patients live with the effects of these acute illnesses and trauma, and thus face chronic illness from which they will never fully recover. In addition, because of the effects of aging, older persons are likely to develop some form of chronic illness. Thus better medical care and demographic trends that contribute to an increase in the elderly population in this country also contribute to an increase in chronic illness. For all of these reasons the problems of the chronically ill deserve special study.

When thinking about the problems of someone with cancer or paralysis, most people focus on such difficulties as physical impairment and pain. However, for the chronically ill one of the most difficult problems (if not *the* most difficult problem) involves relationships with other people [13, 44]. We examine the social and emotional problems of patients with chronic illness in terms of three issues: (a) the crisis of illness, (b) the process of coping with chronic illness, and (c) the importance of social support. We then examine special cases of chronic illness and the particular problems associated with them.

THE CRISIS OF ILLNESS

The onset of physical illness creates a crisis: Consider Mr. James McDonald, a patient who has recently suffered a myocardial infarction. His whole life is disrupted; he was hospitalized for six weeks and out of work for many weeks after that. Not only is his ability to contribute to society limited, but Mr. McDonald must also deal with a variety of problems that are related to his coronary attack. He must cope with pain and with incapacitation, and he must learn to deal with the hospital environment, with special treatment procedures, and with medical personnel. Especially in the initial phases of his recovery from the attack, Mr. McDonald is unsure whether his life is in serious jeopardy.

Mr. McDonald also faces social and emotional difficulties [10, 22]. His relationships with his family and friends are strained; they are worried about him. His family suffers financial hardship. He cannot carry out his usual role in the family as husband and father, and the future of his family is uncertain. Even if it becomes clear that Mr. McDonald will survive his attack, it may not be clear whether he will be able to go back to his former job, whether he will be able to enjoy normal sexual functioning again, and whether he will be able to enjoy the family recreational activities. These overwhelming problems demonstrate the crisis of chronic physical illness. The onset of chronic illness represents an important transition in an individual's life.

Once Mr. McDonald is released from the hospital, he retains the identity of "coronary patient." Having suffered a heart attack, his chances of suffering another attack are high. He must make changes in his usual behaviors and make modifications in his lifestyle. In

take medication, and ease slowly and carefully into sexual activities. He may have to make modifications in his job. Mr. McDonald has become a chronic patient, for he is suffering from a chronic illness—heart disease. He will probably never be "cured," but his condition can be managed [14, 43].

The onset of physical illness represents a crisis in an individual's life. Severe physical illness causes a serious upset in the individual's social and psychological equilibrium. In their daily lives people have certain characteristic ways of behaving, and they use these behaviors to solve minor problems in life. However, when the situation is so new or so major that the habitual coping responses are inadequate, the situation becomes a crisis. Disorganization, anxiety, fear, and other unpleasant emotions may occur, and in the midst of this condition, many matters must be decided. An individual cannot remain in this state of disequilibrium for a long time. Within a few days or weeks after the onset of the crisis, the patient needs to reach some resolution; the equilibrium must be restored. The new balance may represent a healthy adaptation for the person, with personal growth and maturity; on the other hand, it is possible that the result may be psychological deterioration and maladaptive responses. The health care professional and others around the patient (family and friends) can have an important impact on the direction in which this process proceeds.

Adaptation to the Crisis

Researchers Rudolf Moos and Vivien Tsu have suggested that the crisis of illness brings with it seven major adaptive tasks [33]. Some of these problems deal primarily with coping with the physical problems of chronic illness while others are tied to interpersonal relations. The first task involves dealing with the discomfort, incapacity, and other physical results of the illness or injury, including pain, weakness, and loss of control. The second task involves dealing with the medical technology. The patient must adjust to being treated as a medical case and having his or her body invaded for various tests and medical procedures. Encountering medical treatment may in fact be a crisis in itself. A third task for the patient involves the maintenance of adequate communication with health care professionals. Dealing with physicians and nurses can be very trying. Asking physicians for more attention, requesting help from nurses, and so on, can be difficult for a patient whose psychological resources are already being used up in dealing with the physical illness.

The fourth category of tasks for the patient experiencing the crisis of illness involves the preservation of emotional balance. The patient must try to manage the upsetting feelings aroused by the illness, feelings such as self-blame, anxiety, apprehension, and thoughts of failure. There may also be a sense of alienation, feelings of inadequacy, and resentment.

The remaining tasks directly involve interpersonal relations. Moos and Tsu suggest that the fifth task consists of preserving a satisfactory self-image, and a sense of competence and mastery. Changes in physical functioning and appearance must be incorporated into a new self-image. The patient experiences an identity crisis that may bring about a necessary change in personal values and in lifestyle. For example, in order to survive the patient must find a personally and socially satisfactory balance between accepting help when necessary and taking responsibility and action when possible. Some patients find it difficult to resume being independent after a long period of passivity.

A sixth set of tasks involves preserving relationships with the patient's social network—with family and friends. A person who becomes ill may easily become isolated from others and feel alienated both by physical separation and by the new identity as a patient. Seventh, and finally, the patient must engage in a set of tasks that involves preparing for an uncertain future. Particularly when there is loss of a function as critical as sight or speech, or paralysis of limbs, the loss cannot be denied. It must be acknowledged and mourned. This mourning process can be extremely difficult, particularly if the patient has to prepare for a permanent loss of function while at the same time operating under the possibility that future medical breakthroughs may somehow restore the lost function.

Eventually, the crisis of the onset of serious illness is overcome, and the long-term problems of the chronically ill take on increasing importance. We now examine some of these problems.

The Special Problems of the Chronically Ill

People with chronic illness face many social and psychological challenges in their daily lives [39]. The first involves the prevention and the management of a medical crisis. The chronically ill person is someone who is not completely well. The patient's condition may, if not kept in check, actually be life threatening. For example, if diabetes is not kept under control with insulin (injected or taken orally), the patient may enter a diabetic coma. The chronically ill patient and the family must be constantly on the lookout for signs that point to an impending medical crisis. A diabetic patient learns to recog-

identification (such as bracelets or neck chains) so that if they are unconscious, the people around them and medical professionals can immediately identify the problem. Lack of recognition of impending crisis and lack of knowledge about what to do to prevent a crisis can put the patient's life in grave danger. Preventive behaviors require an acceptance on the part of the patient of the *identity* of a chronically ill person. If the patient refuses to accept this identity, the patient may be motivated to ignore impending symptoms of crisis and refuse to carry identification. In addition, the recognition that an acute phase of the illness (a medical crisis) can occur at any time may be a source of enormous anxiety for the patient.

A second important problem faced by chronically ill patients is the need to manage their treatment regimen. Treatment may seem simple: A patient with a chronic illness who wants to control it simply must follow the orders of the physician. However, as discussed in Chapter 3, patients with chronic illness are less likely than patients with acute illnesses to cooperate and follow medical directions. The problem is not that patients are willfully noncompliant or even medically ignorant. Rather, in the management of chronic illness patients must continually juggle the various demands made on them in every aspect of life. The treatment regimen is simply one of many usual demands that are made on the individual.

Whether or not the treatment regimen for the chronic illness is followed depends on a number of conditions. There must be continuing trust in the health care professional who prescribes the regimen. This is difficult to maintain, for it means that the patient must come to value the *control* of symptoms and the *control* of the progress of the disease. Cure is not possible. It is often difficult to convince a patient that the treatment regimen for chronic illness is actually working because the alternative is hidden. In chronic illness, it is often only when the treatment regimen is stopped and a full medical crisis occurs that the patient realizes the connection between the treatment regimen and the control of the illness. In addition, the patient is unlikely to follow the treatment regimen if there are distressing side effects associated with it. For the patient the side effects must be outweighed either by relief of the symptoms or by a sufficient fear of the disease itself. And finally any treatment regimen must produce results that outweigh the negative effect of the treatment on the patient's sense of self-worth [13, 39].

A few additional points about treatment regimens are important. First, when patients initially learn about a treatment, they experience a great deal of anxiety about the change in their life. They need reassurance from a health care professional that they are doing well. Second, patients may be overwhelmed by the initial realization that the treatment regimen is a lifelong undertaking. This is particularly true for patients who are learning to give themselves insulin injections for diabetes, or for patients who are learning to undergo hemodialysis. Even the use of a bronchial inhalator, which clears breathing passages for patients with obstructive pulmonary disease, can be profoundly disturbing, because the patients recognize that use of the inhalator is something upon which their life may depend. Of course, the amount of time required for the treatment and how the administration of the treatment is scheduled also affect whether or not the patient actually carries it out. If a treatment regimen interferes sufficiently with a person's job or other activities, the patient is less likely to follow it. Expense is also an important factor in whether or not the patient follows a treatment regimen. This is something that the health care professional needs to explore before prescribing a specific treatment. Finally, an important aspect of the treatment regimen involves whether or not adherence to it will lead the patient to increasing social isolation. If the treatment is socially isolating (i.e., makes it hard for the person to interact with others), the patient must decide whether to follow the regimen and experience some loss of human contact, or to follow the regimen only partially or not at all.

A third major problem experienced by patients with chronic illness is that of controlling their symptoms, and hiding them from friends and acquaintances. Health care professionals often tend to be so focused on the individual's disease that implications for the patient's social and psychological well-being may be forgotten. It is important, however, for health care professionals to realize that a patient's self-identity with respect to other people may be influenced profoundly by the *symptoms* of the chronic illness and whether or not these symptoms can be controlled. Such control may be difficult if the patient lacks social skills. For example, patients usually do not know what to say to other people about such things as their limited activity, limited energy level, or their inability to go to certain places. For example, a woman who suffers severe asthma may have difficulty telling her friends that she cannot visit them unless they dust their houses. Close friends and family may accept these requests and redesign their environment for the patient, but the management of more peripheral friendships may be extremely difficult for the patient. An example is provided by Anselm Strauss and Barney Glaser [39]. A woman suffering from multiple sclerosis carefully arranged her one-room apartment so that every object she could

they encouraged her to tidy up her apartment. Friends were made uncomfortable by the clutter because they did not understand its purpose.

A fourth major problem of patients with chronic illnesses involves estimating what the future will bring [15]. Different illnesses have different courses, although physical deterioration as a result of the condition is likely. It might occur very slowly, over the span of 20 or 30 years. On the other hand, the decline may be steady and quick. Or it might have a jagged course, in which the patient is fine for short periods, with symptoms disappearing, but then this condition is followed by a relapse. It is often extremely frustrating for a patient when a definitive prediction about the future cannot be made. The health care professional frequently has little idea of the course that the disease will take for the particular patient in question. Because of this factor the patient might view the health care professional as either incompetent or evasive.

Management of social relationships can be extremely difficult without knowledge of the prognosis for the illness. For example, knowing whether someone has two months or two years to live is obviously important to the person in making plans. Knowing at what point severe disability is likely to develop can be also extremely important for the patient. Since no one really knows with certainty what the course of any disease will be, the patient and individuals in the patient's close social environment may be at odds in their predictions. For example, a person with cancer might be considered "socially dead" long before actual biological death. While the patient may expect a remission in the disease (a time during which the disease is arrested or appears cured), others in the social environment may assume the patient's life is coming to a close.

Insecurity about the trajectory of the disease can be particularly distressing for the individual whose symptoms are not obvious to others. For example, a high-level executive who is extremely important to a corporation may decide to retire very early because of a cardiac condition. Without a clear statement from medical professionals about how long this executive can expect to live, and what the chances are for various levels of impairment, the executive is likely to be seen (in the absence of symptoms) as someone who simply does not want to face responsibilities in the corporation. Health care professionals often find themselves frustrated at being unable to help patients in this regard. They sometimes solve the dilemma by helping patients to accept the uncertainty of illness and to live in the present.

Social isolation is a fifth problem that chronically ill patients experience. Social relationships are often disrupted and jeopardized because of the patient's decreased energy, limitations in mobility, communication impairment, or time required for symptom control. In addition, patients, in an effort to hide their disease, may avoid certain friends and associates. Withdrawal from social contacts, therefore, may occur for two reasons: either voluntarily (because the patient has chosen to do so) or involuntarily (because the patient is victimized by circumstances that interfere with social relationships).

Thus people with chronic illness face both a number of short-term (crisis) challenges and many long-term social and emotional difficulties. Now we turn to an examination of the ways in which patients cope with chronic illness. We then also examine the special importance of social support.

COPING WITH CHRONIC ILLNESS

In Chapter 7 *coping* was defined as *contending with physical difficulties*—action-oriented attempts to master, tolerate, or minimize demands of the environment on one's body [13, 23]. The methods that people use to attempt to cope are never *in themselves* adaptive or maladaptive. They must instead be evaluated in the light of the situation in which each occurs. Any given coping technique can be adaptive in one situation and extremely maladaptive in another, as we will see in the following discussion. Moos and Tsu identify various types of coping techniques that patients with chronic illness can adopt [33].

The first type of coping technique involves *denying* or *minimizing* the seriousness of the medical crisis. Sometimes this technique is referred to as a "defense mechanism," because it is a self-protective response to stress. People may, in fact, delude themselves into believing that what has actually happened to them really has not occurred. They protect their self-image. For example, a male patient who has suffered a heart attack might deny this fact to himself, and he might believe that he is in the hospital primarily because of a different condition. So as long as the patient follows all of the requirements of the treatment regimen, takes care of himself as he should, and takes precautions, such temporary denial may be prudent. It may be adaptive for the patient not to believe that he has had a massive heart attack, for this knowledge may increase his anxiety and interfere with his recovery. Denial becomes a *maladaptive* coping mechanism when the patient refuses to follow the treatment regi-

ment regimen, denial may become dangerous. Some degree of denial often accompanies many illnesses, but whether or not it is adaptive depends on circumstances.

A second coping technique involves seeking information. If a person is feeling helpless, gathering information about the particular illness may help to restore a sense of control. However, if the patient insists on extensive information in every step of the treatment, and becomes cantankerous if health care professionals cannot provide or will not provide the chart, results of laboratory tests, and all physicians' opinions, the information-gathering coping technique becomes maladaptive.

Requests for reassurance form a third type of coping technique. Excessive requests for reassurance and emotional support from the concerned family, friends, and medical staff can of course be maladaptive for the patient. They cannot provide constant assurance and support. But suppressing the need for reassurance can also be maladaptive. Patients who keep their feelings bottled up inside them or who withdraw from social interaction and cut themselves off from others also behave maladaptively. A *moderate degree* of expression of feelings can help to relieve tension and help patients open themselves to comfort from others. (We examine this point in more detail when we consider the issue of social support.)

A fourth set of coping techniques involves setting concrete, limited goals. If a patient has something to look forward to, and something to work for, a sense of meaning can be restored to the patient. This coping technique can help the patient to break an overwhelming number of problems into small and potentially manageable parts.

A fifth set of coping techniques involves rehearsing alternative outcomes. According to Moos and Tsu, mental preparation (anticipation and rehearsal) of the various alternatives is important for the patient [33]. The psychologist Irving Janis has called this the "work of worrying" (see Chapter 7) [24]. The patient can learn to deal with eventualities that may arise in the illness by thinking about them beforehand and planning strategies for dealing with possible outcomes. For example, if the patient is facing a breast biopsy, she may prepare ahead of time for the possibility of waking up after the operation and finding that she has had a radical mastectomy (if the one-stage procedure is used). The patient's ability to deal with the mastectomy may depend on her rehearsal beforehand of the feelings and the behaviors that are likely to accompany the experience. This involves an anticipatory mourning process (i.e., the process of mourning ahead of time).

A related technique has recently been employed in coping with cancer. It is called *visualization*. Patients are taught to relax and form a mental picture of the cancer and their body's response to the cancer. Some physicians hope that this process will help mobilize the body's own natural defenses against cancer, but the process also seems valuable solely in a psychological sense. Patients have the opportunity to rehearse the future of their illness and they may achieve a sense of personal control over some of the emotions that are troubling them. In these two ways the visualization process seems to help some patients cope more effectively with their illness [37]. Definitive studies of the role of visual imagery have not yet been done because the existing programs combine imagery with relaxation, social support, self-disclosure, and similar coping techniques, thus making it impossible to determine the effects of each component of the treatment.

A final coping mechanism involves the patient's search for meaning in the illness. This coping technique involves understanding the experience by looking at it with a long-term perspective (with or without a religious orientation). It involves making the crisis work for the good of the patient instead of to the patient's detriment. For example, a woman who has experienced a radical mastectomy may gain from the experience a greater closeness to her family and the ability to share feelings and understanding.

Which People Cope Best?

Different people respond very differently to the crisis of illness. Why? What factors influence their reactions to the illness and their ability to cope? A few individual factors have been found to influence coping. It has been shown, for example, that an individual who has a high level of intelligence and cognitive development may be better able to seek and use information, thus avoiding a sense of powerlessness. This might be true primarily because an individual with high intellectual development and education is more confident in asking for information. It has also been found that the general ego strength and self-esteem of the individual has a significant impact on the ability to adapt to the crisis of illness. On the other hand, people who are insecure or feel inadequate and who are psychologically vulnerable tend to have some difficulty coping with illness. Children and adolescents may have particular difficulty coping with the crisis of illness because of their limited experience in coping

the greater maturity of an individual and the more extensive experience this individual has in successfully coping with crises may make it easier to deal with the crisis of illness [21, 25, 31].

Characteristics of the illness, such as the type and location of symptoms, also tend to influence coping with the illness. For example, if the symptoms are painful, disfiguring, or disabling, the individual will generally have more trouble coping with them than if the symptoms are not at all obvious. In addition, if the body region affected is vested with special importance (e.g., the heart), the individual may feel that his or her entire life is in danger. Patients are often overwhelmed when their illness causes damage to their reproductive organs or to their faces, for there is a great deal of psychological significance attached to certain regions of the body. Amputation of a breast, for example, may have a greater psychological impact on an individual than a very serious chronic illness that is life-endangering (e.g., serious hypertension). In addition, coping can be affected by physiological problems. Extreme weakness may limit the individual's capacity to cope with the problems of illness [13].

Some research has shown that chronically ill patients cope more effectively if they are actively involved in their care. With proper patient education, many patients can be involved in making decisions about their treatment. For example, treatment of hypertension seems to be more successful when patients have an active orientation and endeavor to take some control over managing their condition [36].

Normalization

As Strauss and Glaser have noted in their book on chronic illness, the chief goal of the chronically ill patient is not simply to remain alive as long as possible, under any circumstances [39], but rather to attempt to live for as long as possible as *normally* as possible (see Box 8-1). How "normal" a chronically ill person's life can be, however, depends on a number of factors: the social arrangements that the individual can make; how intrusive the symptoms are; the necessary regimens for treatment; and the knowledge and reactions of other people. The process of *normalization* is the attempt by the ill person to establish and maintain as normal an existence as possible [19]. For example, it involves efforts by patients suffering from chronic obstructive pulmonary disease to rest in certain ways so that bystanders realize that they are tired and not drunk. It involves a patient's trying not to let the symptoms of the disease be obvious [19].

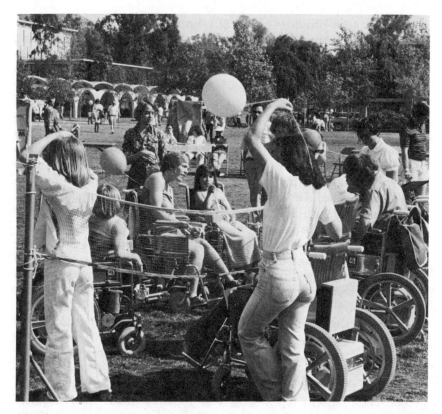

Figure 8–1. Successful adaptation to a handicap: Ann McClellan (center) of the University of California, Riverside. (Photo courtesy of University of California, Riverside, Special Services.)

The ability of patients to control their life and to normalize their illness is partly dependent on the intrusiveness of the symptoms. Some symptoms are immediately obvious, and therefore the sick person cannot choose whether or not to reveal them. Symptoms such as twisted or distorted limbs, a disfigured face, a limp, slurred speech, and disagreeable smells are intrusive and obvious. Unfortunately, sometimes these obvious symptoms are interpreted by others as overwhelmingly pervasive—that is, people view the chronically ill person as incapable of engaging in any kind of constructive behaviors, even though it is not true. This phenomenon is termed "identity spread" [39]. Others tend to overgeneralize, and an insidious stereotype is sometimes at work. For example, blind and physically handicapped people are often assumed to be incapable of work. Or people

chronically ill come to dominate the interaction unless they are able to normalize the situation. Patients may initially try to hide the symptoms and, if it is not possible, to focus attention away from them.

When the symptoms of sick people are invisible or the fact of the disease is not known to other people, they have the option of what sociologist Erving Goffman has called "passing" [19]. That is, these people can engage in normal interactions with others because the others do not know that they are not "normal." Examples are a patient who has had a colostomy and a patient who has had a radical mastectomy. The public is not aware of the patient's disfigurement unless, of course, the patient chooses to reveal it. This passing, however, can cause a great deal of anxiety in the patient. Under some conditions the person may have to reveal the illness condition or disfigurement. This is true, for example, if a woman who has had a radical mastectomy becomes very close to a man that she is dating. At some point, as sexual intimacy develops, the man will discover the fact that the woman has only one breast. The anxiety that builds up as their intimacy level increases can be very distressing for the mastectomy patient. Another problem, in addition to this anxiety, is that the patient who is "passing" is being accepted by others for something that this person is not—that is, a physically "normal" person. The patient cannot disclose feelings about the deformity without acknowledging its existence. Thus the person is, in a sense, trapped, being accepted for something that this person is not. The patient is not sure whether this acceptance will continue when the deformity is revealed.

Goffman discusses passing in his interesting book, *Stigma*. He notes that people, like stage actors, try to manage their identities and present themselves to others in a certain light. In this "presentation of self," people's actions may not correspond to their "true" selves. This acting has implications for the patient's sense of identity. As we saw in Chapter 1, a person's identity comes to some extent from other people. If, however, others have an incorrect impression of what someone is really like, false self-impressions may begin to form. This conflict between self-impression and the impression given to others may be very detrimental to the patients' well-being. For example, if patients give the impression to others that they are physically fine and in turn come to be treated as such, others may be reluctant to give the extra encouragement and support required in times of medical crisis. They may be angry and hurt that these patients were not honest with them.

Box 8-1
The Wheelchair People

People with chronic illnesses that force them to use wheelchairs have traditionally been hidden from society. Three basic factors interfered unnecessarily in the lives of people in wheelchairs: First, the negative perceptions of society, which saw handicapped people as deviant and inferior; second, the negative self-perceptions held by the handicapped themselves, which limited their willingness to venture into the public eye; and third, physical impediments to the mobility of the handicapped. Government programs are eliminating physical impediments in the environment, and handicapped people are now coming together to assert their rights. Together, these two factors are changing the third limitation—the perceptions of the general public.

One of the most progressive programs for handicapped students is at the University of California at Riverside (UCR). Because of its warm, dry climate, numerous ramps and elevators, and small, attractive campus, UCR has dozens of wheelchair students and dozens more students with other handicaps. Because of the special interests and needs these students generate, UCR has a wheelchair repair center, transport vans with lifts, special learning resources and counseling services, and an internship program to help handicapped students train for jobs. The presence of significant numbers of handicapped students active in various aspects of university life has led to a striking absence of stigmatizing perceptions in the university and surrounding communities.

In light of the many problems of passing, why do many patients do so? The reason is that there is a stigma associated with many illnesses. An example is the stigma of cancer. Stigma refers to some characteristic or attribute of a person that is deeply discrediting and takes priority over all other characteristics that the person has [19]. It is important to recognize that stigma is actually a property of interpersonal relations because *people* define what conditions are stigmatizing. Cancer has a greater stigma than heart disease, even though heart disease is a more prevalent killer [44]. Tuberculosis once had a greater stigma associated with it than it does today. Thus what is considered a stigma can change. Some of the many stigmatizing effects associated with breast cancer, for example, were alleviated a few years ago when several prominent women announced publicly that they had had mastectomies. This notion of stigma is important of course because expectations of society are inextricably entwined with how people cope with chronic illness.

Many of the greatest difficulties faced by chronically ill persons result not from their physical disability but from their relationships with others. It is not surprising, then, that successful coping may depend as much or even more on socioemotional resources received from others than on the individual's personal strength. The information, clarification, and reassurance that an individual receives from others is called *social support* [9, 11, 12].

In their daily lives, people are members of various groups that provide the social resources necessary for living. For example, people receive information about the demands of their career from their co-workers; they discuss their feelings with friends and family members; and they form a sense of identity from their ethnic, religious, family, or professional ties. These groups are called *reference groups*. Reference groups help people evaluate their thoughts, feelings, and abilities, and influence what people believe they should or should not do. If a person moves away from these groups (geographically— to a new job in a new state, for example, or socially—by behaving in conflict with group values), psychological and emotional pressures on the person may result. These pressures will be relieved when new group ties are developed.

The chronically ill person is in a position similar to but even more difficult than someone who has moved to a new job. The ill person desperately needs social support but may have trouble becoming "reestablished." For example, a heart patient may no longer be able to play vigorous sports with his or her friends, but may not yet have developed a network of individuals with whom to spend leisure time. Social support is important for three reasons: for medical information, for reducing uncertainty, and for reassurance.

Let us consider the first function of social support. Ill persons need much new information about their medical condition—its physical effects, prognosis, the side effects of drugs given for the condition, financial demands, government services, transportation, nursing care, and many other matters. The range of questions may be enormous: Who sells and repairs wheelchairs? Is insulin easily available when traveling overseas? Is it safe (and legal) to drive a car? Which company makes a good prosthesis? Unfortunately, most pre-illness friends and acquaintances of patients are not likely to know the answers to many of these questions, and therefore chronically ill people need to establish firm ties with new sources of information.

Second, one of the greatest pressures facing a person who has been newly diagnosed as having a condition like epilepsy or cancer is uncertainty [44]. There is uncertainty about how and by whom to be treated, about what friends and acquaintances will think (and who should be informed), and about what the future will bring. Social psychologists have established that in such times of uncertainty, people usually turn to others—to their reference group—for clarification. When they are afraid and uncertain, people generally seek out others in a similar situation to share feelings and compare reactions. However, patients may have great difficulty contacting other people who are relevant. Unafflicted friends may be inappropriate as people with whom the patients can compare themselves because they are too "distant" (in terms of acquaintance with the disease) or the problem may be too embarrassing. Family members may not be knowledgeable about the patient's particular condition. Medical personnel may be too busy or may be seen as able only to treat physical, not social or emotional, problems. Hence patients may be unable to clarify their feelings and unable to reduce their uncertainty. This problem is very important since it may interfere significantly with the patients' recovery.

The third and final reason for the importance of social support involves the patient's need for reassurance. The shock of a medical crisis and the stresses of illness create a need for comfort and understanding. In facing daily problems, people turn to others for the positive feedback, warmth, and caring that helps them deal with life's difficulties. However, patients may have a greater need for such comfort at the same time that their family itself is in need of extra support. In the hospital the role of the nurse is to help fill this need to some extent. But nurses cannot fully replace the supportive role of friends and family.

Although the needs of the chronically ill for social support can be great, the various problems we have considered so far that face the chronically ill may combine to make such support difficult to obtain. In fact, it appears that patients who need the most social support are likely to get the least [9]. Patients with insufficient support may not cooperate fully with their treatment, and this uncooperativeness may in turn reduce the little support that they had been receiving. Fortunately, during the last few years increasing attention has been paid to the problem of social support. Three areas look promising.

The most likely source of beneficial support is the peer group; many patients are put in touch with other patients with similar conditions. For example, the organization called *Reach to Recovery* offers mastectomy patients the opportunity to talk with a volunteer, herself a former patient. This organization provides information, a chance to discuss feelings, and the encouragement of seeing a "re-

recovery, asserts that in reaching out to help others, she helped herself [28].

Today organizations for a wide range of chronic illnesses exist, and in part, they have emerged as a result of the increasing assertiveness of patients. Whereas traditionally physicians had complete control over the information patients received, the increasing "consumer" demands of patients have helped bring about the formation of support groups. Since many of these groups are relatively new and have not been carefully evaluated, it is prudent to be cautious in looking at them. Groups that interfere with necessary medical treatment or that are led by unqualified people might produce detrimental rather than beneficial effects [30] (see Table 8-1 for some examples of support groups).

A second developing area of social support involves the use of psychologists and social workers in medical settings. Although traditionally psychologists have dealt mostly with "mental" problems, recognition of the importance of social psychology to all aspects of illness is leading to the inclusion of social scientists on medical "teams." The social scientist pays special attention to the social and emotional needs of the patient and can facilitate positive interactions with family and friends. Furthermore, such a "health facilitator" can also improve relationships among physicians, nurses, and patients, thereby increasing the social support available from medical personnel [9].

A final source of increased social support is the primary care physician. With the increasing addition of social science to medical school curricula and with the establishment of training programs in community medicine and family practice medicine, physicians are becoming more sensitive to the importance of social support and better able to provide relevant information, treatment, and referral [16].

What Can the Health Care Professional Do?

Throughout the discussion of the process of adjustment to chronic illness, we have focused on the importance of the patients' adjustment to their environment, their management of relationships with friends and family, and their capacity to deal with symptoms. The emphasis has been on the patients' ultimate responsibility for the management of their social and even psychological condition. Remembering that it is the patient's decision and responsibility to carry out the treatment, the health care professional can still pro-

Table 8-1. Self-Help and Support Groups for Coping with Illness

Name and Address	Purpose
American Cancer Society 777 Third Ave. N.Y., NY 10017	A voluntary organization dedicated to the control and eradication of cancer, and to helping patients to cope with the disease.
Cansurmont Program Colorado Division 1809 E. 18th Ave. Denver, CO 80218	A program designed to help people better understand and cope with cancer. This is a volunteer program that serves cancer patients, their families, and those involved with the treatment of cancer patients.
Candlelighters 123 C St., S.E. Washington, DC 20003	An international organization of parents (over 100 groups) whose children have had cancer. Members work for improved medical and social care for children with cancer, their families, and also for cancer research. It serves as an emotional support system for members.
Compassionate Friends PO Box 1347 Oak Brook, IL 60521	A self-help organization that offers friendship and understanding to bereaved parents.
Make Today Count 514 Tama Bldg. Box 303 Burlington, IA 52601	An organization for persons with life-threatening illnesses, as well as for their families and other interested persons. It is a mutual support organization bringing together afflicted persons.
Phoenix Society 11 Rust Hill Rd. Levittown, PA 19056	A self-help, nationwide organization for burn victims and their families. The major goal is to ease the psychosocial adjustment of the severely burned.
United Ostomy Association 1111 Wilshire Blvd. L.A., CA 90017	An organization that provides mutual aid and moral support for people with colostomy, ileostomy, or urostomy. This is dedicated to helping ostomy patients return to normal living by providing moral support, as well as education and assistance.

vide much support in an effort to help patients accomplish their goals.

First, an acute care unit of a hospital may be inappropriate for a chronically ill patient, unless the patient is temporarily in an acute care crisis. The best place for a chronic illness to be managed, and for patients to work at normalizing their life, is at home. Thus part of the support from the health care professional should involve aiding patients to care for chronic illness symptoms at home with the support of family members and friends. The health care professional

should be on teaching the patient as much as possible about managing the illness, and helping the patient to control the symptoms in the home. Furthermore, since an important part of the patient's ability to cope depends on the social support that the patient can obtain, the health care professional should try to assess the family members' acceptance of the patient's condition, as well as assessing the patient's acceptance of the condition.

To aid in communication and understanding, the health care professional must have information about the patient generally, the patient's reactions to the illness, and about the social support system. Although patients often disclose information to health care professionals, sometimes a concerted effort has to be made in order to obtain information from patients. Often, however, health care professionals cannot spend time collecting psychosocial information through lengthy interviews with patients. Strauss and Glaser suggest that the health care professional should engage in "action dialog" or action interviews with patients [39]. This technique involves gaining information from patients (and giving information to patients) *while doing something to them.* For example, when changing dressings on a wound, the health professional might talk with the patient and explore the social psychological and physical resources available to the patient in a program of rehabilitation. Information about the social and physical settings and also the patient's psychological resources can be gained from interviews with family members and friends.

The goal of treatment of chronic illness does not involve care that will end or eliminate the disease completely. Chronic illness generally can be managed and its progress slowed or checked. It is probably because of their inability to cure the disease that the work of people who care for and give comfort to the chronically ill may not be valued as highly as those who provide acute care. Care of the chronically ill is usually somewhat routine, and it is regarded as not as exciting as acute care for trauma. Hence physicians and other health care professionals sometimes become frustrated while caring for the chronically ill. But the care of the chronically ill can be very challenging because of the many social and psychological factors involved. The management of patients and their immediate families demands the skill of professionals well versed in both the social and technical aspects of medicine.

SPECIAL CASES OF CHRONIC ILLNESS

Crisis, coping, and social support are issues that are found in all forms of chronic illness. However, each chronic condition also has various unique problems that must be addressed, and as an illustration, we consider three special cases of chronic illness. The first involves a specific age group—children. The second concerns a specific illness—cancer. And the third case involves a type of traumatic injury—burns. Examination of these three cases also provides a further understanding of the importance of social psychology to chronic illness.

Long-term Illness in Children

The prevalence of chronic conditions in childhood is surprisingly high [32]. Considering serious chronic illnesses of primarily physical origin, American and British surveys find that up to 10 percent of all children are afflicted with chronic illness. The most common physical conditions are cardiac problems, cerebral palsy, asthma, orthopedic problems, and diabetes mellitus. Other serious long-term illnesses in children include hemophilia, muscular dystrophy, rheumatic fever, chronic renal disease, leukemia, and permanent handicaps resulting from physical injuries.

Children with long-term physical disorders tend to be subjected to many stressful situations, but may not have the emotional resources to deal with these stresses. First, children may not have sufficient cognitive development to understand illness. For example, while pain represents an emotional stress to adults, adults are usually able to understand its cause. Children, on the other hand, tend to be extremely confused about the origin of pain and discomfort. They also may not know why they have become sick, and they may feel that they are ill as a punishment for disobedience to parents, or perhaps because their parents were not protective enough. If the condition results from hereditary factors, the child may express a great deal of anger and resentment toward the parents [32, 42].

A second source of enormous emotional stress for the child is the health care system itself [42]. Lengthy hospital stays involve separation from family, school, and friends. Fears of abandonment may arise. This separation is also often accompanied by frightening situations, orchestrated by the physician, not by the parent. The health care system removes much control and chances for self-care from patients. This can be especially troubling to children or young ado-

psychiatrist Ake Mattsson notes that in fact some children may respond to this helplessness by regressing to even more childish or babylike behavior; they may lose some of the achievements that they have attained in motor functioning and social functioning [32].

Finally, surgical invasion of the body may be very difficult for children to deal with because of their fears of bodily mutilation. These fantasies tend to be especially difficult for younger children. Most sick children also find restriction and immobilization particularly stressful emotionally; they are accustomed to freedom of movement in order to express dissatisfaction and to explore the environment. Prolonged restraint of a child may cause anxiety, a buildup of tension, and eventual temper tantrums. On the other hand, the child might respond with withdrawal into an apathetic, depressed condition. This problem can be prevented, however, if the child is given the opportunity, help, and encouragement to channel actions into words—to verbalize feelings.

A third source of emotional stress for the child involves family members. While parents may become more loving and indulgent, siblings may become extremely resentful of the sick child. Or parents themselves may at times reject the ill child, criticizing the child for causing inconvenience. These changes in family attitudes can be extremely confusing to the child who is ill. A good example is childhood diabetes [6].

Childhood diabetes is a chronic metabolic disorder that is treatable but not curable. The child's life depends upon receiving daily injections of the hormone insulin; however, this is not the only responsibility of the person caring for the child. Along with the proper scheduling of these injections, dietary restrictions and activity monitoring are needed. The insulin and the body's glucose (sugar) must be balanced within the child or the child can experience a severe medical crisis. Without a regular pattern of food intake and insulin injection, the child could experience symptoms as simple as confusion and irritability or as complex and dangerous as convulsions and loss of consciousness [6].

The need to schedule injections and to control intake of food can present enormous social psychological problems in the child's family. The parents of the child serve as substitutes for the physician in implementing the treatment regimen and are also responsible for the socialization of the child—that is, teaching the child the rules of conduct and the norms of caring for him or herself. Balancing the usual routine care of a child in the morning (getting the child ready for school) with the extra demands of the illness (urine tests and insulin injections) can be complex. A major problem faced by parents is rearranging their social activities, including the activities of the other children in the family [6]. Much of the scheduling of the family's activities revolves around the needs of the chronically ill diabetic child, especially with respect to the family's eating habits (which may be affected by the requirements of the diabetic child). For example, in order not to tempt the diabetic child, parents may refrain from keeping sweets in the kitchen, thus depriving the other children of sweets. For the diabetic child there are no special occasions on which the child can eat whatever he or she wants.

The operation of psychological factors is peculiar to each specific chronic illness that a child may have. For example, children with a serious respiratory disease such as asthma often express fears of suffocation, drowning, or dying while they are asleep. In contrast, children with chronic heart disease often find it difficult to understand the nature of their illness and the reasons why their activity is restricted, and why extensive medical procedures and perhaps surgery may be required, since they may experience minimal symptoms or none at all. At the same time, these children may be some very frightened when references are made to the importance of the individual's heart to life itself [42].

Children with chronic renal disease experience specific stresses if they are treated with hemodialysis or kidney transplantation. Children may feel overwhelmingly dependent upon a machine, and find it difficult to seek independence from their families. Parents may attempt to exert a great deal of control over children who have received a kidney transplant in an effort to prevent rejection of the kidney. If rejection does occur, the child may blame him or herself for destroying the kidney that was given as a special gift, often by a family member [1, 4, 34].

Children with leukemia frequently become very depressed, upset, and uncooperative. They may refuse to confide in their parents and avoid suggested treatment. Such problems generally result from miscommunication. The parents, trying to be strong and supportive, may act in a friendly, lighthearted manner toward the child, attempting to minimize the seriousness of the illness. However, a hospitalized child is very adept at detecting such attempted deception; it is obvious to the child that something is very wrong. Thus the child may interpret the parents' positive act as evidence that they do not really care about the child's illness and the possibility of death. The child thus feels abandoned and becomes alternately depressed

chological problems experienced by children may be quite complex, and not at all immediately evident.

Many children cope quite well with the stresses of long-term chronic illness. In the proper circumstances, with supportive, understanding adults, children may be very adaptable. In fact, many studies of long-term childhood disorders report surprisingly good psychosocial adaptation of children, usually when the children are provided with emotional support and understanding. In fact, children experiencing long-term disability accept their physical limitations and can often find alternate satisfactions in intellectual pursuits. It has been found that the nature of the child's illness is less important in influencing successful adaptation than are such factors as the quality of the parent–child relationship and the family's acceptance of the handicapped child. The child's adaptation thus tends to depend partially on the parents' ability to master their own reactions of fear and guilt [18].

Some children do not adjust well, and their maladjustment may take any number of forms. In some cases the child experiences extreme fearfulness, inactivity, and lack of outside interests, with a dependency upon the family, particularly the mother. Or the child may become overly independent, often daring to undertake activities that are prohibited and which involve a significant risk to the child's safety. Some children are rebellious. Finally, some children with deformities and handicaps withdraw almost totally and become very shy and lonely. Usually these children were raised in families in which their defects were emphasized [20, 40].

A parent's adjustment to the child's illness can have a substantial impact on the child's adjustment. This fact argues for the health care professional's contribution to the care of *both* parent and child. The provision of information, emotional support, and aid in understanding usual reactions of parents and children in facing illness can help enormously in the overall care of the chronically ill child.

Cancer

It was not by chance that we began this chapter by mentioning cancer. Cancer is an important area of chronic illness. Over 3 million Americans have a history of cancer, 2 million of whom were diagnosed more than five years ago. It is estimated that over 55 million Americans who are now living will have cancer; it will strike two out of three families. At the turn of the century few cancer patients lived very long. Today, however, one in three patients is alive at least five years after treatment. Although some of these people seem completely cured, many of them have a continuing problem or disability: They must face the problems of chronic illness.

A recent study of the social psychological needs of about 1000 cancer patients and their families was sponsored by the California Division of the American Cancer Society [2]. Experienced social workers conducted in-depth interviews with adults who had been living with cancer of varying forms (except skin cancer) for about two or three years. About two-thirds of the sample was female, but otherwise the people were quite representative of the population. A number of interesting findings emerged.

The periods that were reported as being most stressful for both patients and their families were immediately following diagnosis and during hospitalization. Interestingly, a significant proportion of patients reported that *release* from the hospital was the most stressful time. The stress of diagnosis results from uncertainty, whereas the stresses of hospitalization and release from the hospital are in large part due to changed interpersonal relationships. Although people often imagine their pain and weakness are the major problems encountered in cancer, actually the social disruptions are most troublesome for most patients.

One of the significant problems faced by cancer patients is the changes in their physical appearance. Why is appearance so important? First, the physical attractiveness of the patient can somewhat affect the reactions of the doctor [27]. More importantly, however, the patients' appearance affects relations with others. For example, chemotherapy often produces hair loss, and while hair loss in itself is not a terribly severe problem, it can have dramatic effects on family and friends because of its effect on the appearance of the patient. Hence it has been suggested that patients should keep themselves as attractive as possible, including the use of wigs [17]. Mastectomy is also often very threatening to the self-concept of a woman. Negative reactions from a spouse sometimes occur (although they may be in response to the woman's own altered behavior). In such cases the social effects of cancer may far outweigh any physical effects.

In the beginning of this chapter we saw that, after his diagnosis of cancer, Orville Kelley had nowhere to turn for social support. A similar finding emerged from the California survey. On the whole supportive services were missing, inadequate, or unknown. Most people were aware of *no* social services to which they could turn. While only about one-quarter of the patients felt that they could turn to religious leaders, writings about cancer, or other cancer patients for help, the vast majority of patients who knew these services were available utilized them. It was found that there was a tremendous need that could be met but mostly was not being met. Consequently, patients turned mostly to their families for help.

Many people hold stereotyped views of cancer, in which they often see cancer as tied to chronic pain, prolonged weakness, dirtiness, fear, and obsession with death, even though such characteristics are by no means universal. It is also true that cancer patients are often blamed for their illness, much the way people were once seen as "causing" their tuberculosis [38]. Some people assert (although with little evidence) that cancer is caused by a depressed personality and a tendency to "bottle up" feelings inside themselves. Although psychological reactions can affect health, there is little justification for asserting that most cancer patients had a decisive role in producing their disease. A psychological process called *blaming the victim* is at work [35]. Research has demonstrated that many people desire to believe in a "just world" in which people get what they deserve [29]. Seeing a young, active, "innocent" person who is ravaged by cancer is quite difficult for many people to deal with, and therefore they come to believe that the patient somehow deserved to be stricken; the victim is blamed. This process is part of people's general attempt to make sense out of their world, and it appears with other diseases as well; however, the fear and uncertainty of cancer make it a special target. Such reactions understandably interfere with the cancer patient's ability to cope.

In the California survey, many patients saw their communications with their physicians as inadequate. The ability of patients to deal with the stresses of cancer were reported to be hindered by lack of sufficient explanation from medical personnel. Problem areas ranged from diagnosis and treatment, to rehabilitation, to socioemotional matters. We have emphasized the importance of proper communication throughout this book. In this case, however, its critical significance is highlighted by the spontaneously volunteered comments of cancer patients on these matters. In addition to providing much-needed information, medical personnel can warn patients about the psychological reactions of others that they are likely to encounter and suggest ways in which they can try to deal with these reactions. Cancer is not only a biological disease; it also has many significant psychosocial aspects.

The California survey also found that cancer had a considerable *financial* impact on people [2]. About one-sixth of the sample foresaw a problem with their future financial security. Many patients had to make significant adjustments in their pre-illness lifestyle because of monetary problems. Although financial matters are often seen as an economic problem rather than a medical or psychological problem, financial resources are actually directly relevant to the patient's health. With sufficient money, patients and their families are able to maintain their usual lifestyle and concentrate their efforts on dealing with the illness. Adequate insurance makes a big difference. What was noteworthy in the California survey was that the low-income working people (who most needed insurance) were *least* likely to have adequate coverage. This finding is not unusual. In one case costs to the family *after the insurance was exhausted* exceeded $50,000. This means that in many cases the children of the cancer patient had to forego college and the family's house had to be mortgaged or sold. The social and emotional needs of many patients can never be completely addressed so long as the financial burden to families continues to be crippling [2].

Thus there are various problems of chronic illness to be faced by the cancer patient, but again, the problems are mostly interpersonal. Whereas the special problems faced by children with chronic illness resulted mostly from their state of dependency and limited understanding, the problems of cancer flow mostly from the stigma of cancer and its attendant fear, uncertainty, and lack of social support. Additional problems result from changes in the body. This latter problem is discussed next.

The Burned Patient

Hundreds of thousands of Americans suffer each year from burns. In the past most patients died from mutilating burns, but with new medical procedures, many lives can now be saved. Recovery is not simple, however. Being burned is a traumatic experience—it is extremely painful and results in deformity and debilitation. There is also an enormous chance of infection. Furthermore, victims of burns continue to be reminded of the trauma they have experienced, and throughout their lives they have scars to remind them of the experience [5].

There are enormous psychological problems that accompany severe burns. It was found in one study that about half the victims of the major Coconut Grove nightclub fire still experienced severe emotional problems almost a year after the fire [3]. Two years after the initial trauma, most of the patients were functioning interpersonally at about the same level that they had been functioning before the injury. But for many the trauma continued. Since the enormous

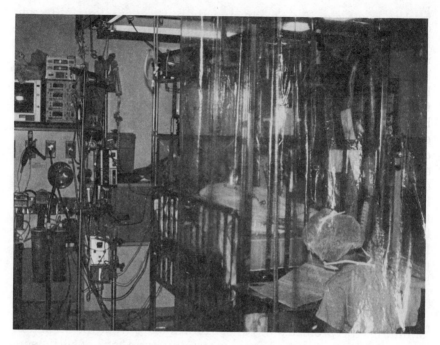

Figure 8-2. In addition to physical problems, burned patients face problems of self-identity and rejection by others. Great stresses may also be placed on their families. (Photo by Howard S. Friedman, © 1982)

negative emotional impact of burns may last for years, it is important for the health care professional to understand the psychosocial issues involved in the care of the burned patient.

A study reported by N. J. C. Andreasen and A. S. Norris suggests some problems that are representative of the kinds of problems usually faced by patients who are severely burned [5]. A major identity crisis usually arises directly from the individual's altered appearance. The patient's body image must be redefined by the patient in order to take into account the scarring, deformity, and weakness resulting from the burns. Strained interactions with other people alter the patient's social identity, and the patient faces a crisis that involves feelings of isolation and estrangement.

While many people attempt to respond to the patient positively, sometimes people respond to the physical deformity of the burned patient with expressions of revulsion and disgust. These reactions can be extremely devastating to the self-concept of the patient.

Furthermore, if patients detect pity in the faces of strangers, a sense of loss at their altered selves can overwhelm them. While resuming a familiar role within the family could help prevent or eliminate an identity crisis, this event usually does not occur because of the prolonged hospitalization that is required after the trauma of being burned. The patient may have trouble fitting back into the usual family role. Family members often treat the patient differently from how this person was treated before the accident partly because of the expectations of the sick role and partly because the burn victim acts differently. An example is the situation of a young woman who is severely burned. As with mastectomy, women who lose their physical attractiveness because of severe burns tend to assume that they have also lost their sexual desirability. In spite of assurances from their husbands, these women may be overwhelmed by the feeling that they are no longer attractive. Their response is to withdraw from their spouses. Of course, burned patients often experience physical handicaps and limitations as well. They may have to wear bandages for a long time, and their skin, which is scarred or recently grafted, may be painful.

Most patients (about 70 percent) eventually adapt reasonably well to the many problems that they face [5]. It has been found that patients who eventually succeed in resolving their identity crises do so primarily by using the following patterns of adaptive responses. In other words, there are specific techniques that patients can use to cope with the trauma, and these techniques tend to be adaptive and successful. The first of these coping mechanisms is called progressive desensitization. Through support and acceptance from people who are close to and love them, patients may begin to believe that what really matters is their "inner selves." The scarred, deformed outer self comes to be seen as unimportant. This denial of the obtrusiveness of the self presented to the world is adaptive in terms of the acceptance of their injury and their ability to continue on with life.

Since the self is partly socially defined, however, problems arise. The patients may unrealistically minimize the obtrusiveness of their appearance. They may consistently underestimate their unattractiveness, and therefore have trouble relating to others. Patients finally adjust if they come to a more realistic self-image (recognizing that they may repulse or scare others who do not know them) accompanied by some kind of rationalization about what has happened to them. A number of patients with severe burns come to the conclusion that what happened to them has made them better people. Patients may arrive at some kind of conversion (although not necessarily religious) and report finding a new direction for their lives. Surprisingly, severely burned patients eventually describe themselves as drawing closer to their spouses and to their families. And after nearly having lost their lives in a fire, they tend to experience a new awareness of life and of their role within their families and their relationships to other people. In addition, patients may take great pride in gradually rehabilitating themselves.

Some of the ways in which patients deal with their disabilities and deformities are quite maladaptive. Some patients withdraw from others and experience a great deal of anxiety about interpersonal relationships. Their shyness and self-consciousness very often reflect their pre-injury personality. This detrimental coping mechanism prevents patients from recognizing that they are accepted by other people, particularly family members and friends. Withdrawal from social contacts and close social relationships prevents patients from reestablishing their identity.

How patients adapt to severe burns is also affected by the amount of deformity experienced, as well as by certain personal factors. The patients' narcissism and extent of their focus on physical attractiveness and personal beauty can make acceptance of the loss of attractiveness very difficult. Probably because our society places such a high premium on attractiveness in women, more female than male burn patients have trouble adapting. Finally, adaptation is facilitated if patients are given an opportunity to ventilate or to express their feelings. If too much emphasis is placed on emotional control and stoicism, the feelings will remain repressed and the psychological pain may continue to trouble the patient.

As with other chronic conditions, there is significant pressure on the family of the burned patient [7]. Many patients experience confusion and disorientation as a result of a temporary acute brain syndrome that often accompanies burn trauma. Relatives find the patient verbally abusive and of course are distressed by this extremely strange behavior. It is important for health care professionals to assure the family that this delirium is common and that it eventually passes. In addition, while the initial response of the family is relief that the patient will live, the family soon begins to feel the stresses of the difficulties involved in the patient's hospitalization. There may be financial drains on the family's resources, and often the family may be temporarily relocated near the hospital. In addition, they must constantly provide emotional support, but there is usually little support provided for them. The burn patient tends to focus only upon him or herself, returning little in the way of support to the distressed relative. Finally, the family member must adjust to the altered appearance of the patient. There is enormous pressure on the family members to monitor constantly their reactions to the patient in order to avoid showing revulsion at the sight of the patient's scars and deformities.

Some solutions to help family members of burned patients might be to give them as much information as feasible about the care of the burned patient. Furthermore, groups of family members of various hospitalized burn patients might meet at regularly scheduled times with the physician, nurse, or social worker (or the entire team) in order to learn together how to deal with the psychosocial issues involved in the rehabilitation of the burn patient, and also to understand their own reactions to the trauma that has befallen the family.

SUMMARY

In sum, a major area for the application of social psychological principles to medicine involves chronic illness. Improved technological treatments for medical emergencies coupled with an increasingly elderly population have made chronic illness a significant health issue. Millions of Americans suffer from heart disease, cancer, paralysis, chronic lung disease, diabetes, and other conditions that create a longlasting, significant physical impairment. For the most part, however, the physical impairments are not the greatest source of difficulty for the chronically ill. Rather, chronically ill patients often face their greatest challenges in psychosocial matters—the crisis of illness, coping with illness, and the need for social support. These matters are an integral part of overall medical care.

Many of the psychosocial issues in chronic illness relate to the individual's sense of identity. Patients may have difficulty obtaining sufficient information about all the implications of their condition, and relatedly, may have trouble finding other people with whom they can share their fears and reduce their uncertainties. In addition, patients with burns, cancer, and other conditions that alter their appearance may experience direct threats to their sense of self. Discovering the new ways in which they must relate to their social worlds is perhaps the greatest challenge facing the chronically ill.

9

Dying and Death

To die, to sleep; to sleep: perchance to dream: ay, there's the rub.

—Shakespeare, *Hamlet*

In your first personal involvement with death, who died? Was it your grandparent, parent, or other family member? Or did you lose a friend or acquaintance? Death is an issue everyone encounters.

What aspect of your own inevitable death is the most distasteful to you? Is it that you could no longer work, or finish something you have started? Do you share Hamlet's fear of future experiences— what dreams may come? Would it upset you most to leave behind dependents for whom you could no longer provide? Do you fear the pain of dying? And what does death mean to you? Is it an end, or a beginning? Is it a kind of endless sleep with rest and peace, a joining of your spirit with a cosmic consciousness? Is there nothing after death?

If you had a choice, what kind of death would you prefer? Would you prefer a death that is sudden, or one that gives you time to prepare for it? Would you rather take your own life than have someone kill you? If you could choose, when would you prefer to die? Would it be in youth, in the prime of life, or in old age? Finally, if you were told that you had a terminal disease and a limited time to live (say, six months), how would you spend the time until you died? Would you complete projects and tie up loose ends? Would you read, contemplate, pray? Would you satisfy hedonistic desires? Would you make no change in your lifestyle? Consideration of such questions helps us to approach the topic of dying and death, for death is a very personal matter.

The following three people are dying:

John: John is 42 years old and has been happily married for 20 years. He has two children, a boy 18 and a girl 12. His son is about to start college. His daughter is a competitive swimmer. John is a research biochemist who is at present doing work on cancer immunization. He has been working for the last four years on a project that may be on the verge of an important discovery. John has many friends, having lived in the same neighborhood for 20 years, and he is an active member of community organizations. His hobbies are listening to classical music, playing the violin, and reading. Until he began to feel ill, John ran five miles a day near his home. Suddenly, John feels very lonely.

Ann: Ann is a 30-year-old housewife who has been married for 12 years. She has five young children. Ann's husband works at two jobs in order to pay for the family's expenses. Ann and her husband have a very close relationship and enjoy bringing up their children. They have just purchased a home in the suburbs where the school system is good and the children can play safely. Ann has just had a breast biopsy, and the discovery of a malignancy has led to a radical mastectomy. Cancer was found in many of the lymph nodes, and Ann's chances of survival are very low.

Mark: Mark is an 18-year-old freshman at an Ivy League university. He is a straight-A student in biology and chemistry. Mark plays the cello in the university orchestra, and sings the bass part in the university madrigal society. Before the diagnosis of leukemia, Mark also played on the freshman football team. His doctors think he has about four months to live. Mark has decided to shoot himself.

Understanding and coping with dying and death are among the most difficult problems that must be faced both by people in general and by health care practitioners in particular [25]. The social psychological management of death and bereavement is an extremely important aspect of the role of the health care professional. Many disturbing questions must be faced and answered. How much should the patient and the family be told about the condition? Should the physician provide an estimate for the patient of how much time there is left to live? Should hope always be offered? How can practitioners best prepare the patient and the family for death? How can health professionals prepare themselves? Finally, what reactions can be expected from patients and what reactions can be expected from family members? How can the health care professional deal with these reactions? In this chapter we consider these as well as related issues.

Thanatology, the study of death, is a relatively new field, but much progress has been made in the last decade [25, 29]. This field provides important information. When reading this chapter, try to look not only objectively at this information, but also concentrate on the intimate, subjective side of the issues considered here. We encourage both an emotional, experiential approach and a scholarly, intellectual approach. Only when we come to grips with our own feelings about death and dying can we hope to help a dying person through the crisis of his or her life's end and help a family to grieve and go on with their lives.

We consider the perspective of dying patients, their feelings about their impending death and their attempts to cope with the crisis. We also examine the impact of impending death on the family and the process of grieving. We examine how family members, friends, and health practitioners treat the dying patient and how they themselves deal with anticipating the event of death. Finally, we also consider the special issues of the response of children to bereavement, children's conceptions of death, growing old and dying, and suicide.

PATIENTS' REACTIONS TO IMPENDING DEATH

Not very many years ago, health care professionals told the families of patients that they were dying, but they did not tell the patients themselves. As recently as the 1950s, most physicians, nurses, and other health care professionals actually denied to their dying patients that they were dying. Information would be given to relatives so that arrangements could be made, but health care professionals saw their involvement with the patient as extending simply to technical medical care. Many providers felt that their only job was to keep the patient alive as long as possible. Within recent years, however, questions have arisen regarding the quality of life and patients' rights to decide their own fate [31].

Dying is a *psychosocial* event in addition to a biological event.

By a psychosocial event we mean that the process of dying affects the patient's thoughts, feelings, and relationships [21]. Even if not told directly, a patient usually knows that he or she is dying [31]. But dying is not usually readily acknowledged by others [3]. Either the family denies the information and refuses to communicate it to the patient, or else the family refuses to deal with the emotional issues that impending death creates for the patient. Dying is a social phenomenon because it affects the way in which people treat the patient [31].

After much research, it has been found that keeping information about death from patients is counterproductive. Research by Herman Fiefel and others reports that over 80 percent of patients interviewed said they would want to know about their terminal illness [14, 16, 17]. In other followup studies, between 82 and 98.5 percent of a group of patients undergoing diagnostic tests at a cancer detection center indicated that they would want to be told the truth even if they had cancer. Yet during the 1950s and 1960s, about 70 to 90 percent of the physicians interviewed said they did not tell patients that they were soon going to die [14]. Thus the patient was enmeshed in an atmosphere of deception. Controlling verbal and nonverbal behaviors was virtually impossible, however, and staff health care professionals and family members were not very good at carrying out the deception.

Patients thus often faced what is called a "double-bind" situation [14]. Conflicting messages such as "you're going to be okay" combined with very sad or depressed facial expressions of family members confused, alienated, and rendered helpless the patient who was already feeling very poorly. The patient would ask him or herself: "Why are the family members visiting for such a short time? Why do I feel like my condition is getting worse? Why won't the doctor look at me and talk to me?" As the inconsistencies recurred, the patient became more apprehensive and suspicious. Eventually the patient would ask, "Am I going to die?" The family members would defer to the nurse, the nurse to the physician, and perhaps only after immense emotional pain would the patient receive the answer that by then the patient already knew [12].

The communication of information (e.g., "The prognosis is poor beyond six months") now occurs with great frequency. However, there are still many social psychological factors at work to render the patient lonely and alienated. While once there was a conspiracy of silence with respect to *information,* today there is a conspiracy of silence with respect to *feelings* [24, 47].

The patients who find out about their impending death face a crisis that is new, and with which they have had no prior experience.

Everything in a person's life is threatened, and extreme anxiety usually results. Often the patient experiences psychological shock accompanied by denial—a feeling that this cannot be happening to him or her—and anger. Finally, when death seems inevitable, the patient may experience some grief, a letting go of people and places, and eventual acceptance of the inevitable. Elisabeth Kübler-Ross has proposed distinct stages in the reaction of the person who is dying [31].

Stages of Dying

In her influential book, *On Death and Dying,* Kübler-Ross proposed that dying patients go through five stages. Based upon her interviews with approximately 200 patients in a Chicago area hospital, she found that the stages are normal ways of responding to the prospect of death. Patients may begin with a stage known as *denial* in which they are not able to face the information. For example, a patient may insist that the prognosis is a mistake, and this patient may seek new tests or even new doctors. According to Dr. Kübler-Ross, denial does not last very long, but patients differ in the amount of time they take in this initial stage. As time goes on, denial usually decreases in frequency of use.

Kübler-Ross claims that in the second stage the patient becomes *angry* and asks the question "Why me?" The patient vents anger and resentment at both family and health care personnel. Concerns of equity may become important as the patient sees other "less deserving" people enjoying good health. The patient may want to assert that he or she is not dead yet and should not be ignored. Anger may also be an attempt by the patient to regain control over his or her life (see Chapter 11).

In the third stage many patients begin to *bargain*. The patient may try to make a deal with fate for more time or less pain. The patient may offer more compliant behavior in exchange for these benefits. The dying person may try to strike a bargain with God, often because of feelings of guilt.

Many dying patients face a number of losses. They may lose their job, financial resources, independence, and even parts of their bodies. There is also the specter of future losses. According to Kübler-Ross, when bargaining does not work these losses lead many patients into the fourth stage: *depression*. The patient goes through a type of self-grieving. If the patient lives long enough, the fifth and final stage may be reached: *acceptance*.

People at the stage of acceptance contemplate death with a kind of quiet acceptance. It is not necessarily a form of giving up, but it is not a happy stage either. Kübler-Ross says, "it is almost void of feelings." For example, John, the research biochemist, may come to an acceptance of the ways in which his family will go on and his work will be taken over by others. At this stage, the dying person often wants to be cut off from the problems of the outside world; they are no longer relevant to him or her. The patient may severely limit the number of visitors permitted. Sitting together with the family in silence is common. Extraordinary life-prolonging measures are not desired.

There has been no scientific demonstration of the existence of these stages. The scheme is a convenient way of looking at different patients' reactions, but there is no clear evidence that there are only five basic orientations among dying people or that people move from one stage to the next in succession. The stages were developed on the basis of psychiatric interviews, and they represent subjective analyses by Kübler-Ross and her colleagues. In this scheme, there tends to be an enormous concentration on the process of dying, but patients' previous usual coping mechanisms are largely ignored.

Other research on crises, including dying, has found that patients respond to the crisis much the same way they have responded to crises in the past [28]. If a patient usually responds to a crisis with denial, this patient is very likely to use denial when facing death. If the usual response is anger, that response will probably appear. Some patients move directly to the acceptance stage. Other patients remain depressed throughout the entire time, from first learning about their impending death to the end of life. The health care professional's prior knowledge of the patient as a person can be important in both predicting and understanding the patient's reaction to the news of impending death. In addition, knowledge of the family system is also important in understanding and helping the patient [41].

Although Kübler-Ross's model of the stages of dying lacks independent confirmation, her work has been important in improving sensitivity to the needs of dying patients. Patients' reactions to impending death were ignored for many years. Yet some practical problems have arisen from Kübler-Ross's stage theory. Patients' behavior may be forced into a mold of expectations, whereas patients differ greatly in their reactions to dying. Patients also react differently to secondary sufferings such as the loss of self-esteem, fears of separation from those close to them, and the anxieties that come with feelings of hopelessness. A patient's response to dying depends upon his or her age, past experience, personality, and lifestyle. A specific disease, treatment, and the expectation of time left to live must be taken into account in understanding the patient as well. Robert Kastenbaum has stated that sometimes people do experience and express similar feelings in their reactions to dying, but they do so within the unique pattern of their own lives. They also do so within a particular environment [25].

Coping with Dying

People differ in the *adaptiveness* of the coping mechanisms that they choose. It may be extremely maladaptive for a person to *deny* the existence of leukemia, since this may lead to refusal to take medication (chemotheraphy) or to undergo other treatment. Hence it is important to consider the overall context of a given patient's reactions.

Through church records, peasant life in the fourteenth century in the small French town of Montaillou has been reconstructed, revealing that an important aspect of life for them concerned death [32]. Death at a young age was very common and saving the soul was very important. Yet it was also of great importance to die surrounded by household and family members—not to die alone. Although today saving their soul is generally less important for many people, dying patients tend to be most afraid of being left alone. Included here is the fear of being left in pain without any control over it. It is very important that patients be given some hope (there is always a chance), and that they be told "We will be with you" (we will not abandon you) and "We will do everything to make you comfortable." Permission to express feelings and permission to die must be granted in open and honest confrontation with the patient. This can be done by the patient's family or by health care professionals. Everything should be done to prevent the patient from becoming lonely as the patient disengages emotionally from the world. Without open, honest communication, the dying patient is likely to be the most lonely person in the world [31].

As we have seen in earlier chapters, the perspective of social psychology emphasizes the importance of other people to our own sense of identity. Our thoughts and feelings are influenced by those around us with whom we compare ourselves. If friends, family, and medical personnel withdraw from a dying person, social comparison becomes very difficult. Without social contact it becomes very hard for a dying patient to validate his or her feelings and even to maintain a sense of identity at this point. The loneliness and confusion may lead the patient to further withdraw from other people who do not understand the difficulty, which may further compound the problem. In short, it is important to remember that all people need regular social contact, and this need is generally especially urgent in the dying [9].

A promising means of preventing loneliness is the *hospice,* a special institutional approach for caring for the dying. The beneficial effects of the hospice movement are discussed in Chapter 11, where we consider the hospital environment in detail.

REACTIONS OF FAMILY AND FRIENDS

We saw earlier that Ann is dying of breast cancer. Ann's impending death will significantly affect her family and friends. Her husband is left to face what is perhaps the major crisis of his life. As we noted in Chapter 7 on life stress, the death of a spouse is probably the greatest source of stress that an individual encounters. The problems that her husband will face are formidable. They involve not only his own loneliness, but also the need to bring up five young children; he is likely to have financial burdens. The social network he has developed with Ann will be partially dissolved, and he will lose his role as a husband and assume that of a widower. He will need to comfort his children and parents-in-law. He will grieve deeply.

Before Ann's death, her husband must deal with making these adjustments at a time when he is still taking care of and hoping to communicate with Ann. There will be financial problems and practical problems as well as emotional problems. He will try to normalize a life that is no longer normal.

The children will be profoundly affected by their mother's impending death. She will be ill much of the time, often too tired to play with them. There will be medical crises, requiring trips to the hospital. Mother and father will often express grief. Few plans will be made for the future, and then one day mother will no longer be with them. The older children at least will try to understand what it means that Mom is dead.

Ann's parents and friends are likely to face their own fears and inadequacies in their attempts to communicate. While they want to understand and to share their feelings, they may not know what to say. Because they may be afraid to dwell on a morbid topic like death, they may avoid the subject altogether. In their visits few people are likely to talk about their own feelings. They may become distressed if Ann becomes jealous of their good health. They may be unable to deal with her anger, pain, and discomfort.

It is very difficult to help a patient work through his or her emotions, and simultaneously accept the silence of a patient who refuses to communicate. Alterness, compassion, and willingness to be completely open to the patient are requisites for family and friends if they are to help the patient. Such communication can also help family and friends. Very often, family members and friends stop touching dying patients. This withdrawal may be a symptom of *anticipatory grief,* but it can leave the patient extremely lonely.

The phenomenon of anticipatory grief is important in understanding reactions to the dying [10, 20, 37, 39]. Anticipatory grief involves beginning the grieving process before the loss occurs. Ann's husband may prepare himself for various aspects of life after the death during the period before her death. Anticipatory grief involves a consideration of the feelings that will occur in the bereavement; it may sometimes help a person to regain a normal level of functioning in a shorter period of time. The opportunity to live with the idea of eventual bereavement may help bring about a more adequate use of a person's recuperative resources.

Bereavement and Grieving

The death of someone close puts a person in a condition of bereavement. *Grief* is the psychological response to bereavement. It involves how the survivor feels and the effects on thinking, eating, sleeping, and other general aspects of daily life. When someone is grief-stricken, this person is experiencing a serious interruption in the total patterning of his or her life [10, 25, 41, 45].

Components of Grief. There are usually five components of grief [23]. First is somatic (bodily) weakness, which includes many of the elements of depression. An individual who is grieving tends to be exhausted and unable to expend energy. Usually there is a marked decrease in appetite. The individual reports feeling "hollow" and having a sense of unreality. The second component of grief is a preoccupation with the image of the deceased person. Bereaved persons often report that they find themselves daydreaming of their interactions with the deceased person. They hear the deceased person talk, may see people who look like him or her, and may have recurring dreams about the person.

A third component of grief is guilt. Bereaved persons think carefully over the period of time before the death in an effort to understand their contribution to the death. If, for example, the friend or relative died in an accident, the bereaved person may think over and over of what his or her contribution to the accident might have been. Or they might say, "I should have taken him to the doctor sooner." Fourth, bereaved people often act with hostility toward others. They

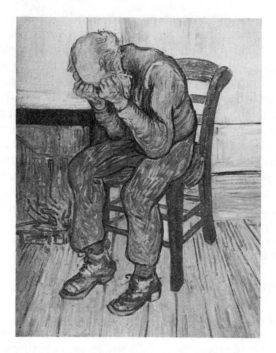

Figure 9-1. *Treurende Man* ("Grieving Man," Vincent van Gogh, 1890. (By permission of Rijksmuseum Kröller-Müller, Otterlo, Holland.)

may express a sense of anger at others who are not bereaved, and they may withdraw from other people or become very formal and stiff in their manner of social interaction. Fifth and finally, the daily activities of bereaved people usually show many changes. They are restless and lack the capacity to initiate and maintain organized patterns of activity. They may be surprised to find how much of their customary activity was done in meaningful relationship to the deceased and how this behavior has lost its significance [22].

The duration of the grief reaction depends a lot upon the success with which a person does what is called *grief work* [34]. Grief work involves the rechanneling of intense feelings of attachment. One of the obstacles to grief work is the fact that many people try to avoid the intense emotional distress that is connected with the grief experience. The length of the grief reaction also depends on the centrality of the deceased individual to the bereaved person, the nature of the relationship, and the degree of dependency of the bereaved person. Interestingly, it has been found that with respect to marital relationships, the more ambivalent the bereaved person's feelings were toward the person who died, the more difficult is the grieving response. There are then contradictory feelings to reconcile. Ambivalence coupled with dependency may make it extremely difficult for the bereaved to work through their grief finally.

The grief process can sometimes be transformed into a meaningful and productive pursuit. If the individuals who are grieving emphasize positive ideals, they can expend their energies in grieving by channeling them with enormous productivity into worthwhile pursuits. They can devote themselves to tasks that were left undone by the deceased rather than dissipate energy in an unstructured, self-pitying way. It is important that they deal with the emotional aspects of grieving, however, and not ignore them [7, 8, 41].

Effects on the Spouse. The issue of bereavement is very significant to the health care professional. Here we consider the deepest form of bereavement—the effects on an individual of the death of a spouse. There are many similarities, however, between the bereavement process when a spouse dies and bereavement in general. Thus many of the issues reported here can be generalized to other settings.

A study of grief conducted at Harvard University was reported in a book by Ira Glick, Robert Weiss, and C. Murray Parkes, *The First Year of Bereavement* [22]. The study focused on the bereavement of young men and women who lost a spouse. The researchers considered both the sociological and psychological side of bereavement. Sociological questions involved the effects of the death on a spouse's place in society and his or her place in the social structure. Psychological questions involved inner experiences, feelings of loneliness, and the length of the grieving process. The researchers attempted to understand the usual or expected pattern of grieving. They looked for processes that would prevent the person from recovering in part or in whole. The primary method of collecting data in the study involved informal open-ended interviews that concentrated on experiences.

People who suddenly found themselves widows or widowers felt overwhelmed. They felt shock and anguish, and it seemed to them that there were no limits to the suffering. They usually felt numb and feared that they would never be able again to move or act or think. Some felt that the pain would never stop. The findings showed that men and women responded somewhat differently to the bereavement. Women's reactions were more intense than men's, and they often emphasized a feeling of abandonment. The men, on the other hand, felt a feeling of dismemberment. The marriage had sustained the men's capacity to work, and they tended to become disorganized in their existing work patterns. The newly widowed women felt more in control once they were able to realize that they could go to work and take care of themselves. These sex differences reflect the differences in meaning of the marriage itself to the men and women in the study.

After the first shock of the death had been experienced, there were feelings of bewilderment and despair. The individuals experienced periods of weeping, although widowers in the study more often reported feeling "choked up" partly because they were unable to express their feelings with tears. Physical symptoms appeared and sometimes lingered for weeks or months. Symptoms included poor appetite, headaches, dizziness, sleep disturbances, and various pains. Controlling the expressions of sorrow was often very difficult, particularly for the women. It was found, however, that while many women who could not control their emotions were afraid that they were headed for a "nervous breakdown," most of them assumed a stance of responsibility and competence and began to trust in their own abilities. Men and women differed in their ability to express emotion, and this factor had an impact on recovery and their ability to come to grips with the death. Whereas the direct expression of emotion by the widows may have seemed at times to be overwhelming, they may have ultimately been somewhat better off than the men who kept the emotion inside. Men were more likely to blame themselves for factors contributing to the death of their wives. The men would say, "I wasn't sensitive enough to her" or "I should have made things easier." The guilt reaction was resolved, however, when friends who knew both the husband and wife helped the husband gain some rational control.

One of the most important aspects of the bereavement process is the *leave-taking ceremony*, which usually takes the form of a funeral. The ceremony establishes the fact that the individual has died, making it an emotional reality both for the widowed person and for others. Social validation of the change, that is, agreement of people in the social network of the bereaved, is necessary [34].

Mourning is the public or ritual display of grief. Like births and marriages, deaths are social events. Community involvement is necessary both to aid the evolution of social relationships and to maintain the psychological health of the bereaved. Funerals, cemetery visits, memorials, the wearing of special clothing, and changed social activities are all rituals that may help both mourners and the community to adapt gradually to a death.

For a short time after the bereavement, the bereaved person receives a lot of attention. However, much of this attention is soon withdrawn; the deceased remains dead, but the practical and emotional problems of everyday life continue. The bereaved individual is left with the realization that he or she must begin to organize life alone. The help that was given in the early days of bereavement is no longer forthcoming, and there is less tolerance among friends for open displays of sorrow.

Many widowed individuals (particularly women) engage in what Robert Kastenbaum calls an *obsessional review* [22]. The bereaved person reviews over and over again the details of the death, and while this activity may seem worthless, Glick and colleagues suggest that the review serves a vital function. It helps the widowed persons to integrate the emotional and cognitive aspects of the loss. Mulling over the loss may be a very painful experience and it may be considered by others to be a useless exercise, but this process is an important component of the work of grieving. The individual must slowly detach his or her intense feelings from the deceased person, which takes time.

Finally, the Glick study found that many of the widows felt deeply immersed in memories of their husbands. They found these memories comforting. At first, they idealized the dead spouse, but as they recovered, they would begin to see the spouse realistically with both positive and negative attributes. Often, however, the bereaved individual would express a fear of "going crazy" because of having extremely vivid visual and tactile memories of the spouse. These memories were often described by the bereaved individuals as similar to hallucinations. Fear of insanity is quite common in the bereaved, and it is important for the health care professional to recognize that these reactions occur and to assure bereaved persons that they are really all right.

The bereaved person must recover both emotionally and socially from the loss. Social recovery includes becoming involved again in activities, making new friends, reestablishing relationships with old friends, and going back to work. Emotional adjustment involves being able to cope effectively with thoughts of the deceased person, only infrequently having nightmares about the person, and no longer expressing or even feeling extreme sorrow. Women tend to recover more quickly emotionally, whereas men appear to recover more quickly socially. A man may appear to be socially recovered from his wife's death—going back to work, making new friends, and perhaps even dating or remarrying. However, he may not have completely coped emotionally with the death. A woman, on the other hand, may actually "feel better" about the death but still refrain from social activities, which are important to her recovery. An understanding of the need for balanced recovery is extremely important.

In the United States, mourning has traditionally been a relatively private affair. Faced with the guilt, anger, and disorientation of grief work, widows and widowers may feel lost in modern society, especially when there are few ties to an extended family [7, 8]. Throughout this book, we have seen the importance of social support for a variety of conditions; such support groups also now exist to help people cope with death. Groups exist for widows and widowers, for suicide survivors and their families, and for those of various religions. Especially helpful are groups for parents who have lost a child. The topic of children and death is considered later in this chapter.

The Amish Way of Death. To examine the importance of family systems to dying and death, the Amish way of death was studied by Kathleen Bryer [5]. The Amish are a distinct cultural and religious group who live in Pennsylvania. To preserve their way of life, the Amish have kept strong family ties and avoided the American cultural mainstream. Many use a horse and buggy instead of an automobile. Since they are a close-knit and separate society, the Amish behavior concerning death provides a good example of the importance of social psychological factors.

The Amish, like most societies before the twentieth century, emphasize the importance of death. The act of preparing funeral clothing (before death) is a type of anticipatory grief. After a death, neighbors notify the community. The body is embalmed and brought home, where it is dressed in white. Women are placed in the same white cape that they wore at baptism and marriage. The body is placed in the center of the house where it is viewed by relatives, neighbors, and friends. The coffin is then viewed again at the cemetery.

Many Amish die at home, where caring for the terminally ill is viewed in a positive light. Many of the ill reach the stage of quiet acceptance before their death and seeing this acceptance helps the family cope with their grief. When a tragic death occurs, other Amish families who have had a similar experience may travel to the bereaved to provide comfort and support. Strong social support is maintained for at least a year after the death; this length of time for continuing support is crucial since grief may last for a year or two. This support may take the form of visits, letters, and handmade gifts. Quilting projects and similar gatherings are a special source of support for widows. Proper concern with death is used to enhance the quality of life.

The Amish way of death is, unfortunately, very different from that dominant in America today [12]. For most Americans, death occurs in an institution replete with restrictions and away from the extended family. Death is hidden and is certainly not a central aspect of life. This orientation often creates great problems for friends, relatives, and health professionals. Even recent attempts to improve care of the dying are often turned over to death professionals.

Some aspects of concern with a "proper" death in our culture may even represent a further attempt to deny death. That is, death is seen as an event that can be managed by hospices and therapists; the stark, challenging fact of death itself can be managed. Instead of hiding death, we may now, to some extent, be smothering death with "therapeutic" intervention. Along these lines, Kastenbaum has called attention to the phenomenon of "healthy dying" [26, 27]. This paradoxical term refers to the quest for a glorious death in which all psychological and social needs are met. A fine line exists between humanized care of the dying (recognizing the fact of death) and unrealistic expectations of death as a very positive experience. These differences must be distinguished [27].

THE CAREGIVER'S REACTION TO DYING PATIENTS

Individuals who work intensively with dying patients must come to grips with the feelings that are stirred in them by their day-to-day contact with death. Without successfully facing these emotions, the health care professional may experience the phenomenon of *burnout,* an emotional exhaustion in which concern for patients as people disappears (see also Chapter 10) [35]. Without a firm acceptance and understanding of their own feelings about death, practitioners may become overwhelmed by the distress that they experience and may develop an unhealthy insensitivity to dying patients [16, 17].

Health care professionals face several stresses when they are dealing with dying patients [17]. First is an identification with dying patients; that is, the caregiver will tend to recognize his or her own limits and mortality. This shared sense of humanity leads to a consciousness of the fact that death is part of life. Second, the process of the disengagement from or "letting go" of the patient can be traumatic for the health care professional. Disengagement tends to be accompanied by a sense of loss, and also a sense of failure professionally. The caregiver's goal is to keep the patient alive and to heal the patient. A death may be seen as a failure, especially if the goals of the medical profession are perceived in a narrow manner. Third, health care professionals may experience confusion, grief, anger, loneliness, inadequacy, guilt, alienation, and a host of other emotions in their care of dying patients. These feelings might be experienced with such intensity that they can lead the health care professional to withdraw from the care of dying patients [17, 18, 43, 48].

Some health care professionals attempt to deal with overwhelming anxiety by intellectualizing the situation and by detaching themselves from a recognition of the patient as a person. This defensiveness allows the health care professional to avoid identification with the patient. For example, the health care professional might perceive the patient's needs as requiring a mechanistic kind of ritualized care. Such treatment would of course be detrimental, both to the patient and ultimately to the professional.

While the reactions of health care professionals to dying patients are in part dependent upon their personalities and their backgrounds, a number of social psychological factors are at work to influence their reactions. Since some health care professionals see the death of a patient as a loss of their own control, they may attempt to gain mastery of the situation by engaging in obsessive-compulsive, perfectionistic technical care. They may find it difficult to recognize and acknowledge that there are many situations in medicine in which there is little or nothing that can be done to save the patient and prevent death. A second way in which the health care professional may attempt to bring about a sense of order to patient care is through emotional distancing from the patient. The practitioner might take refuge in a technical understanding of the disease process. If the health care professional has not come to grips with his or her own feelings about death in general, his or her own death, and the patient's death, these ways of coping may influence reactions to future patients. The physical and emotional distancing might take on larger and larger proportions with each successive patient.

As we have stated, health care professionals often react to dying patients with strong emotions. These feelings, however, are not legitimate or acceptable in health care settings such as the intensive care or coronary care units of a hospital. In the structure of caregiving, there is little acceptance of expression of emotion in response to dying patients or of discussion of the caregiver's personal philosophies regarding dying. The *social setting* in which these health care professionals are required to work may force them to deny their natural emotional responses to dying patients. The action-oriented milieu in which care is provided for dying patients in an acute care hospital prevents the expression of grief among health care professionals who also experience bereavement when a patient to whom they have grown close dies [28]. Thus it is not only the pressures of facing death, but also the need to resolve emotional responses *after* the death of a patient, that are important for health care professionals. Health care professionals can experience a great deal of loneliness and isolation. When the death occurs, the caregiver, who may have had a long-term relationship with the patient, must return to work immediately and be involved in establishing similar relationships with yet more dying patients. The caregiver is, for the most part, denied the opportunity to grieve.

Changes in some institutions in recent years have helped eliminate some of these problems. In many acute care hospitals, physicians, nurses, aides, and technicians working in high-stress settings cannot function effectively within the old system. Therefore a number of hospitals have developed support groups for health professionals working with seriously ill or terminally ill patients [6]. In addition, classes on death and dying are increasingly popular for both medical personnel and laypersons. In hospitals, these support groups, seminar discussions, and experiential group meetings are often led by psychologists or social workers on the hospital staff. These groups allow health care professionals to legitimize and recognize each other's feelings. They work together to find meaning in their care of patients, and they help each other find ways of dealing with the stresses and emotional reactions they encounter. The health care professionals can also help each other overcome feelings of isolation that are brought out by detachment from the family and the patient, which is part of the traditional professional role of the health professional.

Finally, the training of health care professionals should help them see that the prolongation of life is not the only goal of medicine. The meaning of the job of the health care professional is far broader than providing care for the patient solely on a biological dimension. Health care professionals need to realize that some of the care they provide can be purely psychosocial in nature and that this is an important and meaningful activity. In some cases, the caregiver can enter into a mutually supportive relationship with the family and the dying patient. That is, the health care provider may not only *give* emotional support to the family but may also *derive* support from them. The family members can often be very helpful in providing information that is useful in the care of the patient, and in helping the health care professional to communicate with the dying patient, both for technical and psychosocial aims [28].

Box 9-1
Pulling the Respirator Plug

The ethical problems in treating those who are almost dead and the legal questions of the definition of death reached national attention in the case of Karen Ann Quinlan, age 21. In 1975 Karen went into a deep coma. She was placed on a respirator and administered other treatments, including special foods and antibiotics. Karen never recovered from her coma. Her neurologists claimed she had extensive brain damage and had no hope of recovery.

After a good deal of soul searching, Karen's parents decided that she should be allowed to die rather than be kept alive by extraordinary means. But the doctors refused to disconnect Karen from the respirator, mostly because of the legal implications. It was, of course, very costly and very disruptive to keep Karen in special medical treatment even though she showed absolutely no signs of conscious life. Her parents sued for the right to pull the plug on her respirator. After a year, during which Karen never regained consciousness and dropped to 71 pounds, the New Jersey Supreme Court ruled that her parents could turn off the respirator and let her die with grace and dignity. The court's ruling set a legal precedent, establishing a right to privacy for persons who are nearly dead biologically that allows them or their guardians to refuse extraordinary treatment that is deemed hopeless.

Several months later the respirator was turned off. However, the matter was not settled, for Karen continued to breathe on her own. With increasingly more technological means available for prolonging life in terminally ill patients, the ethics of withholding extraordinary treatment is likely to become a more important issue in health care. Some aspects of the problem can be addressed through more modern definitions of biological death. However, the answers to many of the questions will depend on society's evolving conception of the social meaning of dying and death.

Information reported in "Karen Lives On," *Newsweek*, June 7, 1976.

CHILDREN AND DEATH

There are two social psychological issues that are important in understanding children and death. One involves an understanding of parental and other adult reactions to the child who is dying; it involves the feelings of these persons and their ability to come to grips with the child's impending death. The second issue concerns the child's own view of death. For many reasons, we need to understand to what extent children can conceive of death, and how they think of it in different ways at different ages.

These two issues are extremely important to health care. When a child is dying, the entire family needs the health professional's care—not just the child who is ill. Health care professionals can provide optimal care only if they understand the family's reactions. In understanding adult reactions to childhood death, health care professionals can also gain insight into their own feelings about dealing with dying children. The child who is dying can be helped to understand what is happening, and can be encouraged to come to grips with impending death [43, 48]. In addition, understanding childhood reactions to the concept of death and to the death of loved ones helps the health care professional to care more effectively for a child who is bereaved. Let us first look at the issue of adult, parental, and family responses to the child who is dying.

Reactions to the Child Who Is Dying

There are two primary objectives of the health care professional who is dealing with a dying child. The first is to help the child respond both physically and emotionally as positively as possible to the ups and downs that may accompany a life-threatening illness. Health care professionals need to support the child as this child is coping with the crises of illness. The second, but equally important, task of the health care professional is to keep the family together and functioning during this period, which is one of the greatest crises a family can face.

When a child is dying, it may be very difficult for parents to focus on the present instead of the future. Adults tend to see childhood as a preparatory period, rather than as a time in a person's life that is worthwhile in and of itself. Hence the first step in helping the family involves teaching parents that although the child will not have an adult future, the child is alive in the present. There should be a significant concern for the quality of the life the child has left [25].

A reorientation *can* be accomplished, but it is not easy. A dying child places a tremendous stress on a family—on parents and on the other children in the family as well [18, 30]. This stress takes its toll; the family is actually also a victim. In one research study on dying children, about half of the couples involved required some kind of psychiatric care. In another study, a very large percentage of the marriages of the parents either became troubled or failed during the care of a dying child. The stress is accentuated partly because in an effort to construct a more or less normal life for the whole family during the illness of the sick child, parents shelter the child who is ill. The parents withdraw from other people. In their desire to avoid explanations to other people and endurance of their pity, parents may withdraw from close friends and other members of their family. Thus parents of dying children become isolated at just the time when they require the most support. Some members of couples become more alienated from each other at this time. They sometimes cannot understand each other's reactions to the child, and each thinks the other is indifferent or unrealistic in dealing with the problem [20, 30].

In addition to support from others, most parents of dying children need *information*. There is a definite thirst for information that is usually not satisfied even by supportive health care professionals. The parents need some idea of what to expect in the child's reaction to medical treatment. Even though health care professionals cannot guarantee certain reactions, giving the parents some indication of the odds (the bad news as well as good news) can be very important. For example, parents should know about some of the side effects of chemotherapy so that if a child begins to exhibit behaviors that are worrisome, the parents will know that these reactions are to be expected [33]. Second, parents need information to allay their guilt and fears that they are responsible in some way for the child's illness [20]. In the case of cancer, for example, public advertising stresses the importance of early detection. If a child's leukemia is diagnosed late and the child has little chance of recovery, the parent may feel a great deal of guilt as a result. In fact, however, early diagnosis of leukemia often makes little difference in the likelihood of remission.

Parents of dying children need support and guidance in coping with their emotions, and they need information about how the disease and treatment will affect the child. Parents of dying children increasingly address these needs through support groups led by health care professionals. Support groups provide information to the parent, teach the parent to recognize signals of an impending medical crisis, and show ways in which to deal with the illness, all of which gives parents a sense of control. Parents of dying children share information with each other about their emotional reactions. There is some evidence that parents who are able to share their grief over the impending death of a child may stand up better to the burdens of the serious illness than those who are isolated from other people. However, the support groups are not needed by everyone, and some parents may deal with the child's fatal illness better by talking with one person such as the health care professional. Treatment should be structured so that parents have a choice.

The Child's Conception of Death

In a society like ours, in which we strive to put death out of sight and out of mind, children's reactions to death are slighted and children are often left to deal alone with their feelings about death. Adults often assume that children cannot understand the meaning of death and that children do not experience grief during bereavement. But according to various research and clinical findings, children do have very definite ideas about death—ideas that change at different developmental stages in their lives [1, 25, 38, 42]. They think about their own death, and they react with great (although not always overtly expressed) feeling to the death of someone close to them.

It is easy for adults to misconstrue or not even perceive children's responses to death. It is easy to misinterpret behavior that children may exhibit concernig death. Robert Kastenbaum [25] and Maria Nagy [38] (a psychologist, who in the late 1940s studied Hungarian children) have identified three phases in a child's awareness of personal mortality and the mortality of others close to the child. The first stage lasts until about age five. The child at this age does not recognize death as final, but sees being dead as somewhat like being less alive. The young child regards death as a kind of sleep that takes place in an uninteresting place called a grave. Death disturbs the young child, but only because the child sees it as something that separates people from each other and because life in a grave seems uncomfortable and dull.

Between the ages of five and nine, the child develops a second kind of awareness of death. The child sees death as something or someone that strikes people down. Although the child understands that death is final, the child has an important ego-protective feature, believing that death can be avoided. The child believes that by being clever (e.g., never getting hit by a car) he or she can avoid death.

Finally, around age nine or ten the child enters the third stage of recognition of death. The child begins to recognize death not only as final but also as something that is inevitable. Thus it is not until nearly age nine that children can fully understand the concept of death. This is not to say, however, that a child at the age of six does not have visions of a friend, sibling, or parent as dead. And this is not to say that the child does not know the person is missing. Even though the child does not fully understand what death means, the child can be profoundly affected by the absence of the close person.

A child's conception of death is limited by basic processes of cognitive development. As the Swiss psychologist Jean Piaget has noted, most children under age seven cannot take the perspective of another person. They are *egocentric* in that they are able to view the world only from their own point of view. They cannot easily imagine the reactions of others to an impending death and cannot imagine themselves in the place of someone who is dying. Furthermore, it is not until about age eleven that children enter Piaget's stage of *formal operations* and can begin to think about the meaning of death in the abstract [40].

Children at various ages think about death a lot, and they are threatened by it. Children can have very strong reactions to bereavement and can understand something of what it means if they find out they are dying. The child with a terminal illness may experience significant fear and anxiety about eventually being left alone (e.g., in a grave). This anticipated separation from others can be highly distressing. Children need to be assured that they will not be left alone. Parents and health care professionals should do as much as they can to concentrate on living each moment fully with the child while the child is still alive. Of course the approach that involves concentrating on living can be successful only if the parents themselves and other people around the child are themselves successful in concentrating on the present, and they do not withdraw or treat the child in a distressing, ambivalent, or discrepant way [2, 43, 46, 48]. The child's inquiries or desires for information should not be avoided. On the contrary, the child's fears may bring about questioning, which if avoided could increase anxiety significantly. Thus with any curiosity on the part of the child, an attempt should be made to explain what is happening in terms that the child can understand.

The Bereaved Child. What happens when death separates children from someone who is important to them? Children may lose parents, grandparents, or siblings—people who are significant in their daily life. If a parent or grandparent dies, the surviving spouse or children of the grandparent may be temporarily unable to care for the child. If a sibling has died, the parents may be so immersed in their own grief that they may have little energy for dealing with or even recognizing the impact of the death on the brothers and sisters of the child who has died. Thus a child who experiences bereavement is likely to face two sources of stress according to Kastenbaum. First, the child may be deprived of the usual support expected from the parents because the parents are too busy dealing with the death themselves. A child is likely not to eat as well or get as much rest as before, thus placing the child at greater risk for accidents and mishaps. Second, the child must deal with his or her own grief. Adults in this situation often fail to interpret the child's grief response accurately [4, 19].

The child's emotional response (the grief response) depends on a number of factors. First, the child's age is important. It may be particularly distressing for the child to lose someone to death very soon after recognizing that death is final. The child has not had a chance to come to grips with this realization, and it may be profoundly threatening. The quality of the child's personal and family situation before the bereavement is relevant as well. If the child is immersed in a close-knit family and has a strong sense of love and security, the child is probably less likely to be threatened by the death of someone close. However, if a child's life is filled with anxiety and insecurity, the child's entire world can be shaken by the death of someone very close. Thus an understanding of each child's individual situation is important in trying to understand the child's bereavement reaction.

Bereaved children do not always express distress in ways that are obviously related to the loss. Instead the child might experience serious difficulties in school, show behavioral problems, attack people with sudden anger, and express fears of the dark or of being alone. An atmosphere of acceptance must be provided in order for the child to express feelings openly. Children may express their memories of a person that they have lost by acting out specific activities that were associated with the dead person. These acts can be extremely distressing to an adult. For example, a child who has lost a sibling might engage in the very activities that were always shared with that sibling, giving a constant reminder to the parents of the painful absence. Even as young as two or three years old, a child may express longing and sadness over the absence of a parent through actions such as playing with toys that were usually used with the parent who has died, or walking in places where the parent usually took the child [4, 19, 25].

At other times children withdraw and become aloof or seemingly uncaring. This reaction may lead adults to conclude that the child has forgotten the significant death, and the child does not need to talk about it or to resolve the feelings. Research on childhood bereavement suggests that partially because of a misunderstanding on the part of adults, and partially because it may simply be easier for the adult to choose not to deal with the child's reactions, many children bear an enormous amount of pain completely alone with no one to share their grief. At other times a child may not be silent but instead engage in an overt expression of anger toward the person who has died. Some adults find it extremely painful to tolerate a child's feelings of anger that are expressed toward the deceased person. These angry reactions, of course, do not mean that the child did not love or does not miss the deceased person, but rather that the child's reaction to loss is anger.

SUICIDE

At the beginning of this chapter we saw that the college student, Mark, is contemplating suicide. So far in this chapter we have focused mainly on patients who want very much to live. Suicide is, however, another aspect of dying and death relevant to health care. Much has been written in sociology, philosophy, and theology about the subject of suicide. Scholars have long studied the motivations of people who kill themselves, the rightness or wrongness of the act, and the impact that suicide has on society as a whole. Social psychological research on suicide provides us with answers to some of the questions that are relevant to the effective care of patients [13, 28].

Nearly all health care professionals encounter the threat of suicide at some point in their careers. Health care professionals, who are primarily oriented to saving lives, are likely to find themselves experiencing very negative reactions to individuals who threaten or attempt suicide. Such reactions are unfortunate since such people need help. They need emotional support, assistance in dealing with their problems, and sensitivity. Anger and hostility, whether expressed overtly or covertly to a patient, are likely to be counterproductive. Negative attitudes from others are already a source of strain for the person who has found it impossible to cope with life as it is.

If a person does commit suicide, the family and friends are likely to need help to deal with the death. Bereavement, as we have seen, is difficult enough in itself, but the process of grieving for someone who has died by taking his or her own life can be especially hard on family and friends because of their guilt. They wish they had understood, heard the warning signals, and provided support for this person. The process of adjustment of family and friends to a suicide is difficult. Thus health care professionals have to dissociate their feelings of anger toward the individual who committed suicide from the feelings and behavior toward the people who remain. Only by resolving this anger and making sure that it is not transferred to the bereaved survivors can effective health care be provided for the survivors. Since the health care professional is often the first person encountered by the family and friends of the suicide victim (or by the individual who has attempted suicide), it is important to understand what has been learned about suicide in years of research.

Myths About Suicide

A number of *myths* have developed over the years regarding suicide. First, while it is often believed that someone who talks about suicide will not attempt it, research has shown that about three out of every four people who eventually committed suicide had given some kind of hint ahead of time to others. An individual's threat of suicide is a cry for help [15].

It is also a misconception that suicide is specific to any particular group of people. People in all income and social status brackets commit suicide, and not only depressed people commit suicide. While people with a psychiatric diagnosis of depression do have a higher suicide rate than those with other psychiatric disorders and those with no known psychiatric disorder, suicide is not a risk only with depressed people. A person may not even seem particularly unhappy before attempting suicide [25].

Another myth about suicide is that people are "out of their minds" when deciding to kill themselves. While some suicides are obviously related to mental disorders, others have no relationship to psychosis at all. It is also not true that only a psychiatrist or mental health professional can prevent a suicide. There is much evidence that human resources of a community including people without any professional training can help to prevent suicides simply by providing emotional support and caring.

When someone who has attempted suicide recovers, this person is in particular danger. After the first attempted suicide, the individual has received a lot of attention from family members, friends, and health care professionals. After recovery (and discharge from the hospital), however, the person may again feel lonely and detached from others, and may attempt suicide again.

Preventing Suicide

Robert Kastenbaum has suggested some guidelines for understanding and dealing with suicide [25]. Many suicides can be prevented, although there is no general formula for dealing with a person who is suicidal. All suicidal threats should be taken seriously, but it does not mean that someone hearing the threat should panic. An individual who verbalizes a threat of suicide may be trying to get attention, and it is important to be sure that the individual who has threatened suicide is not dared to carry it out. Sometimes goading is done on a very subtle level. If an individual's troubled state of mind is belittled, this person will respond with a heightened need to do something desperate to have others recognize the seriousness of the threat.

Value judgments should not be made about the person's intentions. Telling someone suicide is wrong is likely to be responded to negatively. An individual may not only be unconvinced not to attempt suicide, but may realize that another's value system is very different from his or her own, and therefore may come to value the act positively. It is very important to note that many people end up being successful at suicide when their intention was actually only to get attention by providing an obvious threat. The person's motives may be meant only as a gesture, signifying "I will show them. I'll make them wish they had appreciated me."

Fortunately, resources are increasingly available in most communities from schools, religious groups, and mental health centers. Community crisis intervention lines and services are often available to help people who are responding to a crisis in their lives with a threat of suicide. Friends of potential suicide victims will also be better able to cope with the situation if they know that additional help is available by telephone.

Justifiable Suicide?

Is suicide ever justified? Many people fear suffering or old age more than they fear death. This fact was dramatically demonstrated recently when a British organization produced a manual on how to kill oneself. For example, it described the lethal combinations of common drugs. Many thousands of people tried to join this organization and obtain the book *(A Guide to Self-Deliverance)*. Since both the United States and Great Britain have laws against aiding and abetting suicide, a host of legal and ethical issues arise concerning such matters. Do people have the right to such medical information? Or is it better, for example, to risk having people live with extensive brain damage that can result from a botched suicide attempt? As people gain more control over their health care, such questions will join the traditional questions (e.g., "Is suicide always wrong?") in the public's interest [44].

Especially problematic is the so-called passive suicide by the chronically ill. Many hemodialysis patients may ignore their diet and refuse dialysis, and diabetes patients may refuse insulin and cancer patients may turn down chemotheraphy. There are two ways in which such cases differ from other unhealthy behaviors like smoking and from the refusal to treat acute illness like an infection:

First, the natural process is already one of serious deterioration, and second, there may be severe problems, such as extreme discomfort, associated with the treatment. However, just as active suicide is influenced by psychosocial forces, so too is passive suicide. In the right social situation even the chronically ill can hold a positive outlook on life (see also Box 9-1).

Suicide Among the Elderly

Geriatric suicide is a surprisingly common phenomenon in this country as well as in many other countries. In 1975 people over 60 represented 18.5 percent of the population, but committed 23 percent of the suicides. And while the suicide rate for women in the United States reaches its peak by the age of 55, male suicide rates rise steadily with age through the eighties. Between the ages of 65 and 69, male suicides outnumber female suicides by 4 to 1, and by age 85 they outnumber female suicides by 12 to 1 [36].

While younger persons attempt suicide as a means of manipulating others, a cry for help, or as a reaction to an overwhelming but temporary crisis, older persons attempt suicide in a determined effort to bring their life to a close. Older persons use more violent and obviously effective methods to kill themselves than do younger persons. They shoot, hang, or drown themselves, or they jump from high places. Firearms represent the major means of elderly suicide. Rarely do the suicide attempts of older people fail; they are usually saved only by an accidental, unanticipated occurrence (such as someone coming home unexpectedly). They rarely use suicide prevention services available in the community [36].

Older people commit suicide for a wide variety of reasons, most of which have to do with *loss*. Losses may be economic or social (loss of income, financial insecurity, or job status), physical (loss of health and vigor), emotional (loss of spouse), or psychological (loss of self-esteem and confidence to cope with distressing or challenging events or loss of enthusiasm and resilience). Older people often suffer more than one loss at once [11]. Whether or not an older person is able to cope with the stress of the many problems he or she must face is partly a function of patterns developed in the past. It is important to recognize, however, that many of the problems faced by the elderly are not resolvable (e.g., loss of a spouse a person has had for 60 years or terminal illness), and the elderly person in question simply makes a judgment about whether or not he or she is willing to live under the new circumstances [36].

What can be done? Little is being done about the issue now, partly because a general societal attitude is that older people are not pro-

Box 9-2
Is Your Body Your Own?

A controversial issue of increasing importance involves the extent to which a person retains control over what is done to his or her body. Some of these cases involve extraordinary life-preserving equipment (see Box 9–1). But many cases concern questions of medical judgment and the quality of life. In one case, a 72-year-old woman with gangrenous feet refused to have an amputation. The gangrene was almost surely fatal, but with the operation she would have a 50-50 chance to live; the doctors went to court to have her declared incompetent to make this decision. In another case, parents of a child with leukemia refused to allow chemotherapy since they believed they could better treat the disease through diet and other means. In still other cases, members of certain religious groups refuse promising treatment because it is against their religion to receive blood transfusions, take certain medication, or engage in certain other modern medical treatments.

Should such patients be forced to be treated? Should such parents of ill children be prosecuted as criminals? Are medical personnel who respect a patient's wishes guilty of malpractice or other crimes? Questions like these often end up in the courts. In many cases, however, they are not legal questions but ethical questions instead. It is up to patients, medical personnel, theologians, as well as lawyers, to decide such issues. Each individual must participate in the decision and share in the responsibility.

For further reading: R. Hunt and J. Arras (eds.), *Ethical Issues in Modern Medicine* (Palo Alto, Calif.: Mayfield Co., 1977).

ductive members of the community. Because they have little ahead of them, people believe that they ought to be allowed to die if that is their preference. The suicide of an older person, however, can have profound effects on the people closest to that person and on other old people. Geriatric suicide itself reflects the sad plight of older people in our society, and their devaluation as human beings. Interestingly, most older people who have committed suicide visited a physician within a month of the suicide. Many of them visited the doctor within the space of a week. Rarely, however, do physicians even bring up the issue of how a person is feeling about him or herself [11]. The prevalence of geriatric suicide is unlikely to be reduced unless we provide the elderly with something worthwhile for which to live (see Box 9-2).

SUMMARY

Death is the greatest crisis of life. In our society the fact that each of us must die someday is met with profound denial by many people. As a result, dying patients, who exemplify human mortality, are often rejected by the living, and their needs are ignored. The dying frequently become angry, depressed, afraid, and, most of all, lonely. Dying may be made easier for the patient and for family, friends, and health professionals if the emotions surrounding dying are brought out into the open and dealt with knowledgeably. For the survivors, bereavement can be an experience of emotional growth.

Dying as well as bereaved children require particular attention because of their limited understanding of the meaning of death. The parents of dying and bereaved children need special support from health professionals to help them deal with the children's responses. In this chapter, we have suggested some solutions to the psychosocial problems surrounding death and dying.

10
The
Health
Care
Professional

Many people hold a stereotypical image of the health care professional. Doctors are often imagined to be attractive and wise white men who are able to solve a tremendous variety of health problems. This image is exemplified by such television characters as Dr. Kildare and Dr. Marcus Welby. The doctor's role may be thought to resemble that of Dr. Albert Schweitzer, the Nobel Peace Prize winner who spent many years ministering to poor people in Africa. Nurses may be imagined to resemble Florence Nightingale, the nineteenth-century female English reformer who improved the training of nurses and the care of patients. In actual fact, however, the role of health care professionals is rarely glamorous, but is instead stressful and difficult. The Albert Schweitzers with a consuming dedication to help humanity are quite rare. Furthermore, health professionals themselves are various types of people with various problems of their own.

Physicians, nurses, physicians' assistants, nurse practitioners, and others on the medical team usually experience intrinsic rewards in helping people, in doing socially useful work, in being exposed to a wide range of human experience, and in facing problems that are intellectually challenging. Some health care professionals also gain the rewards of high income. In general, studies of physicians, nurses, and physicians' assistants suggest that health care professionals are satisfied with their careers. However, health care professionals pay a price, for there is a great deal of emotional distress inherent in the health care occupation and a high suicide rate. There are great pressures in training and in practice, and there is a tremendous psychological drain in taking responsibility for other people's lives and encountering disease and death.

Throughout this book we have discussed how health practitioners examine patients, but in this chapter we turn the tables and examine health care professionals themselves. We consider characteristics of training and of practice, and special problems that health care professionals experience, including "physician impairment." We suggest possible solutions for dealing with these problems, both on an individual and on an aggregate level, and examine what structural changes in the medical care system might help to minimize these stresses. Relatedly, the stress of decisionmaking under uncertainty—which health professionals experience every day—is analyzed as are the factors influencing medical decisionmaking. Finally, we consider the special role of women in medicine.

There are two important reasons why an entire chapter is devoted to understanding the position of the health care professional. First, individuals in the health care professions who are reading about the social and psychological aspects of medicine will recognize that the social and psychological aspects of their *own* lives affect their work. Second, students of social psychology need to understand the experiences of health care professionals in order to work more effectively with them. A social scientist who works in the health care field cannot work in a vacuum; communication between the social psychologist and the health care professional can be effective only if they understand each other.

Most of the research conducted on health care professionals has focused on physicians. However, many of the issues that surface in studies of physicians are relevant to all health care providers, particularly dentists, nurse practitioners, nurses, physicians' assistants, and pharmacists. Many of the research findings on physicians can be generalized to other health care professions (see also Box 10–1).

The quality of health care that is provided to patients depends in part upon social psychological aspects of the lives of the providers of care—of which there are at least 5 million currently. Health care providers are likely to find it very difficult to communicate with their patients or to be very empathic when they are themselves very anxious. There is even some evidence that shows that health care providers under stress are less effective in the technical care that they provide. They may become rigid and make inaccurate diagnoses, or they might even consider patients' complaints trivial because they are so overwhelmed by their own problems [10].

The stresses of health care begin with medical education, and for this reason that is where we begin our discussion.

MEDICAL TRAINING

Medical School

Medical students enter training with high expectations; they have reached the pinnacle of their student careers after having prepared for years for this experience. Often reality does not coincide with these expectations, however, and the resulting problems and stresses may be serious. This situation is not peculiar to medical students; nurses as well as other health professionals also face a stark reality very different from what they hoped it would be.

A popular stereotype of the beginning health student is someone who is highly idealistic and deeply concerned with the physical, emotional, and social problems that people face. Entering medical students generally hope to be interpersonally sensitive and to "help people" [42], but actually by the time the student has begun the first year of medical school, the potential physician has been through many anxiety-provoking experiences that have begun to erode this idealism [3, 4].

Premedical education is highly competitive; at present over 60 percent of the applicants to medical school are rejected. The distress brought about by the competitive pressures of premedical education is often compounded by the fact that some admission criteria are of questionable validity. While the medical profession espouses the belief that a physician should be humanistically oriented and exhibit a sensitive interpersonal approach to patients, almost all of the formal criteria used by most medical schools for admission are academic criteria, such as MCAT (Medical College Admission Test of the Association of American Medical Colleges) scores and grades in science courses. The admission interview is important in some schools, but initial screening is solely on the basis of scientific promise. The successful applicant to medical school can insure being included in the first wave of the admission procedure by becoming heavily technically oriented. A different admission model—under which students are evaluated first on social and interpersonal grounds and *then* screened for scientific competence—is quite rare.

Medical school applicants learn that there is a division between

Box 10-1
The Physician's Assistant

During the past ten years a new health profession has emerged that may cause significant changes in the structure of medicine and nursing; this is the physician's assistant. The physician's assistant is a trained health worker, neither a physician nor a nurse, who is qualified to provide primary health care services to patients. The range of services that can be provided is stringently defined. The physician's assistant receives both academic and practical training and cares for patients under the supervision and direction of a licensed physician, although the physician remains ultimately responsible for the care of the patients.

The physician's assistant differs from the nurse practitioner in that nurse practitioners may operate independently from physicians, whereas physician's assistants work directly with physicians. Until recently, physician's assistants were found primarily in underdeveloped nations, and in the U.S. military, where medical services could be provided in an efficient manner amidst shortages of health manpower. Perhaps the best-known system of using the physician's assistant is in Russia, where the "feldsher" provides a large volume of the medical care to individuals in rural populations.

The number of physician assistant training programs in the United States today is almost 100. Length of training varies. About 1000 graduates of these programs are now in practice and many more are about to be graduated. The average physician assistant in the United States is about 30 years old, usually white and male. About 77 percent of them are engaged in primary care. The physician's assistants function primarily to alleviate health manpower shortages—particularly resulting from the maldistribution of physicians. More primary care professionals are needed, especially among low-income patients. Since there is a shortage of general practitioners, the physician's assistant is important in meeting this need.

The physician's assistant has also been used extensively in an effort to increase the productivity and quality of health care while decreasing its cost. The cost of the physician's assistant's time is about one-sixth that of the physician. The physician can concentrate on more serious cases while the physician's assistant can deliver routine care. It has been found that the quality of care delivered by the physician's assistant is equal to that of the physician, and patient satisfaction is as high as with the physician. When the physician does not have time to spend with patients explaining, counseling, educating, and guiding them, the physician's assistant can take over these tasks. Many of the suggestions made throughout this book about the importance of psychosocial care of patients can be implemented by physician's assistants.

For further reading: E. C. Nelson, A. R. Jacobs, and K. G. Johnson, Patients' acceptance of physician's assistants. *Journal of* the *American Medical Association*, 1974, *228*, 63–67.

their own expectations, or image of the physician's role, and the realities of admission. However, the successful applicant to medical school expects that constant attention to technical issues is a phenomenon of premedical days and that, once in medical school, an orientation toward people can once again be resumed. Unfortunately, idealization of the professional role is once more frustrated in the medical student. During the first two years of medical school, the major goal of most medical school faculties is to teach as much technical information to the medical students as possible. This goal has an unspoken corollary—that the medical students recognize their ignorance. Few students receive A's in medical school, although nearly all have received A's as long as they can remember. This overwhelming onslaught of material presented by the faculty humbles many medical students and encourages caution. This approach is considered important in making a physician. However, it demands enormous adjustment on the part of the medical student. This process continues for the first two years of medical school (the preclinical years) in which the academic work is concentrated. After a full year of learning a tremendous amount of basic material about a normal human body, and another year of learning all of the possible diseases a patient can experience, the medical student is then thrust into the world of patient care.

During the third and fourth years of medical school, the medical student serves as a clinical clerk. The student works on the wards with interns and residents attempting to make diagnoses and helping to plan and administer treatments. Feelings of inconsistency are often experienced by medical students who, in learning a new role, must come to grips with the fact that their self-image as a medical student does not always coincide with reality. Researchers have referred to the realms in which inconsistency is experienced as the *zones of discontinuity* [3, 4].

The first conflict or discontinuity for the medical student arises in the first year. The student has to resolve the problem that there is more material to be learned than is humanly possible in the time given. First-year medical students often complain that there is more material to be memorized in a particular period than can even be read. Furthermore, medical students experience anxiety when thinking about taking care of patients later and realizing that they might be missing a critical piece of information, something that was taught but that they failed to grasp and memorize. And as they begin to recognize their own limitations, students eventually have to understand that medical knowledge itself is limited. There is disagreement among even the most prominent physicians as to how to treat patients; and medicine does not have all the answers. Students find that their faculty members do not always know what to do about a medical problem, and, in addition, some diseases are incurable [21].

Second, medical students often become enormously frustrated when they recognize that they may be becoming cold and calloused toward their patients in dealing with the patients' emotional problems. Students focus on a central goal of finishing the necessary laboratory tests and completing the charts. They may begin to cut corners and save minutes in order to be able to sleep during nights on which they are on call. They may recognize that they are developing unhealthy attitudes toward patients and their feelings, but when the demands of clinical work are high, idealism is threatened. This loss of idealism, with the resultant change in expectations, is a significant source of anxiety for medical students.

Another psychological strain for medical or nursing students is their initial contact with human suffering and death. When a medical student is first faced with a patient who is severely ill or badly hurt, the anxiety can be overwhelming. The student may fear not being able to handle the situation and care for the patient appropriately. Conflict arises within the student for the only stance the student can take with the patient is that of calm assurance. This calm assurance is *expected* by patients and also by colleagues. Consequently, regardless of how much anxiety a student is experiencing, assurance and confidence must be projected. As responsibility increases for the student, there is less time to pay attention to internal fears and emotions. The need to play the part of the assured professional with competence and confidence causes the student to begin eventually to feel very much in control [35].

Finally, student physicians often experience identity crises, which is understandable since the medical student has a dual identity. Among peers and in the eyes of the faculty, the medical student is a "student." But to patients, the medical student is a "doctor." While working with patients, the medical student begins to feel like a doctor, but then the student receives constant reminders from faculty and fellow students that a medical student is *not* a physician. This dual identity or "role conflict" is a common source of anxiety to the medical student.

The stringent medical curriculum often strains the personal lives of medical students [10, 45]. To survive academically, some students have to become compulsive about their work, leaving little time for recreation, friends, and family. Without ties to the "outside world," students lose perspective on what they are doing and miss the emotional support that friends and family can provide. Perhaps the most serious consequence of medical education is the violence done to the self-image of the medical student. The medical student's self-image is systematically broken down by faculty members, who then proceed to build it up again in the mold of the profession. Many faculty members place a major emphasis on purely intellectual values, research activity, and on becoming scientists. This is sometimes in direct conflict to the needs of students for relevancy and for caring for patients. Many students feel abused in the hierarchical system of medical training, and the treatment they receive from others often translates into their own overall feeling of disrespect for patients. Students tend to treat patients as they are treated. Thus, according to some authors, aspects of the medical school experience may actually foster cynicism and a lack of recognition of patients' emotional and social needs [3, 12, 25, 45].

In sum, the traditional medical school milieu brings about conflict and stress in the medical student, stress detrimental to both students and patients.

Suggestions for Improving Medical Education

Student culture involves communication and shared understanding among students in a medical school class. Through informal means students provide information and support for each other—particularly in assessing and validating the demands of the faculty. Most medical school classes, depending on their size, quickly become either one cohesive group or break down into a few smaller groups. In facing the tension experienced during medical education, many students are able to turn to their group members. Students support each other and help each other solve problems. "Student culture" facilitates the adjustment of medical students and develops their ability to cope with the stresses inherent in medical education [4]. At some medical schools discussion groups for medical students are organized by counseling services, and they often receive heavy use.

A second mechanism by which medical students cope with the stress of medical school is through their identification with the faculty. Students learn the role of the health professional by watching physicians and sharing a sense of collegueship with them. As they gain clinical experience, follow in their teachers' footsteps, and are given responsibility for patients, students are rewarded by the fact that they are trusted by others to be competent enough to handle important situations. A new identity is developed through comparison and interaction with established professionals. Appropriate role models are essential for healthy development.

A third and final influence on student coping involves the structure of medical training. The biomedical disease model, which has, up until recent years, been part of the socialization process for the medical student, is now slowly being replaced by what the medical educator Dr. George Engel calls a bio-psycho-social model of medicine [19]. Slowly, medical school training is beginning to incorporate into the study of medicine an understanding of how the social forces, lifestyle preferences, and maladaptive behaviors of patients affect their health. It has been proposed that a biopsychosocial model that emphasizes the issues we have discussed in this book might be of overall benefit for the physician in training as well. In receiving understanding and caring themselves, medical students would learn to develop the same qualities in the care of their patients. It is probably when the faculty has tolerance for the psychological and social aspects of the lives of medical students that medical students can most effectively learn to deliver appropriate care to their patients [10].

Personality and Specialization in Medicine

Medicine is a diversified field that allows a broad spectrum of activity. However, the trend in medical education is toward specialization (including the new "specialty" of primary care). Hence decisions must be made by physicians-in-training (particularly during the last two years of medical school) regarding which of a number of specialty areas (surgery, pediatrics, radiology, etc.) they will enter. In addition, the student must choose whether to perform research, patient care, teaching, or a combination of these things. The choice of specialty is an important decision; each specialty carries with it specific pressures and specific requirements [10].

The suitability of a physician for a particular specialty may be an important factor in the physician's eventual ability to cope with specific stresses of the chosen specialty. Improper specialty choice may produce dissatisfaction with and poor competence in a given field of medical practice [26]. Unfortunately, there is no comprehensive theory of proper specialty choice; no investigator has yet been able to understand completely the factors that affect it. But although the research is in fragments, we do understand some of the factors that influence a physician to choose a particular specialty.

Environmental factors are an important influence [22]. In a number of studies it has been found that faculty influence is important, particularly in recruiting physicians to less prestigious and little known specialties. The popularity of different specialties varies with the times. Before entering medical school, students usually have some idea about their relative preference for surgery, medicine, psychiatry, or general practice, but these preferences are often based on stereotypes, which may be for the most part inaccurate. While they are in medical school students are heavily influenced by faculty members, and therefore the current setting takes on enormous importance in influencing future career choice [4]. At a medical school heavily oriented toward research, students are likely to choose research-related specialties.

A second factor affecting specialty choice involves student characteristics such as personality, values, and academic achievements [24, 48]. However, the research findings are mixed. For example, while popular stereotypes depict psychiatrists as emotionally unstable but interested in intellectual problems, research has found this is not true. Individuals who are attracted to psychiatry are less authoritarian than other students, and they do have higher anxiety about death; but they are not generally unstable. In addition, social and aesthetic values are held in greater esteem by students who decide on psychiatry.

Students who choose surgery tend to have high economic values. Would-be surgeons also tend to prefer treatment and research issues as opposed to the problems that demand dealing with people. In terms of background, it has been found that students from lower-class backgrounds are more likely to choose general practice or family medicine rather than specializing. It has also been found that students from medical families gravitate toward more specialized areas such as ophthalmology, dermatology, and surgery, and that they are less likely than others to choose psychiatry, pediatrics, and obstetrics. Women physicians have traditionally chosen certain specialties like psychiatry, pediatrics, and anesthesiology (also see the section on women in medicine in this chapter).

A "good" choice of specialty is one in which the physician feels comfortable. The choice should be based both on self-knowledge and an awareness of the satisfactions and limitations of the particular specialty. A good choice of specialty involves the appropriate utilization of an individual's talents and abilities. For example, a physician who wants close and reciprocal relationships with patients will do well to choose a specialty such as internal medicine, psychiatry, or family practice, all of which entail continual and intense contact with patients. On the other hand, individuals who need some distance from patients do best to choose surgery or other consulting subspecialities. A particularly stressful situation will occur if, for example, a physician who is prone to isolation and withdrawal from people chooses a specialty that demands intimacy. Such factors should be made explicit to the student when choosing a specialty.

Internship and Residency

The years of internship* and residency (usually three to five years after medical school) are the last major steps in the socialization and professionalization of the physician [39]. It is the last direct influence that the medical profession has on the physician. The intern and resident are no longer medical students but neither are they full-fledged practicing physicians. Their work on the house staff of a hospital is supervised by attending faculty members. The intern and resident deliver nearly all of the care that the patient in a teaching hospital receives, but they generally do so only with the final approval of the attending physician. Any new problems they encounter can be discussed with the attending physician; thus the intern and resident spend a good deal of their time learning and studying [36].

Because they are not completely trained to deal with all medical eventualities, interns and residents experience anxiety about the possibility of not handling the patient's situation appropriately. After years of being almost continuously supervised in carrying out every procedure, the intern now feels alone in caring for the patient (even though the faculty physicians must provide final approval). The need to deal effectively with the patient's problems may motivate the intern to rely continuously on the advice of the attending physician. However, since the goal of this training period is for the intern and resident to learn to think through problems that are encountered in the care of patients and to take responsibility for patient care, the young physician is discouraged from relying too heavily on consultations. Striking an appropriate balance is difficult and often stressful.

*"Intern" traditionally referred to a student physician in the first year of post-medical school training. With the development of extensive formal residency programs, however, many schools now use the term "first-year resident" rather than "intern."

Lack of time and the overwhelming amount of clinical work required can also be a significant source of anxiety for the intern or resident. The on-call schedule of the residency program may involve 36 hours of work with 12 hours off in a 48-hour period. Many physicians are unable to cope with the enormous fatigue that results from this schedule. Interns and residents may find that their lack of time causes them to cut corners by not talking to patients. This behavior may lead to unhealthy attitudes toward patients and their emotions. Furthermore, interns and residents fear that their fatigue might lead to serious errors in the care of patients. When they are off duty, many report that they are unable to leave their work behind and truly relax [9].

Despite these challenges, in residency as well as in medical school, there are few formal mechanisms for the delivery of emotional support to the physician. A formalized biopsychosocial training orientation with respect to the care of residents may be a pragmatic as well as humanitarian change [39].

NURSING

So far we have discussed medical education in terms of its many pressures and the effects of these pressures on the medical students, interns, and residents. Becoming a doctor is intellectually and emotionally challenging, but no less can be said about becoming a nurse.

Nurses have enormous responsibilities in their care of patients, for they take on complete care of the patient when the physician is not available. This is particularly true in emergency situations, of which there may be many in the day-to-day hospital routine (e.g., cardiac arrests). Nurses are usually responsible for making the important decision about whether or not a particular situation is actually an emergency. Nurses are also primarily responsible for reducing fear and emotional upset in patients—factors that could interfere with recovery. Nurses may be directly involved in maintaining a patient's will to live. Such responsibility for the socioemotional aspects of care can produce as much stress as the pressures of technical care [2].

A significant source of stress for nurses is the gap that exists between their training and their professional lives. This gap does not exist for physicians, whose training generally matches their professional responsibilities [25]. For nurses, however, "role training incongruities" arise [34]. There is often a reality shock for the nurse when it becomes apparent that there is a disparity between professional values and norms learned in school (such as the need to spend time talking with patients) and the bureaucratic norms set in hospitals (such as time limitations). Because of economic pressures, attitudes and work habits developed in nursing school may not be held in high esteem in the workplace. Such conflict is said to be the primary cause of nurses leaving the profession [34].

STRESS AND ITS EFFECTS ON PRACTICING HEALTH CARE PROFESSIONALS

Physicians and dentists are more prone to die of coronary heart disease than the average person. In a large cross-cultural study of professional men, it was found that American physicians have a higher incidence of heart disease than other professionals [33]. This exaggerated risk is a factor in the lives of dentists too [16]. The daily pressures and stresses of work result from long hours with many and varied patients, as well as many demands on the technical and interpersonal skills of these health professionals [29]. Recurrent emergency calls for physicians also bring about special stresses. The most important factor, of course, is the emotional response of the health care professionals to the events in their lives; but many are lacking the time and skills to cope with the demands of their profession in an adaptive way.

Many studies have examined the stresses that health care professionals are likely to experience. This research suffers from methodological problems, however, because distressing symptoms tend to be underreported by health care professionals. When asked whether they experience various symptoms, many health care professionals who in fact do suffer these impairments simply deny that they do. It is particularly true that colleagues and family members overprotect the stressed health professionals instead of referring them to rehabilitative treatment. Yet classic symptoms of occupational stress are highly prevalent among physicians and dentists.

Suicide

Suicide is perhaps the most drastic response to stress. Suicide has been found to be more prevalent in medicine, dentistry, and pharmacy than in the general population even though many suicides of these individuals are not reported. Medical students are also more prone to suicide than are members of the general population [43].

Some interesting sex differences have been found in the research on physician suicide [14, 20, 50]. Women doctors are significantly more prone to suicide than are male doctors. One study found that female physician suicides are 3.2 times greater than the general population whereas the suicides of male doctors are only 1.2 times greater. Interestingly, there are also high numbers of suicides among women psychologists and women chemists—but not among women nurses—something that suggests that women in male-dominated professions may be at high risk.

Pharmacists have an unusually high suicide rate as well [43]. It is about 3.5 times higher than that of other professionals (nonmedical) sampled. It is assumed that this high rate is because drugs are readily accessible to pharmacists.

In attempting to explain these findings, it has been suggested that members of the health care professions are not necessarily more likely to *attempt* suicide than are members of the general population, but owing to their access to drugs and their knowledge of anatomy and physiology, they are more likely to *succeed* at suicide. It may be that the differences in suicide rates reflect a greater ability to complete the suicide. Overall, however, there is still not enough information about health professional suicide. Why is it that nurses (as well as other helping professionals like social workers, teachers, and clergy) are not at risk, while physicians, dentists, pharmacists and psychologists are?

In this country about 28 percent of the deaths among physicians under the age of 40 are suicides. This figure probably involves underreporting, for many suicides of physicians are not recognized as such and may be termed "accidents." In the general population, however, only about 5 percent of deaths under the age of 40 are suicides. There are at least 100 physician deaths each year from suicide, which means that every year about one average medical school class is needed to replace the physician suicide victims.

There are of course special environmental stresses on physicians and nurses. Nurses and physicians are more likely to contract infectious diseases such as hepatitis and tuberculosis, and they also catch viruses and bacteria that are part of the hospital environment. It may take health professionals who work with patients (particularly children) a few years to develop an immunity to the everyday viruses and bacteria to which they are exposed, and while developing this immunity they are often ill.

In addition, health care professionals involved in anesthesiology sometimes develop lymphomas and leukemias from the gases used in anesthetizing patients, whereas those who work closely with x rays may suffer the effects of exposure to radiation. These physical occupational hazards can also lead to stress-related problems.

Impaired Health Professionals

Drug abuse among physicians is a problem. Of all the physicians who are now licensed, 2 to 3 percent of them may be drug abusers, and this percentage may be an underestimate because of the problems of underreporting. Among health professionals in general, it is estimated that the incidence of drug abuse is 30 to 100 times that in the general population [38]. Alcoholism is also a serious problem. Although the estimates vary, it is believed that 8 to 12 percent of the total physician population in the United States are hardcore alcoholics [13, 40].

Health care professionals, particularly physicians, often strongly resist recognition of the fact that they (or any of their peers) are impaired. A cloak of silence is the usual reaction to the problem [6]. Impaired physicians and other health care professionals deny that their problems are real and avoid assistance. It is usually only after alcoholism or drug abuse has severely interfered with a physician's practice and personal life that the problem comes to the attention of someone who can help.

There are a few positions in society in which direct and immediate danger to other people can result from the inability of the individual to function effectively; one of these roles is that of airline pilots. Federal Aviation Administration regulations prohibit pilots from drinking or taking drugs before a flight; careful precautions are taken to assure that pilots comply with these rules. But no immediate, direct regulations or controlling mechanisms exist for the medical profession. Medical professionals are relatively autonomous in their work. Significant numbers of health care professionals operate every day under the influence of alcohol and drugs, and there is abundant evidence of the harm that has come to patients as a result of the inability of health care professionals to function effectively because of the influence of drugs and alcohol. A classic example is that of the Marcus twins—two New York gynecologists who were addicted to barbiturates and died of the addiction. However, this addiction was concealed from public view during the time they were practicing in a large New York hospital.

It is extremely difficult to identify a physician as an alcoholic or drug abuser and take steps to rehabilitate this physician. Not only do physicians tend to deny that they have a problem, but fellow physicians and other health care professionals may cooperate by

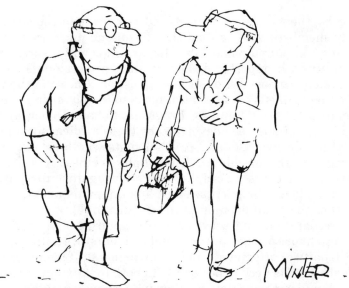

"I felt rotten this morning, but on a hunch I took a couple green pills I found in my bag--and it's amazing. I feel good now."

Figure 10-1. Physician drug abuse. (Reprinted by permission of Robert Minter.)

covering up for them. Why does this happen? Part of the problem lies in the unwillingness of physicians and other health care professionals to interfere with the freedom of physicians to treat patients in their own way. It may also be difficult to understand the source of the impaired physician's strange behavior. Accusations are unlikely to be made. Therefore colleagues attempt to normalize the behavior of the physician until something drastic happens—such as a patient recognizing that the physician in unable to deal with the task at hand or severe consequences befall a patient. Colleagues then fulfill their moral and legal responsibilities and remove the doctor from practice.

Treatment. There have recently been attempts to identify and treat impaired physicians and those in danger of suicide. The American Medical Association and various state and county medical associations have begun programs that make it possible for physicians to request help for themselves or for their colleagues. An information telephone number and a help hotline are available within various state medical association headquarters (e.g., the California Medical Association) to allow physicians to report suspicious behavior by their colleagues or else to ask for help themselves [6]. Family members also can call the telephone numbers to request help for an impaired physician. This arrangement insures the confidentiality of the report and allows trained professionals to contact the physician whose behavior is in question. Care can then be offered on a completely confidential basis to the physicians and also to members of their families. Programs for alcoholism and drug detoxification have been developed by these medical societies, and referral to psychiatrists and psychologists who have expertise in working with the special problems of physicians can be arranged. Sometimes, of course, disciplinary action against the physician must take place. The purpose is usually not punishment, however, but rather the rehabilitation of the physician [6].

The recognition and prevention of impairment in medical students and house officers (interns and residents) are critically important. Reports of attempted suicides by house staff members and by medical students need to be dealt with both in the stage of crisis and also in long-term psychiatric followup. Alcoholism and drug abuse among interns and residents need to be recognized—not only by fellow students and house officers but also by faculty members, to whose attention the problem must be brought. Preventive action is necessary. The approach, however, should not be punitive or disciplinary; instead, help in coping is essential. The grueling work and study schedules that place stress on physicians-in-training usually become worse in medical practice. Thus the problems need to be solved early. Certain steps have been suggested as important elements of faculty responsibility [10].

First, in residency or in medical school programs should be designed to promote adjustment and the sharing of problems among physicians-in-training. Instead of an atmosphere of competition, physicians-in-training should develop a sense of personal responsibility for their own and their colleagues' well-being. Support groups, even including spouses or significant others, could do much to strengthen the feeling among the physicians-in-training that they are not fighting an uphill battle alone.

Second, residents, interns, and medical students should be encouraged to utilize existing mental health facilities for support as a preventive measure instead of only to resolve a crisis. Part of the physicians' training in behavioral science and psychosocial issues in medical care should include understanding psychosocial issues in their own life. Third, each residency and medical school program should identify faculty members who are visible and available to help with problems at their early stages. Fourth, this professional help should be confidential. Finally, physicians-in-training should be given a chance to participate in making decisions about the structure of their educational programs.

Causes of Professional Impairment

The bulk of the research on the causes of health care professional impairment involves physicians. The probable causes of physician impairment have been suggested as the physical and emotional demands of the profession and the enormous amount of time required for training and practice; the easy availability of drugs; and professional autonomy. Empirical research suggests another factor that may override all of these factors; that is, the presence or absence of such problems as drug addiction, attempted suicide, and suicide tends to be correlated primarily with life adjustment *prior* to medical school [54]. There are limits on the effectiveness of social support itself, although support for "at risk" individuals is important.

In a longitudinal study of physicians George Vaillant and colleagues found that emotional adjustment before medical school, even as early as childhood, was highly correlated with adjustment to the pressures of the physician's role [54]. In short, there is evidence that physicians who develop psychiatric illnesses do so because they are already psychologically vulnerable. Individuals who go into the medical field unprepared emotionally because of their backgrounds and early adjustment have a great deal of difficulty adjusting to the pressures and strains of a medical career.

The very traits that make an individual a successful applicant to medical school can actually become liabilities if these traits are further cultivated and come to dominate the individual. Throughout premedical training, medical school, internship, and residency a physician is rewarded for long hours, intense competition, and overwhelming involvement. The physician can easily become locked into a life pattern in which personal and social reinforcement comes primarily from overzealousness in work. There is always enough work to do in the medical field, of course, and a physician can very easily become overcommitted. Being a wise "parent figure" to patients can be extremely flattering to physicians and give them a sense of command. But the overwhelming responsibility for patients who become dependent can prevent physicians from caring for themselves. It is easy for physicians to engage in self-destructive behaviors, such as poor nutrition, smoking, passing up exercise and relaxation, and thinking about nothing but medicine. This kind of behavior can quickly become the dominant pattern in the physicians' life [10]. If physicians have not developed adequate coping mechanisms the stress and strain of day-to-day effort may begin to take its toll. They may be unable to accept imperfections and limitations, and will begin to view their professional role unrealistically. From their roles as the rescuers of patients they can easily become victims themselves.

As we have mentioned, one of the major factors contributing to the problem of psychiatric illness among physicians is their reluctance to ask for help when they are encountering difficulty. Vaillant has suggested that many physicians use denial as a defense when they are not dealing very well with the problems of practice that they encounter [54]. They also have a great deal of difficulty in relinquishing control, and while under treatment, physicians present outstanding difficulties. Physician addicts often ultimately commit suicide, and many physician patients leave the hospital against medical advice. Physicians on the whole make very poor patients [5].

Burnout. One of the major psychological causes that has been posited for health care professional impairment is the phenomenon of *burnout* [37]. As described by psychologist Christina Maslach, burnout involves a loss of concern for people, an emotional exhaustion resulting in cynicism, and a dehumanized perception of patients. Maslach claims that many physicians, social welfare workers, and even childcare staff experience this phenomenon.

Burnout may be at the root of many problems of health care professionals such as drug abuse and alcoholism. Burnout results from difficulties encountered primarily in the emotional care of patients. When health care professionals are fully involved in caring for patients who have difficult or life-threatening illnesses, strong emotions are produced. But these emotions need to be denied or repressed in order to carry out the job. Health care professionals may thus be forced to split off feelings and emotions from the intellectual and technical care of the patient, with this detachment possibly resulting in fragmented, dehumanized perceptions of patients.

Burnout can be prevented by support groups among health providers; by teaching providers to disclose their feelings; by helping them face problems with a perspective gained through humor; and by providing opportunities for stressed professionals to escape from the difficult situation for a needed rest. These measures can be particularly important among health care professionals working in environments such as the intensive care unit, coronary care unit, burn unit, or chronic renal unit (in which patients receive dialysis) of a hospital. Nurses in these units are particularly prone both to burnout and to stress-related problems. Institutional policies that make room for staff emotions can do much to prevent these disorders among health care professionals. Of course, better communication with patients is also valuable in many ways.

Abortion. A special source of stress for health providers, especially nurses, comes from the performance of abortions. Abortion is a relatively simple and safe medical procedure. In the United States abortions have been legal throughout the country since 1973 and are easily obtainable. Research shows that, contrary to earlier views (which were tainted with personal opinions and which reflected the cultural taboos associated with abortion), there are few if any major negative psychological effects on women who have abortions [1].

Abortion often has strong negative effects on medical staff, however. According to social psychologist Nancy Adler, social workers and counselors are usually able to identify with the woman patient and her difficulties; they can therefore cope with their involvement with abortion [1]. However, nurses and doctors, who have to physically abort the fetus, tend to identify with the fetus [11, 32, 44]. Late in the pregnancy (the second as opposed to the first trimester), the performance of an abortion can be highly stressful for medical personnel, and they report feeling physical and emotional exhaustion as well as an absence of positive feelings, sympathy, or respect for patients. They may develop a cynical, dehumanizing attitude toward patients.

Because of the cultural taboo that continues in our society, nurses and doctors who perform abortions often encounter hostility from the general public and also from their patients. Reports suggest that health professionals may experience depression as a result of these responses [32].

Although most women feel relieved after an abortion, two factors are important in increasing the stress that the woman may experience. One is the meaning of the pregnancy to the woman (whether she really wanted the baby). The other factor is the social environment surrounding the abortion; this includes the medical environment, the support or hostility of the medical staff, the reactions of significant others in her life, and the influence of culture and religious sanctions. Major problems in any of these realms can increase the chances that the woman will experience more pain or discomfort as well as psychological difficulties. It is easy to see that the distress health professionals feel in performing an abortion can significantly interfere with their ability to maintain a caring and supportive atmosphere for the patient. As Adler has pointed out, staff uneasiness can contribute to the patient's feelings of distress and guilt. What the woman undergoing an abortion needs most is support, respect, and a neutral person with whom she can discuss her decision.

A final great source of stress on physicians is the necessity of making many decisions, some of which involve life and death. The process of decisionmaking and its results are a key aspect of the life of the health professional. It is a topic worthy of separate consideration.

DECISIONMAKING IN HEALTH CARE

Uncertainty

In September 1951 Renée Fox began a study of the reactions of physicians and patients to medical uncertainty [21]. The research took place in a 15-bed metabolic research ward in a university teaching hospital. Fox, a medical sociologist, was conducting a participant observation study of physicians and patients in a setting in which medical experimentation on the patients was part of everyday life on the ward. Most of the patients were ill with diseases that were not well understood and could not be effectively controlled by medical science in the early 1950s. These patients had agreed to act as research subjects for a team of eleven physicians because it was their only hope for prolonging their lives. The physicians had a dual role: One was to care for their patients and try to keep them alive as long as possible; the other was to conduct clinical research on them.

The physicians were attempting to assess the activity of newly synthesized steroids as clinical agents in the treatment of metabolic and endocrine, cardiovascular, renal, and other diseases. Hence the procedures were radical and still largely untried. These procedures were attempted only on patients who were acutely, seriously, and often terminally ill. The physicians were all relatively young and in early phases of their professional careers; many of them had completed internships and were serving as residents or fellows. They were seriously interested in careers in academic medicine and were trying to strike a balance between caring for patients, teaching, and research.

Fox's sociological research is reported in a book, *Experiment Perilous* [21]. The physicians who were part of the metabolic research group were confronted with major problems of uncertainty in caring for their patients. This uncertainty sometimes resulted from their own incomplete mastery of the medical knowledge that was available, their limited skills, and their inability to synthesize completely all the relevant material. Their uncertainty, however, also derived from limitations in medical knowledge at the time. There was also stress resulting from the physicians' *inability to distinguish* between their own personal inadequacies and the limitations of medical science.

In her research, Fox found that the physicians reacted with a considerable degree of feeling to problems of uncertainty and to problems concerning the ethics of human experimentation. These physicians came to terms with the stresses and pressures of the uncertainty. To begin with, they found deep personal and professional gratification in being associated with each other. The atmosphere of working together helped them to counterbalance some of the strains to which they were exposed. Their unity provided social support and a chance to exchange both opinions and feelings about common problems that were associated with the research. They also were able to share responsibility for what happened to the patients—something that made the awesome responsibility for patients easier to handle. A number of group meetings took place in which the physicians could express their mutual problems and talk about how they felt about them. The physicians "sounded off" a good deal to one another about the strains that they experienced in the uncertainty and unpredictability of their professional situation. They listened sympathetically and gave active encouragement and support to each other.

Another way in which the physicians dealt with the stresses of their experimentation on human beings involved humor. A highly patterned and intricate form of humor served as a protective device. The physicians' humor and jokes focused on the major problems they faced as a unit. They joked about the problems of uncertainty with which they were confronted:

Dr. D: Mr. Goss is still alive.

Dr. S: Is he putting out urine?

Dr. D: No.

Dr. S: Is he having hemodialysis?

Dr. D: No.

Dr. S: Then how is he alive? *(Laughter)* [21, p. 78]

They also joked about the trial and error nature of their scientific pursuits:

Dr. G: Are you *sure* Mr. Stark's adrenals are out?

Dr. H: They *must* be. His carcinoma got better. [21, p. 78]

Others joked about the moral ambiguities and conflicts that conducting research on patients involved:

Dr. G: Mr. Powers' test will be over on Wednesday. What are the plans for his management after that?

Dr. S: Why, I suppose we'll finally get around to *treating* him. [21, p. 79]

The physicians' humor reflected the recognition of the fact that in their roles as clinical investigators they were operating under conditions of extreme uncertainty, limitations, and conflict. The humor of the physicians in the metabolic groups was cathartic as it enabled them to express and dissipate the tension they felt over the problems they faced. To some extent their humor was deviant. By laughing at events that were extremely serious, the physicians were able to express their refusal to accept the poor prognoses of their patients as inevitable. They were able to make light of their own feelings and to achieve a more detached attitude toward the pressures of their work. In sum, by freeing them from some of their tensions, humor helped the physicians strengthen their resolve to deal with the problems.

Another way in which the physicians from the metabolic group were able to deal with the stresses of uncertainty involved becoming close to the patients and getting to know them as individuals. The relationship between the physicians and their patients was usually more personal than professional in nature. The physicians provided special privileges for their patients such as a television set, books, and games. They tried to select nurses who would give special attention and consideration to the patients. Patients were given privileges such as permission to move about freely in the ward and visit other patients in the hospital when they were well enough to do so. A close association with the patients after they went home was maintained by the physicians through followup visits. The patients were also given a considerable amount of information about their disorders, and the procedures that were done to them were explained in detail. The patients were considered working members of the research group. The physicians expressed indebtedness and gratitude to their patients for the role that they played in facilitating research.

Could some of the techniques for coping with stress used by these physicians be adapted for effective use by physicians undergoing the usual pressures of uncertainty? In a book, *Adaptation to Life,* the psychiatrist George Vaillant noted that one of the most effective mechanisms for coping with stress is altruism [53]. We saw this phenomenon at work in the behavior of the physicians of the metabolic group. They were better able to cope with the uncertainties and stresses in their care of these seriously ill patients by attempting to make the patients feel better in other ways, for example, by providing social, emotional, and physical support. In addition, the treatment of patients as colleagues helped to relieve some of the physicians' responsibility. By providing patients with information about their own treatment, the physicians were able to engage the patients' cooperation more readily. The enthusiasm that the physicians generated by developing these cooperative relationships with their patients helped them to overcome the stresses of research [41].

Reaching Rational Decisions

Health care professionals must consistently perform their duties under conditions of uncertainty, and therefore they have to weigh various probabilities and courses of action and make decisions. These decisions are not straightforward, for medicine is not an exact science. The factors that affect decisionmaking are not only matters of evidence, but social and psychological issues also influence how medical decisions are made and what form they take.

When a physician hears a patient's complaint, the physician conducts an examination and makes a decision about what is wrong. This diagnosis is based on answers to questions asked of the patient and on tests that are performed. Even at this stage a physician has to weigh the risks inherent in a particular diagnostic procedure against the risks of following a treatment plan without the information that would result from performing the diagnostic procedure. In prescribing treatment, the physician also knows that the treatment for one illness may aggravate another illness. Furthermore, many factors must be taken into account, such as the patient's health, body build, medical history, psychological and social characteristics, ability to tolerate pain, and so on. In addition, diagnosis and treatment decisions are subject to systematic biases [18].

Physicians and other health care professionals usually develop judgment from two sources. First, during medical training they observe assessments made by people more experienced in their field. Second, health care professionals learn directly through trial and error—they make a diagnosis, prescribe a treatment, and observe the results. It is important to recognize, however, that there is a great deal of disagreement among experts in medicine regarding particular treatments. For example, physicians often do not agree about the use of certain drugs for particular illnesses.

There are many forces that account for these disagreements. One of them is that physicians make different value judgments on the question of risk. If a particular procedure has a mortality rate of 2 or 3 percent, some physicians would advise against the procedure because the risk is too high. Other physicians may believe that the patient would encounter an acceptable risk by having the procedure. Some physicians are also more conservative than others with regard to any given treatment.

Physicians, too, differ among themselves in their approaches to various treatments. This is because each works from a different data base. Some physicians are more experienced than others with relevant cases. The propensity of physicians to use a particular treatment often depends upon their positive experiences with it. Although a long-term research program may have established that a particular treatment has a mortality rate of 50 percent, physicians will often tend to rely more on their *own* experience with the treatment. Few physicians will jump to any conclusions if the treatment works one or two times; but if among six patients, the treatment helps five with one dying (i.e., there is a mortality rate of only one out of six), the physician may begin to believe that the mortality rate is much lower than 50 percent. The doctor's data represent only the *short run,* however. Psychologists D. Kahneman and A. Tversky have studied such errors in estimating odds [30, 31]. They reported that people tend to develop confidence in a treatment that works four out of five times. This result is *not* significantly different from a 50–50 chance. But this problem of the "belief in small numbers" may lead the physician to place undue confidence in a small amount of data. People believe that their samples, even if very small, are representative of the population from which they are drawn. That is, they extrapolate the findings from a small set to an entire population and judge the probabilities of success accordingly. Faulty inferences result.

It also has been found in work by Tversky and Kahneman that people judge the probability of an event by the *salience* of previous instances of that event—that is, how easily instances of that event come to mind [52]. Thus physicians may conclude that a treatment is better than it actually is (i.e., has a greater probability of working than it actually has) if they can easily remember patients who succeeded after having had the treatment.

Emotions also affect decisionmaking. Physicians often have difficulty in deciding whether to give patients bad news; for example, telling a patient that the patient is dying is one of the most difficult tasks many physicians must face. Apparently there are two reasons for this hesitation. First, people prefer to avoid the unpleasant feelings that occur in sad situations [51]. Second, the physician who bears bad news is sometimes held responsible for the bad news; that is, the physician is unfairly blamed for the patient's condition [27]. Such influences on decisionmaking are emotional rather than rational approaches to patient management, however.

The values of the health provider also influence decisionmaking. A victim of his or her own drunken driving or a destitute old person is more likely to be classified as "dead on arrival" by emergency room personnel than would a child upon whom resuscitation would still be attempted [46]. Similarly, decisions may be subtly affected by the costs of treatment and whether the patient's case is useful for research or teaching purposes [55]. To reduce such biases, health professionals might acknowledge their relevant values as explicitly as possible and then analyze them outside the pressures of a specific decision.

Groupthink. Sometimes decisionmaking is affected by the pressures of the group. In the case of special medical teams or units, a special team spirit may develop. This closeness and liking for the group are called group *cohesiveness*. Members of a cohesive group work well together, feel secure, and each member feels good about belonging to the group. Unfortunately, cohesive groups also have a strong tendency to subtly force members to conform to the group norms and therefore may interfere with rational decisionmaking. The social psychologist Irving Janis labels poor group decisionmaking, which can sometimes replace independent critical thinking, *groupthink* [28].

Although Janis primarily analyzed political decisionmaking, groupthink can also occur in a medical setting. Symptoms of groupthink are such phenomena as the group's unquestioned belief in its own morality, collective use of the defense of rationalization, stereotyped views of outsiders, and pressure on dissenters. As each member goes along with the group, there is suppression of personal doubts and a shared illusion of unanimity. Groupthink might occur if a medical team is challenged by an outsider such as a friend of the patient, a family member, or even an outside health professional. If the medical team comes together to oppose this common "enemy," rational decisionmaking may be distorted as the group gathers to protect itself. A physician may transmit his or her expectations to another physician who in turn reassures a nurse who in turn helps another nurse rationalize away doubts, and so on, until an unintentional self-deception occurs. To protect against groupthink, each member should be *encouraged* to express any doubts about a particular procedure, perhaps even playing the role of devil's advocate. Most importantly, outside experts and qualified colleagues who are not directly involved should be consulted extensively about any controversial medical situation. In this way the isolation of a cohesive "ingroup" is minimized.

Clinical Versus Actuarial Predictions

Statistical or *actuarial prediction* involves the method of reaching diagnostic decisions by using formal quantitative (mathematical) techniques. For example, a physician may make a prediction about the probable effect of a certain treatment on a patient based on the statistical probability of the success of that treatment. This probability would be based on the findings of research studies done on that treatment. *Clinical prediction,* on the other hand, involves the informal, qualitative techniques that are usually employed by clinicians. In this case a physician would make a prediction about the probable effectiveness of a certain treatment based on the physician's knowledge of the patient as well as some intuitive hunches. The clinician (physician) will be unable to identify precisely what pieces of information entered into the decision and exactly how the decision was reached. For many years in psychology, there has been debate about the relative effectiveness of the two approaches. Proponents of the statistical method say that their method is objective, reliable, and sound, whereas proponents of the clinical approach have called their method dynamic, meaningful, and genuine [17].

Many people oppose the clinical approach on the grounds that it is vague, hazy, subjective, and unscientific. On the other hand, some people oppose the statistical approach because they consider it is artificial and pseudoscientific. Debate revolves around the following question: If a given level of diagnostic or predictive accuracy can be achieved by applying rules of thumb or by relying on statistical formulas, how much can an experienced clinician's artful (but expensive) combination of data contribute? In any given prediction situation, which of the methods will be more accurate overall? Translated into medical terms, these questions become as follows: Is the physician's clinical, intuitive judgment necessary to determine the probable efficacy of a treatment for a particular patient if the effectiveness of that treatment is known from past research? In other words, are the physician's experience and judgment necessary? Could a diagnosis be made by a computer? How much would a physician with years of experience add? When faced with diagnostic information about a patient are the data best combined by a computer or by an individual who makes an intuitive judgment?

These questions are important, for some of the research in both clinical psychology and medicine has suggested that the statistical (actuarial) approach is better [15]. In medicine it has been found that programs for computer-assisted diagnosis may exceed the accuracy of the diagnosis of clinicians. But there are limits in this kind of research. For one thing, the methods of the research may favor the actuarial approach. The importance of clinical activity may be slighted primarily because studies tend to ignore the fact that most clinicians view decisionmaking as a sequential process; that is, as new information is added the clinician continually changes and updates the decision. Furthermore, it has been argued that clinical judgment aims to do what is best for a particular patient, and since no two patients are alike, findings describing entire populations have inherent limits. An exceptional treatment devised by an experienced clinician might save a patient's life, even though the treatment might not work in general. It is also argued by those favoring the clinical approach that a more formal statistical approach cannot deal sufficiently with the aspects of a problem that make it unique. Some physicians hold that medical judgment is more an art than a science.

The two approaches are actually not disparate, and they can be used in conjunction with each other if a number of points are kept in mind [23, 47]. Clinical and statistical predictions have similar characteristics. First, in both approaches the data must be combined in a way in which a decision can be reached. Second, the same observations should be used in both methods. Third, the relationship between the disease and the symptoms is one of probability rather than logical necessity. Because the physician's mind is more adaptable than most computer programs, it is probably true that decisions can be improved upon by employing statistical procedures *in conjunction with* global clinical judgments—judgments that involve more art than science. On the other hand, in unfamiliar situations the physician has a tendency not to draw all the inferences that are possible with the set of data, a weakness of the clinical method. In addition, human inferences are subject to the biases described earlier.

Good clinical judgment is also needed because a physician must be sensitive to the emotional needs of patients, which are hard to define. Clinical sensitivity is necessary to deal with the social and psychological problems that frequently arise when a patient must cope with illness and the consequences of certain therapies. Social and psychological information forms a part of the stuff of clinical judgment and is rarely included in the statistics concerning the efficacy of various treatments. The issue of values is also relevant. A decision about treatment must often be made in the context of the peculiar value system of the particular patient, which is a difficult task for a computer program.

More research is needed in this area. The effectiveness of different decisionmaking approaches has yet to be examined completely. At present diagnostic recommendations should probably be based both on mathematical decisions (e.g., computer diagnosis) and on subjective judgments.

WOMEN IN MEDICINE

You may have heard an old but very interesting riddle, which goes like this:

> A man and his son went out fishing on a Sunday afternoon. Driving home, they were in a car accident with a drunk driver and the man was killed instantly. His son was rushed to the hospital, needing surgery.
>
> When the boy arrived at the hospital, the attending surgeon exclaimed, "I can't operate. He's my son!"
>
> How can this be?

Even today, many people do not know the answer to this riddle, or else take quite a while to solve it.* Our expectations about the roles of women in medicine are deeply ingrained.

Sex roles are shared expectations we hold about the appropriate behavior of men and women; they are stereotypes applied to sex. For example, in America men have traditionally been expected to be aggressive, strong, athletic, dirty, and insensitive, whereas women have traditionally been expected to be emotional, dainty, talkative, sensitive, and neat. These expectations are shared by both men and women [49].

Sex roles are important in all areas of social relations, but they are especially important in medicine. Inferior roles for women date back thousands of years to biblical proclamations about the superiority of men and the uncleanliness of women. The ancient Greeks also viewed women as biologically and emotionally inferior. Church laws and Greek philosophy continued to exert a strong influence on the development of the roles of women in medicine until recently.

Sex roles affected both the possibilities for women as health pro-

---

*The answer of course is that the surgeon is the boy's mother.

fessionals and the treatment women received as patients. As scientific medicine developed in twentieth-century America, women were, on the whole, limited to positions as nurses; even the role of midwife was denied to them.

Women as Professionals

In 1965 only 6 percent of beginning medical students were women. By 1975, three years after the passage of an amendment to the federal Health Manpower Act and of the law that prohibited educational discrimination according to sex, about 20 percent of the nation's incoming medical students were women. Today the percentage has leveled off at about 30 percent [10].

In the early 1970s most of the women physicians followed very similar career paths. About 22 percent of the pediatricians in the United States were women, about 20 percent of the public health physicians, and about 25 percent of the child psychiatrists. Altogether about 65 percent of the female physicians worked in pediatrics, public health, child psychiatry, or internal medicine. Perhaps surprisingly, only 3 percent of the obstetrician-gynecologists in the United States were women. There were very few women in surgery (see Box 10–2).

Until very recently, female physicians were likely to have parents with high education, and professional fathers. They tended to marry physicians or other professionals, but often they made less money than their physician-husbands. It was also true that a large percentage of them did not marry, and those who did had few if any children. Women physicians who married encountered a tremendous workload; 76 percent of the women physicians in one survey reported that they handled all the cooking, shopping, childcare, and money management in their houses. Most of the women physicians surveyed reported that they had the ultimate responsibility for almost all the household tasks, whereas the male physicians who were studied had none. A significant number of professional women in medicine reported that they experienced a conflict between their work and home life. They experienced great stress because of working too hard [8, 9].

Women were (and in fact still are) underrepresented in seats of power in medical education and in medical practice. At this writing, it is still true that there is not one female dean of a U.S. medical school, and less than 3 percent of the full professors in medical schools are women [7].

There are special problems related to being a woman in medicine,

Box 10–2
Female Surgeons

There are fewer women practicing surgery than any of the other major medical specialties. From 1970 to 1976 there was a "dramatic" increase in female surgeons—from 2.5 percent to 3.4 percent. In recent years the percentage has slowly edged even higher.

There are various obstacles to women who want to become surgeons. In the 1960s it was common for women to be flatly refused entry into surgical residencies. Male surgeons have sometimes asserted that women are not strong enough to withstand the strains of surgery, although there is no evidence that women have less stamina in this situation. Some doctors also oppose having a woman in charge of a surgical team.

When they do become surgeons, women encounter special strains because of the extraordinary time demands of surgery. Many female surgeons do not marry. Female surgeons may have difficulty establishing a practice because they do not have the right connections, and without close friends who are surgeons, women may also have difficulty entering certain professional societies or gaining access to certain hospitals. They also have difficulties receiving referrals. Unfortunately, this system is self-perpetuating. Only when there are sufficient numbers of female surgeons will it become easier for females to become surgeons.

For further reading: M. A. Campbell, *Why Would a Girl Go into Medicine?* (Old Westbury, N.Y.: The Feminist Press, 1973).

most of which have to do with role conflicts. Many women physicians try to integrate the demands of a career with a role as wife and mother [8, 9, 10]. Some women, particularly during their childbearing years, take part-time, salaried positions or leave the professional workforce for a time, and as a result their income and professional development suffer [7].

It is sometimes argued that women make less effective use of their medical training than do men because they are in practice for a shorter period throughout their lives. This claim is erroneous. Female physicians live longer than male physicians, and therefore can practice longer. In addition, male physicians are more likely to have their professional careers interrupted by military duty, which may result in less than optimum career development.

Many women physicians experience role ambiguities in which they are torn between doing what their training has prepared them for and what they believe they must do to fulfill their personal goals.

Because of these uncertainties, women physicians are more prone than the average woman and than men to divorce. Women trained during the 1960s are at a very high risk for suicide.

The relationship between the professional and personal behavior of women physicians is beginning to change, and these changes may have a significant impact on the future of medical practice. Women currently entering medicine are more likely to choose private practice, and they are working longer hours than in the past. These younger female physicians are insisting on equal pay, and they are moving into disciplines such as surgery and its subspecialties. In recent surveys both women and men ranked family practice, pediatrics, internal medicine, and psychiatry as their most preferred specialty, in that order [22, 24].

Women physicians trained recently are different from how women physicians were even a few years ago. They are more vocal in protecting themselves from the slurs and prejudices against women that they experience in the academic environment. They do not endure, for example, slides of *Playboy* centerfolds during anatomy lectures, and they challenge professors' sexist remarks. They tend to make demands on the system of medical education and practice to bend to what they consider legitimate needs of their own.

Is medicine better off with women in the profession? Some clues come from studies done by psychologist Lillian Cartwright [8, 9, 10]. It has been found that women are more sensitive than men to values concerned with interpersonal relationships and are more willing to consider interpersonal issues in health care. Probably because of this orientation, women physicians are more likely to be aware of the patient's psychosocial environment. With encouragement to hold on to what are considered traditionally "feminine" values, women physicians may be likely to have a strong and positive impact on the psychological aspects of medical practice. They may also improve the treatment received by female patients.

In the United States about 70 percent of the health care workers are women. Most of them are in ancillary worker positions; they are not physicians. Over 95 percent of nurses in the United States are women. Few of them (at most about one-fifth) are in any kind of administrative position within medicine [2].

Nursing is a very old and honored female profession, and for a long time, it was one of the few professions open to women. Nursing dates back to the time of Hippocrates. During the dark ages, nurses were considered "the healers" because they used homeopathic remedies more readily than did physicians, and the invasive therapies used by physicians sometimes did more harm than good to the patient. Women nurses took care of people with dietary prescriptions, poultices, and herbal preparations. As a result they were often burned at the stake for being witches, privy to the devil's secrets of healing.

Life for the female nurse is considerably better now, although she still faces discrimination, stereotyping, and expectations for her performance lower than that of which she is capable. One example of this attitude is a commonly held belief that nurses are simply women who are preparing to be doctors' wives. Even women with advanced degrees (M.A. or Ph.D.) in nursing are thought to be "just nurses" and not at all serious about the job. Although nurses are known to provide the socioemotional care of the patient—that is, they are comforting and supportive—the nurse's therapeutic, technical care of the patient is often minimized. In fact, however, the nurse's contribution to technical patient care and to prevention (such things as bathing, massaging, turning patients to prevent sores, arranging diets, changing wound dressings, etc.) is a critical aspect of technological medicine. Though perhaps not obvious at first, the nurse is central to the care of the patient, in both the technical and socioemotional senses.

We consider the issue of women patients in the next chapter.

SUMMARY

Social psychological issues are not only relevant to the care of patients, but these factors also impinge daily on the role of the health professional. The care of patients is stressful, and in response to uncertainty emotions are often strong. Health professionals suffer high rates of suicide, divorce, and addiction. For the good of both the patient and practitioner, these emotions must be successfully managed. Thus understanding how health professionals can learn to cope with pressures on them is extremely important. This chapter has dealt with these issues by considering the sources and effects of stress in the training and practice of health professionals. Attention has also been focused on the process of decisionmaking by health professionals, and on the classic controversy between clinical and statistical prediction. Finally, the special problems faced by women health professionals have been examined.

11
The
Health
Care
Environment

Throughout this book we have hinted at the broader implications of a social psychological approach to medicine—that is, the total health care environment. Specific issues of communication, illness definition, coping, and so forth, all occur in a social environment. In this final chapter, we consider directly the psychosocial factors in the promotion of health and the structuring of healthy medical environments.

In 1979 the U.S. Surgeon General issued a report on health promotion, *Healthy People* [78]. The remarkable conclusion was that further improvements in the health of Americans were most likely to result from efforts to prevent disease and promote health. In this chapter we describe some of the results of the report. We briefly consider the social psychological aspects of such issues as nutrition, drug abuse, sexuality, and the matter of women patients.

Thus far we have primarily concentrated on outpatient care in which patients live at home and are primarily responsible for taking care of themselves. The doctor's office and the neighborhood medical clinic are outpatient settings. In this chapter we consider the *hospital* environment, examining some of the problems faced in hospitals by people who have become "inpatients." In the hospital, matters of personal control and dehumanization may have a significant influence on health.

Although people of all ages may be hospitalized, this fate is especially likely for the aged. The problems of the elderly as well as the special problems of hospitalized children are considered in this chapter. In Chapter 9 we examined the many psychosocial problems faced by the terminally ill, some of which are created or aggravated by the hospital environment. In an attempt to address these matters, the *hospice* movement has recently been gaining momentum. This movement is also examined in this chapter.

Many books have been written about each topic discussed here, and of course such work cannot be condensed into a few pages. Instead, this chapter focuses on the social psychological aspects of healthy orientations and environments, especially as related to the other ideas in this book. For example, in discussing sexuality we focus on the psychosocial causes of certain sexual problems and suggest a general approach to dealing with them; however, to deal with disease-caused sexual difficulties or to manage severe psychological disturbances in sexuality, information must be obtained from other sources. In this way we hope to present the general philosophy of promoting health that emerges from social science research.

NUTRITION

Although diseases caused by a deficient diet are now quite rare in the United States, there is increasing evidence that diet may still have important links to health and illness [78]. Most obviously, it is unhealthy to be extremely overweight or extremely underweight. Perhaps more importantly, diet has been linked to everything from heart disease to hyperactivity. Since the development of germ theory in the nineteenth century, the perceived importance of the human host to health and illness has been low. That is, disease is usually conceived to be the result of the invasion of the body by an external organism rather than a failure or breakdown of the body's defenses. In recent years, however, the importance of the body's "environment" has been increasingly recognized, and nutrition is a key aspect to maintaining the healthy body environment [3, 20, 78] (see Figure 11-1).

An obvious role that can be played by the health provider is in the area of patient education and nutrition advice. For example, patients can be warned about foods containing high sugar (contributing to dental caries and obesity) and high salt (contributing to hypertension) contents but very little protein. Similarly, diets can be modified to deal with problems in digestion and elimination. How-

RISKO

The purpose of this game is to give you an estimate of your chances of suffering heart attack.

The game is played by making squares which — from left to right — represent an increase in your RISK FACTORS. These are medical conditions and habits associated with an increased danger of heart attack. *Not all risk factors are measurable enough to be included in this game; see back of sheet for other RISK FACTORS.*

RULES:

Study each RISK FACTOR AND its row. Find the box applicable to you and circle the large number in it. For example, if you are 37, circle the number in the box labeled 31-40. After checking out all the rows, add the circled numbers. This total — your score — is an estimate of your risk.

IF YOU SCORE:

6-11 — Risk well below average	**25-31 — Risk moderate**
12-17 — Risk below average	**32-40 — Risk at a dangerous level**
18-24 — Risk generally average	**41-62 — Danger urgent. See your doctor now.**

HEREDITY:

Count parents, grand-parents, brothers, and sisters who have had heart attack and/or stroke.

TOBACCO SMOKING:

If you inhale deeply and smoke a cigarette way down, add one to your classification. Do NOT subtract because you think you do not inhale or smoke only a half inch on a cigarette.

EXERCISE:

Lower your score one point if you exercise regularly and frequently.

CHOLESTEROL OR SATURATED FAT INTAKE LEVEL:

A cholesterol blood level is best. If you can't get one from your doctor, then estimate honestly the percentage of solid fats you eat. These are usually of animal origin — lard, cream, butter, and beef and lamb fat. If you eat much of this, your cholesterol level probably will be high. The U.S. average, 40%, is too high for good health.

BLOOD PRESSURE:

If you have no recent reading but have passed an insurance or industrial examination chances are you are 140 or less.

SEX:

This line takes into account the fact that men have from 6 to 10 times more heart attacks than women of child bearing age.

AGE	1 — 10 [illegible] 20	2 — 21 [illegible] 30	3 — 31 [illegible] 40	4 — [illegible] 50	6 — [illegible] 60	8 — [illegible] 70 [illegible] er
HEREDITY	1 — No [illegible] own his[illegible] of heart [illegible] isease	2 — 1 [illegible] with cardio[illegible] scular [illegible] Over 60	3 — 2 rela[illegible] s with cardio[illegible] scular [illegible] Over 60	4 — 1 rel[illegible] with ca[illegible] scular [illegible] Under 60	6 — 2 rel[illegible] es with ca[illegible] cular [illegible] Under 60	7 — 3 re[illegible] s with cardi[illegible] scular [illegible] ease Under 60
WEIGHT	0 — M[illegible] an 5[illegible] s. [illegible] ow [illegible] rd weight	1 — −5 t[illegible] +5 lbs. st[illegible] dard w[illegible] ght	2 — 6-2[illegible] lbs. ov[illegible] weight	3 — 21-[illegible] lbs. over [illegible] ight	5 — 36-[illegible] lbs. over [illegible] ight	7 — 51-[illegible] lbs. ov[illegible] weight
TOBACCO SMOKING	0 — [illegible] on-[illegible] r	1 — Ciga[illegible] and/or [illegible] e	2 — 10 ci[illegible] rettes or [illegible] a day	4 — 2[illegible] rettes [illegible]	6 — 3[illegible] ettes [illegible]	10 — [illegible] are[illegible] s [illegible] day [illegible] ore
EXERCISE	1 — In[illegible] sive occu[illegible] tional and re[illegible] eational exertion	2 — [illegible] ate occu[illegible] ional and [illegible] ional exertion	3 — Sedent[illegible] work and [illegible] ense recre[illegible] onal exertion	5 — S[illegible] tary oc[illegible] tional and m[illegible] erate re[illegible] tional exertion	6 — Sede[illegible] ry work [illegible] ht r[illegible] nal exertion	8 — Co[illegible] lack [illegible] se
CHOLES-TEROL OR FAT % IN DIET	1 — Cho[illegible] sterol below [illegible] 0 mg.% Diet [illegible] ntains no a[illegible] mal or solid fats	2 — C[illegible] terol 181-2[illegible] mg.% Die[illegible] ntains 10% [illegible] al or solid fats	3 — C[illegible] terol 206-2[illegible] mg.% Diet c[illegible] tains 20% [illegible] mal or solid fats	4 — Che[illegible] terol 23[illegible] mg.% [illegible] ins 30% [illegible] mal or solid fats	5 — C[illegible] terol 25[illegible] mg.% Diet c[illegible] tains 40% [illegible] mal or solid fats	7 — [illegible] erol 281-[illegible] mg.% Di[illegible] ontains 50% animal or solid fats
BLOOD PRESSURE	1 — [illegible] 0 uppe[illegible] eading	2 — [illegible] up[illegible] ding	3 — upper [illegible] ading	4 — up[illegible] ding	6 — up[illegible] ding	8 — 2[illegible] over up[illegible] ding
SEX	1 — F[illegible] ale [illegible] der [illegible] 0	2 — F[illegible] le [illegible] 50	3 — F[illegible] ale over 50	5 — M[illegible]	6 — [illegible]	7 — [illegible] d [illegible] ocky male

MICHIGAN HEART ASSOCIATION 69

Figure 11–1. Health promotion game, RISKO. (Copyright © Michigan Heart Association)

ever, few medical providers include questions about daily diet in medical examinations, although almost all would admit the importance of diet to health [78]. The general expectations of the medical environment do not yet give sufficient attention to diet. Nevertheless, although there is still a long way to go in improving diet education and diet advice, severe limits exist on how effective such educational techniques can be. A good example is obesity.

Obesity

About one-third of middle-aged women and about one-tenth of middle-aged men are obese. Although precise causal pathways have not yet been proven, obesity is related to diabetes, gall bladder disease, and high blood pressure [78]. In addition, obesity can affect a person's self-concept and physical attractiveness. A "cure" for obesity in many cases involves a proper, restricted diet. Yet obesity remains one of the most stubborn health problems. Obesity is intimately tied with social psychological issues.

Feelings of personal control and responsibility are very important in successful control of obesity [51, 52, 66]. There are often many opportunities for people to eat throughout the day or the night. People who are aware of when and how much they are eating and who have a sense of control over this behavior are more likely to be successful in controlling overeating. Of course, gaining such a sense of control is not easy. For many people, social support groups, a dieting "buddy," and encouragement by a health provider may prove effective.

Part of the problem in helping people to gain control over their overeating and other unhealthy behaviors involves explanations or attributions for behavior. As discussed in Chapter 6, attributions are social psychological phenomena: They are explanations for behavior that arise out of social situations. People who blame their obesity on their genes or metabolism, their cooking partners, or their personalities are likely to experience difficulties in controlling their weight. While all of these factors may indeed influence the tendency to eat, placing the blame on the environment or on heredity makes it next to impossible for someone to control overeating [65].

Despite the importance of diet to health, it is difficult to get people to change their eating *habits*. Aside from its biological necessity, eating is partly a social and cultural phenomenon. First, meals, especially dinners, are often social occasions in which friends or family gather together. The kinds of foods eaten depend in part on the desires of others. Similarly, eating is often tied to holidays like Thanksgiving and to various celebrations and parties. In America, what is a birthday without a birthday cake? Second, eating certain kinds of foods involves habits from childhood; foods are often part of a family's tradition. People may learn that a breakfast is incomplete without buttered toast or that a dinner is incomplete without meat and potatoes. Or a family may take pride in its Sunday morning omelets. Finally, eating habits are part of a general cultural influence. Only certain foods are available in local markets, certain foods are heavily promoted through advertising, and certain foods are proscribed because of religious or other moral grounds. For example, in American culture red meat is a highly prized food. Furthermore, there is a social consciousness about what foods are "healthy." For example, in recent years "organic" foods have become faddish in some circles.

Because of their strong ties to social factors, eating habits are most effectively changed through a general shift in social norms rather than through an individual's efforts. For example, it is easier to help an individual cut down on beef consumption if there is a general social belief that too much beef is a bad idea for health or economic reasons than it is to try to change the attitudes of an individual person solely on the basis of logical argument. Advice from public health officials and influences in economic policy will, in the long run, have a significant impact on eating habits [78].

For people who must change their diet for health reasons, there are certain specific techniques that may be helpful [37, 40, 78]. First, it is useful if they keep a written record of both the type and quantity of all food eaten each day as well as their daily weight. These objective records promote awareness of the need for change and help prevent rationalization of poor eating habits. Second, diet can be modified by controlling the external or environmental cues. To eliminate unnecessary snacks and overeating, for example, meals could be confined to the dining room at mealtimes; dieters could be instructed to take the proper portion of food on their plate all at once and then eat and chew the food slowly. Similarly, shopping can be controlled by using shopping lists or being influenced by others, and unwanted foods can be kept out of the house. Third, diet modification on the individual level can be encouraged through the use of rewards. For example, people could buy new clothes as they lose weight, or they could buy gifts with the money saved on food. Finally, as with other situations in which stress may arise, eating may be controlled through participation in social support groups such as Weight Watchers.

Anorexia Nervosa

Imagine a young woman who eats one Cheerio for breakfast each day. People who suffer from extreme malnutrition and loss of weight caused by insufficient food intake are diagnosed as having *anorexia nervosa*. Such people are generally young women, with no known medical disease or other psychiatric disorder, and then often have a very strange attitude toward food and weight. Many patients report a desire for an extremely thin appearance that they perceive to be attractive [5]. They have a distorted body image.

Although it is well documented, anorexia nervosa is still a controversial medical syndrome, probably because social psychological factors are heavily implicated. In most cases there is no simple "germ" or "disease" that can be isolated, and therefore the traditional medical model may have a difficult time addressing the problem. Yet it is unquestionably a serious illness. Estimates of mortality rates range from 3 percent to 25 percent [5].

Regardless of the origins of anorexia, it is clear that family interactions are or become an important part of the illness. Most anorexic patients are teenagers who live with their parents, and of course, a severe weight loss produces worry and strained relations within the family. Family reactions often lower the patient's self-esteem and sense of control, which may be very low to begin with. For patients who enjoy the attention given them by their new illness, family worries may serve as a reward for maintaining the poor eating behaviors. Family therapy, which addresses the patient's needs for independence and self-identity, is thus sometimes helpful [58].

As with other nutritional matters, information about proper diet, causes of weight loss, and the relationship between various foods and health can have a positive effect in curing anorexia, but the effect is often limited. It is important to note that severe weight loss and other accompanying symptoms (such as amenorrhea in women) have a significant impact on self-concept and family relations even if a "medical" cause for anorexia nervosa is eventually discovered. A vicious circle often develops in which physical problems, family concern and worry, low self-concept, patient's excessive concern with food, and strained interactions with health providers all become related as causes and effects of each other. Aside from the specific treatment regimen for any single individual, it is important for all health providers to understand the complex nature of the various psychosocial factors in this health problem.

DRUG ABUSE

Society is filled with contradictory messages about drugs. On the one hand, people are urged to take various pills to feel better, control pain, aid them in sleeping and relaxing, stay alert, and so on. At the same time there is a stigma attached to relying on drugs, and the dangers of drug addiction are well known. This contradiction was well illustrated several years ago by the case of Dr. Peter Bourne, an advisor to President Carter on drug abuse. Bourne was well known for his opposition to the abuse of common drugs like sleeping pills, but when asked for help by a distressed colleague, Bourne wrote a prescription for Quaaludes [61]. To protect his colleague from embarrassment, Bourne wrote the prescription in a phony name, thus violating the drug laws. When the story became public, Bourne was forced to resign from his position.

To prevent drug abuse, it is useful to have some idea of the predisposing social psychological factors. In general, there are four main influences on whether or not someone is likely to use illegal drugs [25]. First, parents seem to have a significant influence on whether their children will become drug abusers, and parental influence operates in two ways. On the one hand, the warmth of the parent–child interaction and the cohesion of the family unit are often related to a child's sense of identity and self-esteem; this is in turn related to whether the child will turn to drugs. Parents also influence their children through modeling. If parents use, encourage the use of, or abuse drugs, their children are likely to follow suit. Second, the use of drugs is clearly related to the influence of peers, and this factor also operates in two ways. Both the lack of involvement in healthy groups in which drugs are not used and direct involvement in drug-abusing peer groups will lead to an increased likelihood of drug abuse. Third, general social adjustment is related to the potential for drug abuse. People who are heavily involved in normal social activities and have close relationships with others are less likely to become drug abusers. Finally, initial experiences with drugs may affect subsequent drug use and abuse. If the initial experiences are unpleasant, dangerous, or troublesome, there is less likelihood of subsequent abuse. Of course, some of these general factors may not hold true in a specific case. However, it is clear that overall the best means of preventing drug abuse involves basic and far-reaching social and societal factors rather than any specific limited action. If the family, social structure, and culture all combine to frown on drug abuse, the incidence of drug abuse is likely to be quite small.

Smoking

Cigarette smokers are about twice as likely to die from heart disease as are nonsmokers. Cigarette smoking causes more cancer than any other single element. Smokers are much more likely than nonsmokers to develop lung cancer, cancer of the mouth, and cancer of the urinary bladder. Cigarette smoking is also associated with many other diseases, especially various lung diseases. Smoking is therefore a major health problem [78].

Traditional medical approaches have been relatively ineffective in dealing with this health problem. For example, medical and surgical interventions for lung cancer are mostly ineffective. People begin smoking because of the influence of other people in their culture. Smoking is thus a major issue in the field of social psychology and medicine.

Adolescents are especially susceptible to the social pressure of their peers, and it is during adolescence that most people begin smoking. About 4000 American adolescents begin smoking cigarettes each day [78]. Once a person begins smoking, it is very difficult to quit; hence smoking should be a major focus of pediatric medicine and primary care medicine. Yet many physicians and dentists do not even discuss smoking with their patients and do not urge them to avoid or quit smoking. Following the traditional medical model, many health care practitioners wait until a disease develops before addressing the problem. However, physicians, with their prestige and credibility, could be influential in preventing smoking.

Cigarette smoking is a complex issue because certain aspects of our culture glamorize smoking. For example, advertisements for cigarettes may promise sex appeal. Although research is still being conducted, it seems likely that young people will avoid cigarettes if their peers believe it to be an unhealthful and undesirable addiction. An important first step is to make it clear that nonsmokers are in the majority and have taken an active decision to protect their health.

While there are currently many efforts to help people quit smoking, evaluations generally show mixed results. Certainly, information about the ill effects of smoking, encouragement from valued others, and appropriate advice from medical practitioners are all helpful steps. However, the primary emphasis must be placed on prevention of smoking. Just as most people learn to avoid accidents and eat nonpoisonous foods, so can people learn to avoid cigarette smoking.

HUMAN SEXUALITY

Twenty years ago, most health practitioners were woefully ignorant about human sexuality. First, training about sexuality was absent from most medical education programs. Second, most medical students, busy with long hours of studying and pressured to uphold high moral standards, were likely to be less sexually experienced (in a personal sense) than many other people their age. Not only were they ignorant, but also many health students and practitioners held erroneous beliefs, for example, that masturbation leads to insanity.

Most people have some kind of sexual problems at some time in their lives. Often they are related to psychosocial issues, but they are also commonly caused by disease states. In our society most of these people turn to physicians for assistance. Yet many physicians have traditionally not only been ignorant about sexuality, but have also been uneasy talking about the subject and unwilling to bring it up as a part of a routine medical history. Today, most American medical students, during their first year of medical school, are exposed to vivid sexual films including scenes of masturbation, intercourse, homosexuality, and oral-genital sex. Nevertheless, research by Dr. Harold Lief shows that health personnel have a long way to go before they become proficient in promoting healthy human sexuality [45]. In this section, we sketch some of the major themes that have emerged from careful research over the past two decades on human sexuality [19, 31, 42, 43, 47].

Because of ties to issues of morality, religion, family structure, tradition, and the social implications of intimacy and pregnancy, matters of human sexuality have been difficult to view in an unbiased scientific manner. However, research by Alfred Kinsey, William Masters and Virginia Johnson, and others has produced two general facts about sexuality [42, 43, 53, 54]. First, it has been found that there are various means of sexual arousal and none is superior to the others in a biological sense. Masturbation, oral-genital contact, stimulation through mechanical means, sexual intercourse, and other activities may all lead to the same sexual arousal and to orgasm. The different activities may have different meanings or implications for different people, but the biological response is the same. Second, research has shown that sexual response is heavily influenced by learning and by technique. There is a tremendous range of sexual activity. People can learn to become aroused or to lose their desire by various activities and may choose various objects as sexual goals. It is impossible to say that these activities are more or less healthy in a biological sense; of course, some activities have implications for other issues such as the rights of others.

Research has shown that many sexual difficulties are due to psychosocial issues rather than being caused by disease states. Many of these problems can be dealt with in a simple and straightforward manner, and consultation with a sex therapist is often not necessary.

For males the two most common sexual problems are attaining or maintaining an erection and premature ejaculation. Often, these problems are due to anxiety and negative sexual experiences. Because of certain societal pressures that sexual enjoyment may be immoral, the lack of information about sexuality, social embarrassment about discussing sexual matters with one's partner, and pressures to "perform" like an expert, many men are very anxious when becoming intimate. These same factors and the resulting anxiety often lead to distressing early sexual encounters. Anxiety may then increase even more, and sexual problems result [19, 47].

What can the health professional do to help men with sexual problems? First, the health provider can give *permission* to someone to fulfill his sexual needs, assuring him that he is completely normal and that everyone has sexual urges. This reassurance itself is often enough to break the cycle of anxiety and start the patient on the road to a more fulfilling sexual relationship. Second, the health professional can provide information about sexual activities, their prevalence, common techniques, and the wide range of sexual responses. Third, the practitioner can urge the patient to practice the development of good sexual feelings. Often, advice to engage in touching without sexual intercourse proves helpful in reducing anxiety and developing more control over ejaculation [38, 47].

For women, common sexual problems involve difficulty in becoming aroused, especially to the point of orgasm. Here, too, decreasing anxiety and increasing practice are often helpful. Urging women to explore their bodies and their genitals when they are by themselves is often quite important. Telling couples to communicate with each other about what feels good—either verbally or nonverbally—is also often helpful. Another common problem found in women is painful intercourse. Sometimes it is because of inadequate lubrication and can be cured either through increased foreplay or through use of an artificial lubricant. In other cases, however, it is a learned response and professional treatment by a sex therapist is required. Finally, some of the sexual problems of women result from a traditional unconscious discrimination against women patients by the medical establishment. We consider this problem in the following section.

WOMEN AS PATIENTS

The Greek word *hystera* means uterus. Hysteria or "wandering womb," an emotional "craziness," has long been expected of women. Psychiatry has been heavily influenced by the writings of Sigmund Freud, who believed that "anatomy is destiny" and that a woman's anatomy often led her to a troubled destiny.

As in other fields, sex stereotypes have led to certain detrimental effects in the treatment of female patients. Before the turn of the century, some women were forced to have their clitoris removed as a "cure" for sexual enjoyment, and hysterectomies as treatment for psychiatric disorders were especially common. As such cultural expectations continued in one form or another, unnecessary hysterectomies continued into contemporary times and may still occur in some settings. The health care environment is often unhealthy for women [22, 26].

Some people become needlessly defensive when the topic of sex discrimination arises. In discussing the effects of sex roles in medicine, two important points should be kept in mind. First, sex roles like other roles are generally very subtle and unintentional. For example, the fact that women were kept out of many professions for many years does not mean that men, or anyone else, conspired against women or indeed that anyone recognized what was happening. Sex roles then were just "the way things were." Second, it is important to note that there is a methodological limitation in designing simple laboratory studies to test the effects of people's sex role expectations. To use an extreme example, if it is asserted that pregnant women are not given enough pain relief, we cannot test the possibility of sex discrimination by examining the pain relief given to pregnant men. Nevertheless, problems can slowly be uncovered, and careful examination of indirect evidence must be undertaken.

Many physicians expect women to be more troublesome as patients than men. They also expect to find more symptoms with psychological links in women than in men. Such expectations may interfere with the physicians' judgment. For example, women are much more likely than are men to receive prescriptions for mood-modifying drugs such as tranquilizers [14, 22, 26, 46]. An important unanswered question involves the extent to which these sex differences are physiologically based or result from the expectations of physicians and of female patients. Part of the difference may lie in the greater tendency of women to report symptoms. Females are generally expected to monitor their family's health while males are expected to ignore "minor" pain; or perhaps women are more attuned to the feelings of their bodies than are men. Only a health practitioner, either male or female, who is alert to the long history of differential treatment of men and women can attempt to avoid errors in medical diagnosis that result from unjustified expectations.

Rape

A special problem involving women as patients is rape. Rape is a crime of violence and aggression in which a man asserts his power over a woman, vents his anger, and demonstrates her helplessness in the face of his strength. It is relatively uncommon for rape to be a purely sexual act, for rape involves domination. In as many as two-fifths of the cases, rape is a group phenomenon in which two or more assailants attack a woman [2, 28].

A woman who is raped may be hurt physically, but her physical wounds often heal long before her psychological wounds. Women who have been raped are often plagued by feelings of guilt, shame, humiliation, and the loss of their self-esteem. They feel overwhelmingly vulnerable, and are usually afraid to be alone. These feelings may last for a very long time, and they may significantly interfere with the woman's life.

Until recently, many women who had been raped avoided reporting it to the police and medical authorities because the physical and psychological treatment of the rape victim was so distressing in itself. Women who had been raped were interrogated with harshness and insensitivity, and the burden of proving their own innocence and lack of consent to the rape was upon the women themselves [28]. Women who had been raped were often examined by physicians in such a way that they felt powerless and physically abused. Many women described the medical examination as much like another rape.

Many communities and college campuses today have groups of men and women engaged in rape prevention and in rape crisis intervention. These groups sponsor escort services for women who would normally have to walk alone at night. They also sponsor courses instructing women in self-defense. Nevertheless, in many areas and on many campuses, rape still occurs all too frequently.

Changes in rape treatment and investigation have come about in recent years, primarily as a result of the women's movement. In many communities methods for treating rape victims differ greatly from that of the past. For example, today a specially trained rape counselor can be called at a rape crisis intervention organization; she stays with the woman throughout a rigorous physical examination designed to secure evidence for identification and prosecution of the assailant. The health professionals are taught to give a woman control in everything that happens to her. For example, she is asked permission to be questioned and to be touched or examined. This is done in an effort to reverse her feelings of helplessness and invasion. Psychological counseling is provided for the rape victim and for her close male friend or husband. This counseling can help to prevent a common occurrence—the breakup of the woman's ongoing emotional-sexual relationship [82]. The woman's husband or lover is counseled to deal with his anger, and the woman is counseled to overcome her fears and to begin to trust men again. She is likely to need to overcome nightmares, a fear of being alone, and feelings of intense vulnerability.

While there are no reliable statistics on its frequency, rape against men also occurs. Rapes are common in correctional facilities; they are a fact of prison life. Inmates use rape partly as a method of establishing masculinity and a hierarchy of dominance. Physically small or muscularly underdeveloped men are particularly vulnerable. For men, too, rape is a serious health care problem because of its often devastating psychological consequences [44].

Pregnancy and Social Support

Another aspect of a healthy medical environment for women involves childbirth. The birth of a child, particularly the first child, presents a major life change for most couples. There are new financial, emotional, interpersonal, and physical strains, and it is normal for many couples to feel overwhelmed and to have trouble adjusting to this event [29].

In the past in our society, social support, esteem, assistance, and information were readily given to the couple by their parents or grandparents and other relatives who lived nearby. But new opportunities for mobility make it likely that a couple may live far away from family and friends who could provide this kind of support and help. Consequently, the health professional is often called upon to fill this role.

During pregnancy, couples need assurance to allay their fears and anxieties over the course of the pregnancy and the upcoming delivery. The initial postpartum months are among the most stressful times the couple is likely to ever face. Health professionals may find that new parents call them frequently to check on the most minor detail in the care of their infant. The new parents usually also want to ask questions relating to their own feelings, adjustment, and health, but tend to do so only if they are given the opportunity [13, 54].

Health professionals are in an excellent position to provide support for new parents and to help them avoid some of the problems that can result from the stress of having a new baby—marital discord, sexual problems, or the inability to control emotional outbursts.

The new mother and father are unlikely to immediately and openly verbalize feelings, fears, and problems, but rather may "beat around the bush," hedging and hinting at what the problem is.

One of the best things that the health professional can do for a couple is to provide information, especially about what is likely to happen to them. In addition, including the husband in aspects of the prenatal visits, during labor and delivery, and in postpartum visits and childcare are important in establishing the importance of the father to the child, both from the point of view of the mother and the father.

Thus far we have considered aspects of the health care environment on which the health provider can have an impact but over which the practitioner has only limited and indirect control. There is, however, a significant health care environment over which health providers have complete and direct control—namely, the hospital.

THE HOSPITAL ENVIRONMENT

In the early part of this century hospitalization was dreaded. Hospitals were seen as unpleasant and costly places, and most importantly as places where people went to die. With the advent of medical "miracles," however, hospitals cure millions of seriously ill people each year. Yet hospitals still suffer a negative reputation; the problem is not merely their association with disease.

The words *hospital* and *hospitality* come from the same Latin root. The Latin word for hospitality refers to the way in which guests should be received. Yet hospitals are often not very hospitable and patients are rarely treated as guests. Of course, there are some medical benefits that accrue from this discrepancy, but there are also negative effects.

The word *hospice*—a place where the terminally ill may go to die—also comes from the same Latin root. As we shall see, the hospice movement in America is growing [59]. Despite their association with terminal illness, hospices may evoke more positive feelings in many Americans than hospitals. The difference lies in the social psychological nature of the hospital environment.

There are more than 7000 hospitals in the United States [1]. People no longer go to hospitals only when they are seriously ill as in the early days of this century. The performance of most surgery, many laboratory tests, and procedures requiring expensive medical equipment necessitates hospital admission. In addition, when a patient needs to be observed for a while, the hospital is where this patient should be, often for the convenience of the health care professionals.

Hospitals are *total institutions* [24], which means that they manage every aspect of the patient's life. The hospital is one of the few places where people forfeit almost all control over their life. (Other examples of total institutions are prisons and mental hospitals.) Patients relinquish their clothes for hospital gowns; they are rarely addressed in familiar terms, are highly restricted in where they can go, encounter a fixed schedule of eating and sleeping, and have little privacy. Patients are usually unable to make even the smallest effort to help in their own treatment. Patients must operate according to the schedule of the hospital and follow its rules, with little chance for individuality. Patients may begin to lose their identity in hospitals.

Institutionalization is a special concern for the elderly. Aging is a physiological phenomenon; the cells die and tissues wear out, losing their resiliency. Healing takes longer and bodily processes slow down. However, aging is also a *social* phenomenon. It has been said that older persons have two kinds of problems—the problems they actually have and the problems that others think they have. Social expectations strongly influence the course of aging, and they often define the situation of the aging person. Consider the example of

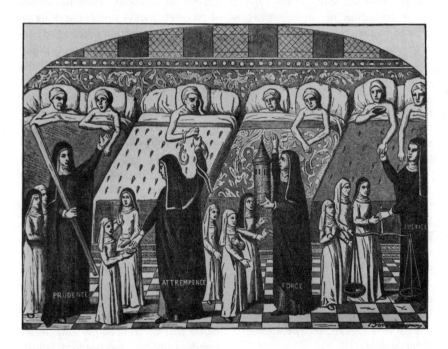

Figure 11-2. The hospital environment: a fifteenth-century French hospital. (Courtesy of The Bettmann Archive, New York.)

Box 11–1
The Elderly in the United States

Approximately 81 percent of aged individuals (over 65 years old) in the United States suffer from some condition of chronic illness. About 33 percent of the aged have no physical limitations on their activity, but about 16 percent are totally unable to carry out major activities. Overall, only about half the elderly are somewhat disabled because of chronic illness. It is interesting to note the nature of the problems; more than 30 percent of the elderly have trouble walking up and down stairs. Thus, in a society in which individuals (at least those with limited incomes) must use stairs all the time, a major limitation on their activity is created by the *environment*. Estimates of the rate of mental impairment of the elderly very, but are usually around 10 percent (some estimates are as high as 25 percent). This means that most elderly people are completely capable of thinking clearly and making decisions for themselves as well as contributing to the society.

Forced dependency among older people stems primarily from the fact that most older people in the United States have some financial problems. This is especially true for widowed women who may have no economically viable skills. Older persons have about half the income of younger persons. And while inflation threatens the lifestyle of younger persons, it threatens the very lives and independence of older people.

Loneliness is a significant problem for the aged, although probably not as great as might be expected. For example, 15 percent of aged women and about 10 percent of aged men report feelings of loneliness. These feelings may result from the changed pattern of their lives in retirement and the loss of old friends and spouses. However, the facts that most older people live within about one hour's drive of their close relatives or their children and that they receive at least a weekly visit from them suggest that loneliness for physical contact may not be the major problem. The problem involves the quality of relations. Visits from children often involve simply checking on the physical condition of the aged person and not really intimately talking with the person. Of course, loneliness can also result from not having a spouse: widowhood is very common. Between the ages of 60 and 64, more than a quarter of the women and 6 percent of the men are widowed. Between the ages of 70 and 74, half of the women are widows; and by age 85, half the men are widowers.

People face another problem as they age, that is, a change in their usual social role. The aged experience a transition from a career as a worker, or as a homemaker and parent, to a position in society that demands no contribution, and which seems purposeless at times. Roles taken up in later life include that of "retired person," independent institutional resident, volunteer, or sick person. These roles do not enhance the self-esteem of the persons involved. Compulsory retirement, for example, forces the role of "pensioner" on a worker who still feels useful and productive. Besides experiencing the financial worries that come with the decreased income in retirement, retirees are prevented from performing work that they consider useful. Feelings of being degraded may be experienced by residents of "retirement communities," who are expected to be comfortable and content to spend their time engaged in "arts and crafts."

For further reading: M. M. Seltzer, S. L. Corbett, and R. C. Atchley (eds.), *Social Problems of the Aging: Readings* (Belmont, Calif.: Wadsworth, 1978).

Grandma Harper, who is 75 years old. She lives with her daughter and son-in-law and two granddaughters. While working one day in the kitchen of her daughter's house, Grandma left a doll's dress that she was knitting on the kitchen table, and went to answer the phone on the other side of the room. While there, she cleaned the kitchen counter and then went to the front door to pay the newsboy. When she returned to the kitchen, her knitting was nowhere to be found: She concluded that she must have misplaced it. Her 18-year-old granddaughter came in, and Grandma asked her if she had seen her knitting. The granddaughter suggested that Grandma had been very forgetful lately, and the lost knitting is thus understood in terms of Grandma's advancing age. Both Grandma and her family may believe that she should gradually undertake fewer responsibilities and that eventually she will have to enter an institution. Such facts as Grandma's 10-year-old granddaughter taking the knitted dress to try on her doll are never discovered. We return to the problems of the aged later in this chapter (see Box 11–1).

Control

Hospitals and nursing homes are generally regarded as unpleasant places to be as patients. A prime reason is lack of control. People generally wish to maintain some individuality, to have some control over their environment and their schedules, and to gain information about what is happening to them. However, inmates of hospitals and other health institutions quickly learn that this is not the way they are expected to behave. Instead there is an obligation to be a "cooperative" patient. Most patients learn that they should not try to play a "consumer role." They should be quiet, submissive, obedient, and not distinguish themselves as individuals [48].

The social psychologist Shelley Taylor has analyzed the hospital patient role. Most patients assume the expected role; that is, they behave in ways that make them "good" patients. However, a significant number of patients are considered "bad" patients; bad patients play the consumer role, insisting on their rights, including the right to know everything that is happening to them. Consumer patients (who may be seen as "bad" from the perspective of certain health care professionals) insist on their own autonomy, and the right to help take care of themselves. These patients may become angry, particularly if freedoms are withdrawn from them for the convenience of the staff. They also resent the hospital bureaucracy [48, 77].

The patient's angry reaction to the seemingly arbitrary withdrawal of freedom is a common psychological reaction. It has been termed *reactance* [8]. Reactance theory proposes that people try to reestablish or regain freedoms that are lost. Patients may react with anger primarily because they have not been prepared for the withdrawal of freedom that they encounter in the hospital, and because they see the restrictions as having no significant purpose.

Patients may rebel by failing to take their medications. This petty mutiny may actually function as a form of self-sabotage. Patients in an angry state are experiencing a physiological arousal that may be detrimental to their recovery [23, 41]. Staff attempts to mollify irascible patients with condescending comfort may increase this anxiety. On the other hand, staff members may ignore angry patients and avoid listening to their complaints; in so doing, they may overlook a complaint that has medical significance [48].

While it is probably true that most so-called bad or angry patients receive negative reactions from staff members, are treated poorly interpersonally, and may be punished in some ways, they may often be in *better* physical and emotional shape than good, compliant patients, and may actually get better faster. Their fighting for control may be a psychologically healthy response.

Very submissive patients, on the other hand, often have given up control. Because they have received very little information, these patients may remain in a condition of anxiety. These individuals are exposed to aversive stimulation over which they have no control. They may question nurses who do not have the information they need, or turn to family members, who have little idea of what is happening to the patient. They may receive an assortment of misconceptions and contradictory information. Most of the time, submissive patients are highly regarded by the staff because they do not complain and are not demanding [48]. Their passivity, however, puts them in a position where they are unlikely to do much that will improve their health. These patients not only do not ask for information, but also they do not divulge it; they have learned to be quiet. These passive patients may be in a condition that is referred to as *learned helplessness*. People may learn to give up and do nothing in response to challenges to their well-being [71, 76].

Helplessness and Control. Anna Jones was a 75-year-old widow who lived along in a tiny New York City apartment. Although it took her all day to perform her chores, she did her own shopping, cooking, and cleaning. She saw her friends a few times a week, and she entertained herself by knitting, talking on the phone, and watching her favorite television programs. Her only son lived in California.

The low-rent apartment building in which Anna had lived for 20 years since her husband's death was sold one day to developers, who planned to build a group of high-rise condominiums in its place. Anna was sent an eviction notice. Since she lived on meager social security checks, she was overwhelmed at the thought of searching for affordable housing. Even though she was independent with respect to her daily living, Anna was unable to cope with the thought of making a major transition to a new place to live. She needed help. Her son, however, wishing to settle things as soon as possible and also recognizing that his mother's faculties would soon be failing, arranged to place her in a modern nursing home. Despite Anna's protestations, her son argued that he knew best. Anna was moved to the nursing home, where all of her meals were cooked and served to her. Her clothes were washed; her room was cleaned every day, and she was allowed to go to the TV room to watch whatever happened to be on television. Within three weeks of her arrival, Anna gave up doing anything, went to bed, and died of heart failure.

Helplessness, according to psychologist Martin Seligman, is a psychological state that frequently results when a person encounters events that are uncontrollable [71]. Uncontrollable events are events about which the person can do nothing. Anna, for example, experienced many of these events. She could do nothing that would have any impact on her environment. No one needed her in the nursing home, and none of her actions had any consequence. She could not leave, for she had nowhere to go.

Although it occurs in many aspects of life (e.g., in business where one's actions may have no effect on the evaluation of the boss), helplessness is a particularly salient characteristic of old age. As people lose their physical capabilities and their financial resources, they become more and more dependent upon other's decisions for them, and less and less able to control their own fate.

In his research, Seligman found that people may lose the motivation to control many other events in their lives once they experience significant loss of control in one realm. They also have difficulty in recognizing that any successful responses they have actually are successful in affecting the environment. That is, experience with uncontrollable events can result in learned helplessness. Learned helplessness can lead people to emotional disturbance, and also to serious depression. Seligman has presented many cases in which he believes even sudden death has resulted from helplessness.

Helplessness is partly a function of the situation. But people differ in their basic beliefs about how much control they can exert over their environment. *Locus of control* refers to an individual's belief about what determines what happens to him or her [67, 68].

People with an *internal* locus of control believe that their fate is in their own hands; those with an *external* locus of control believe that they have no power to determine their fate and that it is up to chance or luck. This personality trait represents a continuum on which a person can be described as more or less internal, or more or less external.

A considerable amount of research has been devoted to this aspect of personality. People with extreme scores on either end of the locus of control continuum tend to be maladjusted. Those with a predominantly internal orientation are likely to seek constructive solutions to frustrating problems instead of giving up on them. They are more active, ambitious, powerful, achieving, independent, and effective. Some studies show that people with an internal locus of control are more willing to make changes in their own behavior to correct personal shortcomings if they are given the opportunity to do so. This suggests that a person with an internal locus of control would be more likely to put health recommendations to use.

The Rotter I-E scale measures locus of control. In a number of interesting research programs, locus of control has been utilized to predict health behaviors [79, 80]. A study done after the release of the U.S. Surgeon General's report in 1964 implicating cigarette smoking as a major cause of lung cancer showed that those who continued to be smokers were significantly more external in orientation than nonsmokers, and that heavy smokers were more external than those who smoked less [32].

In studies of unmarried female college students it has been found that there is a significant relationship between locus of control and the use of birth control, such that more internal women tended to be more likely to use some form of birth control [49]. In a study of hospital patient behavior, it was found that internal patients knew more about their condition, were more inquisitive with doctors and nurses about their illness, and indicated less satisfaction with the amount of information they received than did external patients. Internal patients attempted to gain a greater degree of control over their health by gaining information [70].

Rotter himself suggested that the locus of control orientation in specific situations like health might best be measured by a test instrument tailored specifically to assess the issues at hand. Researchers have adapted the Rotter I–E scale to a health locus of control scale [81]. This scale is an initial attempt to operationalize health-related locus of control beliefs, and to look at the relationship between them and health behaviors. Research is still relatively sparse, but some results show that people who were internal *and* who placed a high degree of value on health exposed themselves to more health information than did others.

The hospital environment may overwhelm even a healthy personality. Patients with an internal locus of control may be especially upset by the sense of helplessness created by the typical hospital environment. It is especially difficult for patients who must institute and carry out self-care after being discharged from the hospital to overcome the lack of control induced by the hospital. Patients may have trouble assuming the tasks necessary to take care of themselves.

Thus the degree and nature of control exercised by hospitals and the various resulting reactions by patients can have both short-term and long-range impacts on health. Strict, arbitrary, unexplained hospital rules may harm the very patients they are trying to help.

For a number of reasons, older people are more likely to become submissive in the hospital and to try to fulfill their perceived expectations of the health care professionals who care for them. They may also attempt to show that they are grateful for the care given them. Thus old people in institutions are prone to helplessness, dependency, and resultant depression. We examine the institutionalized aged later in this chapter. First, however, we consider another psychosocial danger in hospital care.

Dehumanization

The hospital patient is sometimes treated like an inanimate object by most of the staff [24]. Things are "done to" the patient. The patient may have a great deal of trouble acquiring information or respect. Questions from the patient may be put off onto others. Many different people enter the patient's room throughout the day, few of them even bothering to identify themselves. Patients are often referred to by their symptoms, diseases, or conditions. Thus a patient may become "the gallbladder case." Medical staff making rounds usually talk about the patient in highly technical terms in front of the patient. For whatever reasons that the staff may have, patients are usually told little about what is happening to them [12, 15, 48]. This phenomenon is called *dehumanization*. Dehumanization is the process of treating a person as less than a whole human being [6, 69].

Dehumanization is often associated with instances of mass violence in that it helps ease psychological restrictions on murder. Terms like "redskin," "heathen," "nigger," and "gook" reduce people to objects and reduce the psychological restrictions on eliminating such "menaces" [69]. Unfortunately, sometimes an equally insidious epithet is "patient." How can this be? Interestingly, dehumanization produces an emotional detachment that may sometimes be useful in medicine. For example, it may be beneficial for surgeons not to be emotionally involved with their patients during an operation.

Although it is sometimes helpful, dehumanization produces a decreased awareness of the human attributes of the patient and a loss of humanity in dealing with the patient. The health care professional may stop perceiving the patient as also having feelings, thoughts, and impulses, and instead deal with the patient only on an intellectual level [72, 83]. Dehumanization in medical settings puts the patient in a position where he or she is responded to with objective, analytical responses, but the responses are lacking in emotion or in empathy. Health care professionals may engage in dehumanization partly to protect themselves emotionally from having to deal with pain and illness.

A particularly severe and unnecessary form of dehumanization in hospitals has traditionally surrounded childbirth. Expectant mothers are often isolated in labor rooms, wheeled into sterile-looking delivery rooms, and anesthetized. The baby is delivered and sent to the nursery, the mother wheeled to a recovery room, and the father notified so that he can go home to pass out cigars. In rare life-threatening births, strict environmental control is obviously necessary. However, with most births such dehumanized procedures may interfere with the natural birth process [4, 9, 50].

There is increasing evidence that more humane treatment benefits the mother, father, and the infant. Pleasant surroundings and the presence and assistance of the father at the birth may reduce the anxiety and difficulty of the mother and so facilitate the birth. A calmer entry into the world may produce a more relaxed infant.

Perhaps most importantly, humanized maternity care may increase the psychological bonds within the family. By sharing in the birth experience, many fathers may become more attached to both their wives and their children. Furthermore, a special parent-infant attachment—sometimes called "bonding"—may be fostered [29].

Obedience

Hospitals and similar institutions have very clearly defined authority hierarchies; that is, there is a well defined power structure that ranges from the directors at the top to the orderlies at the bottom. There is a clear expectation that each member of the institution will obey a perceived legitimate authority, for obedience helps the institution run smoothly. However, like other aspects of an institution, obedience can also produce deadly side effects.

A traditional ranking in hospitals is that nurses are subordinate to physicians. This status difference has traditionally been further supported by sex roles since most physicians have been men while most nurses have been women. The implications of this status difference are well illustrated by a dramatic study by C. K. Hofling and associates [30]. In this study doctors telephoned nurses in a hospital and instructed them to administer a dose of medicine to a patient on the ward. (Prescription by telephone was against hospital policy.) The drug was a "new" drug, unknown to the nurses, but the prescribed dose was an overdose according to directions on the label. Out of 22 nurses who received these telephone orders, 21 of them attempted to administer this potentially fatal overdose to the patient. To protect the patients, the experiment was set up so that the drug was actually harmless and the nurses were intercepted before they could administer it. This study dramatically demonstrated the extent to which nurses would obey authority. Interestingly, many of the nurses reported that they had encountered similar (real) incidents in the past.

A followup study helped isolate the factors that produced compliance on the part of the nurses [63]. First, the nurses were unfamiliar with both the drug and the doctor; they had little previous information on which to evaluate the order. Second, the nurses were instructed not to discuss the order with other medical personnel. In fact, the Hofling study was done with nurses on the evening shift when staffing was minimal. If in doubt, the nurses would usually consult with other nurses or endeavor to recontact the doctor. Still, in a replication study in which an overdose of valium was prescribed while other options were available, some nurses obeyed the order completely and few directly challenged the order [63].

The point of such studies is *not* how many nurses will obey dangerous orders. The point of the study is also *not* weaknesses in the nurses' personalities or training. Rather, such studies demonstrate the tremendous power of a legitimate authority in an institution. Such instances of well-intentioned but dangerous obedience to authority are found in many social situations.

The classic studies demonstrating the tremendous power of the social situation to elicit obedient behavior were done by the social psychologist Stanley Milgram [57]. Milgram created a laboratory study supposedly on the effects of punishment on learning. When someone arrived to participate in this study, this person was assigned to the role of "teacher" in which he or she was supposed to teach another person a list of paired words. The learner was hooked up to electrodes, and the teacher was supposed to administer an electric shock to the learner as punishment whenever the learner made an error. As the study progressed, the "teacher" (the experimental subject) was instructed by the experimenter to administer a continually higher dosage of shock to the learner. The shocks became quite painful and eventually very dangerous. The learner, who was in another room and connected to the teacher by an intercom, called out and demanded that the study be stopped. However, the experimenter insisted to the teacher (subject) that the experiment continue. On orders of the experimenter, more than 50 percent of the teachers kept administering electric shocks even at a level marked extremely dangerous. Fortunately, unknown to the teacher, the learner was a confederate of the experimenter and was not actually receiving the electric shocks.

When Milgram asked a number of psychiatrists what percentage of people would obey orders in this situation and administer dangerous shocks to an innocent victim, the psychiatrists estimated that less than 1 percent of the population would comply fully. However, we have noted that most people did comply. It is difficult even for trained psychiatrists to understand the great power of the social situation in producing obedience. This pervasive willingness to follow orders helps us understand such shocking episodes as the massacre at My Lai in which American soldiers in Vietnam shot innocent civilians. Just as the teachers in the Milgram study and the soldiers in Vietnam did not desire to do any harm but felt they had no other choice, many nurses and medical assistants feel they have no choice but to obey the orders of a doctor.

Some safeguards can be instituted to help each individual recognize his or her own personal responsibility for actions, but the problem cannot be completely eliminated so long as an authority hierarchy is in place. Such power structures are an integral part of most hospitals, and therefore all medical personnel should be alert to the dangers that may result. We cannot rely on a health professional's "common sense" to avoid the dangerous consequences of erroneous medical orders.

Nosocomial Infection

Should patients remind doctors and nurses to wash their hands? Of the more than 30 million Americans who will be admitted to hospitals this year, over 1 million will develop *nosocomial* infections—infections that are acquired *in* the hospital. Thousands will die because of entering a hospital. Of course, for most patients the benefits to be gained from hospitalization far outweigh the risks; but nevertheless the problem is still serious, although mostly avoidable [16, 64, 73].

Since the discovery of germs, most nosocomial infections have been controllable in theory. Sterilization of equipment, disinfection of the environment, and isolation of certain patients all help control the transmission of bacteria. Also important is the simple act of handwashing. Yet the biological problem of killing bacteria has become the psychosocial problem of controlling the attitudes and behavior of hospital personnel. How can weakened patients, often with open wounds, be protected from those trying to help them? Will doctors wash their hands? (See Box 11-2). A number of social psychological issues come together on this question. First, simple precautions like handwashing may lose their importance if the emphasis of the overall hospital environment is on the technological wonders of medicine and miracle drugs. Second, authority hierarchies may preclude a nurse or patient from questioning a doctor about simple infection-preventing measures. Relatedly, people in a hospital may wish to avoid "insulting" a health care practitioner by implying a lack of cleanliness, even though their lives are at stake. Such matters of embarrassment and manners are psychosocial phenomena. In some hospitals, expectations make it perfectly permissible, perhaps even desirable, for everyone to work together to prevent nosocomial infection. Just as errors in technical treatment are pointed out, so too are lapses in cleanliness. If the people around the health professional are very conscious of nosocomial infection, it is likely that he or she will be also, and will adopt the values and procedures of the surrounding people [64].

We have singled out nosocomial infection for attention because

Box 11-2
Study Finds Hospital Personnel
Fail to Wash Hands Frequently

(The following UPI article appeared in the Riverside, California Press on June 11, 1981.)

Boston (UPI)—Patients in intensive-care units risk contracting new diseases because hospital personnel often fail to wash their hands, it was reported today.

"We found that, on the average, hospital personnel washed their hands after contact with patients less than half the time," Dr. Richard K. Albert wrote in the New England Journal of Medicine. He is head of the intensive-care unit at the University of Washington Veterans Administration Medical Center in Seattle.

"Physicians were among the worst offenders."

He said patients in intensive-care units are particularly susceptible to infections transmitted by hand because of the frequent use of catheters, wires, tubes and other "invasive" procedures.

Such infections are common, Albert said. They could come from hands carrying an infection or from another patient.

"You might even liken it to seatbelts," he said. "It's very difficult to say after an accident if that person had been wearing a seatbelt, would that injury have been prevented. And yet how many people don't wear seatbelts?"

Albert said he doesn't believe physicians are consciously ignoring the need for hand washing—they probably just don't realize it is important even after contact with a patient where infection isn't obvious.

Infections contracted in hospitals are a common problem caused by all kinds of bacteria, said Albert and a research assistant, Frances Condie. These infections can be fatal.

The Centers for Disease Control in Atlanta and the American Hospital Association have said hand washing is the single most important step in preventing hospital infections, the study reported.

Albert and Condie secretly watched hand-washing habits at an unidentified university-affiliated teaching hospital and a private hospital under the guise of studying medical personnel traffic patterns.

They found hands were washed 41 percent of the time at the university hospital. At the private hospital, hands were washed 28 percent of the time.

Respiratory therapists ranked the highest in the study, washing their hands 76 percent of the time at the university hospital and 48 percent at the private hospital.

Nurses washed their hands 43 percent of the time after patient contact at the university hospital, and 28 percent of the time at the private hospital.

the danger of disease and death from improper behavior of medical personnel is so obvious. However, in a total institution like a hospital, the general expectations and standards for behavior are extremely important in many areas. Expectations about patients' chances for recovery, their sensitive treatment, the role of family, and the dignity of the dying are all social psychological factors that are a key part of any hospital.

INSTITUTIONALIZATION OF THE AGED

If a 25-year-old woman forgets to pick up her husband at the train station and later burns the roast chicken, she is not assigned to a nursing home. But what if she is forgetful at age 75?

There are many popular stereotypes of aging, many of which are inaccurate. In health care many of these assumptions have implications for institutionalization. First, many people believe that intelligence declines with age, and therefore they believe that a person at 70 is likely to be less intelligent than at 60. In some poorly designed research, older people of one age were compared with younger people of another age—a research method referred to as *cross-sectional* analysis. For example, a group of people in their twenties are compared with a group of people in their sixties. The assumption is that any differences between the two groups can be attributed to age changes. However, this assumption is wrong because people of various ages differ in many ways. They belong to different generations and have had very different life experiences and different levels and quality of education. Thus, although some studies found that people in older age groups had lower intelligence than people in younger age groups, much of this difference had to do with the low quality of the schooling that the older people had received. Furthermore, the elderly were inexperienced in taking the kinds of standardized tests that were used to measure intelligence [7, 60, 74].

Only recently have we begun to see the results of *longitudinal* studies. In these studies individuals are followed over long periods to discover if there are any changes in their intelligence levels. The same persons are measured at age 30, 40, 50, 60, and 70. It is only then that valid scientific conclusions can be drawn about age changes. As can be imagined, these long-term longitudinal studies are very costly. They require the continued interest of the researchers, continued funding, and the ability to keep track of the subjects over a long time. Nevertheless, such studies are necessary. The results of longitudinal studies of intelligence show very different results from cross-sectional studies. People do *not* decline significantly in most of their mental abilities. While there are physical changes, there are few intellectual changes. Most of the aged can cope intellectually on their own in the modern world. With failing health and the loss of visual and auditory faculties, individuals may lose some intellectual capabilities. However, with proper steps taken to assure visual acuity (e.g., eyeglasses) and auditory acuity (hearing aids), most people can continue to be active intellectually until well into their eighties and nineties [18].

Interestingly, it has also been found that physical activity can continue throughout a person's life and institutionalization can often be avoided. Lifestyle, environment, and culture, rather than age, tend to be the primary determinants of a person's activity level. With proper diet, exercise, and other healthy behaviors, aging persons can maintain high levels of physical activity and health.

Sexual activity can also continue among the aged. The belief that older people have no desire for sexual behavior is a dangerous myth, for it can become a self-fulfilling prophecy. Fortunately, in recent years there have been a number of books written about the myths of aging and sexuality [11, 84]. The supposed loss of interest and development of problems in sex are often *social* phenomena, not biological. Recent studies have shown that people can usually remain sexually active into their eighties. Eroticism in the aged requires primarily a comfort with and acceptance of a leisurely, sensuous activity. Such behavior may be difficult in an institution.

There is no doubt that some older persons become what is called "senile." Senility may result from a chronic organic brain disorder that produces poor memory, an inability of the individual to orient in time and place, and a general marked decline in intellectual functioning. Institutionalization may be necessary. Although we know that learning can occur throughout life and that most older persons need not decline significantly in their intellectual abilities, many people still cling to the myth that senility is inevitable. A self-fulfilling prophecy may result. Attitudes of other people are probably the most significant determinant of the development of senility in most persons [17].

"Senility" is also a label, just like "mental illness." The organic condition actually exists, but it is not as prevalent as it seems. Applying the label to someone can make his or her behavior fulfill the expectations of the role of the senile person. These behaviors might be inappropriate displays of affect, the person being confused about where he or she is, and so on. Some health professionals use a convenient label of senility to explain this kind of behavior, and the temporary confusion that the person is experiencing can thus become permanent because the person is then confined to a nursing home and custodial care. Furthermore, because health professionals expect the elderly to be senile, they may therefore overlook many acute diseases that may actually occur in the elderly.

Thus many of the attributions that are made about older people can be very detrimental to their ability to remain independent and to care for themselves. The temporary difficulties that they experience and for which they need help can be interpreted as indicating that they can no longer take care of themselves. Their family members or physicians may then decide that institutionalization is the best approach. But it is actually with institutionalization that many of the aged begin to fulfill the many stereotypes that exist about them. Individuals in nursing homes often experience a significant decline in their physical and mental capabilities [17, 56].

If we look at the social characteristics in an average nursing home, we see a picture that makes it very difficult for the aged person to be anything but dehumanized [56]. These problems are a product of the institution, not the caretakers. Aged people who live in institutions tend to live communally with a minimum of privacy. They have little in the way of close relationships with each other or others outside the hospital. The staff members lead a separate existence, and members of the staff change often. Individuals in nursing homes must submit to an orderly routine and have almost no opportunity to exercise self-determination. They have little opportunity for sexual expression. Residents of nursing homes may be forced to consume special diets. They are usually not allowed to walk outside of the facilities because of the fear that they might injure themselves. These practices may be "medically" sound, but they tend to control the patients and their environment to the point where the inhabitants of nursing homes relinquish all control and responsibility for their own destiny [10].

The human environment in nursing homes can be changed in order to prevent significant deterioration among the aged. Psychological support needs to be created, social interaction with the outside world is necessary, and procedures that encourage humanization of the aged are needed. A sense of independence and direction in life need to be part of the institutional setting in order for the aged patient to cope adequately.

A successful rehabilitation program for aged patients in institutions includes having realistic expectations for what they can do. Some may reenter the community. For others, however, successful rehabilitation may involve learning to dress, feed, and groom themselves. A popular form of rehabilitation therapy for aged patients in institutions is called *milieu therapy,* which involves an attempt to alter the behavior of patients by changing their environment as well as the expectations held of the patients. In most nursing homes, residents are shaved, bathed, and dressed by attendants, simply because these things can be done more quickly by the attendants and it is less trouble. But milieu therapy involves patient self-care to the maximum extent possible. Staff members give assistance to the inhabitants only when absolutely necessary. Allowing residents to spend their own money for the various services available to them can also give them added responsibility. Studies of milieu therapy show that positive behavioral changes among the inhabitants of nursing homes can result. Furthermore, the patients in the nursing homes begin to know each other better and to express feelings for each other. Intellectual impairment and delusions tend to decrease [17].

We now turn from the aged to the young and examine the special problems faced by another group in institutions—children in hospitals.

CHILDREN IN HOSPITALS

A child of age four was contacted through an intercom by a nurse from the nurses' station. After a number of calls with no response, an answer was finally received in a tiny, very frightened voice. The child asked, "What do you want, wall?" The child did not understand that the nurse's voice was coming through the intercom [27].

There is a growing awareness of the traumatic effects of hospitalization on children, particularly children in their preschool years. Studies have indicated that much of the trauma results from *separation anxiety*—the anxiety experienced by the child in being separated from parents, particularly the mother. Coupled with this separation anxiety is an intense fear of bodily mutilation. Even though physicians and nurses involved in the hospital care of sick children recognize that it is often extremely difficult to care for children who are hospitalized, they often show little active professional interest in anything beyond the children's physical needs. This situation is slowly changing, however. It is important to understand the problems of caring for children in hospitals in order to reduce their anxiety and to prevent long-term effects of the trauma of hospitalization [27].

The major problem occurs with children from the ages of three to five who are hospitalized for the first time since birth. Hospitalization is a threat to most young children, primarily because they feel betrayed and deserted by their parents. These children are usually too young to understand assurances that their parents will return for them and they will soon be able to go home. Children may also become quite anxious at the sight of hospital equipment. Toddlers may react to hospitalization with developmental regression—that is, regressing to earlier behaviors. These behaviors include nighttime fears and screaming, clinging to and being dependent on their parents, intensified thumb sucking, and loss of bowel and bladder control. Many doctors now advocate that parents remain in the hospital with the child who is under the age of five. In addition, attempts are made to avoid voluntary hospitalization and elective surgery on young children.

Sometimes hospitalization is necessary and other measures must be taken to reduce the serious emotional problems that can result. Whereas not long ago children were taken into the operating room unaware of what was going to happen to them, it is now believed that giving the child some control may be the best approach (as it is with adults). While it was once believed that it was better not to excite fearful expectations in the child, research suggests that avoidance of the issue proves too traumatic and produces too many long-lasting effects. First, the child should be given information about what is happening. Providing information to the child is something that can be done in the context of storytelling or play acting. The child can be given a demonstration of the frightening equipment. Second, the child should be encouraged to express emotion, and there must be a relationship of trust established with the hospital staff. It is not uncommon for a child to feel that he or she is being sent to the hospital as a punishment for being naughty. Furthermore, children should be forewarned about pain that will accompany medical procedures. Telling children "It won't hurt" and then inflicting pain in various procedures that actually do hurt destroys the trust that the child has in the health care professional.

It is also important for children to maintain links to home. If parents cannot be at the hospital to reassure preschoolers, telephone calls with the parents and other siblings can be a very important means of communication. It is helpful for children to look through the windows of the hospital and see their parents leaving and arriving.

Finally, it is important for the staff to promote autonomy and independence in children. As much as possible, aspects of the child's environment should be child sized. Between the ages of one and five, children develop skills of eating, washing, dressing, and controlling their bowel and bladder functions. In the hospital setting it is very easy for the child to be fed, washed, dressed, and changed and to be required to assume no responsibility. But just as an adult may become helpless, so can the child. Regressive behavior could easily make the child lose a sense of responsibility and self-esteem. If the child is given psychological preparation, some control, and is supported in the ability to respond emotionally, hospitalization can become a meaningful learning experience for the child instead of a time of trauma.

THE HOSPICE

All of the problems of institutionalization may come together to plague the terminally ill in an acute care hospital. The dying may be too weak or come to care too little to attempt to assert any personal control. They may have their various physiological needs met on schedule by constantly changing members of the medical team. They may be cut off from friends and family. The terminally ill may be studied by medical residents learning their profession and occasionally may be observed by large classes of medical or nursing students. Simple requests may be denied because of hospital rules. In its extreme, such treatment may be so "efficient" that there are extremely negative consequences for the patient. Some of these problems arise from the fact that the patient is dying, as discussed in Chapter 9. However, many of the difficulties arise from the hospital environment itself.

The *hospice* movement attempts to improve the institutional environment for care of the terminally ill. As we saw earlier in this chapter, both "hospital" and "hospice" are related to the word "hospitality." Hospices endeavor to improve the psychosocial care and the quality of life of terminally ill patients.

Traditionally, a hospice has been a place of rest for travelers, the elderly, or the sick. Hospices took on their modern meaning from St. Christopher's, a London hospice founded by Cicely Saunders [75]. The hospice movement has spread to the United States, although the precise characteristics of a hospice have not yet been formalized [59].

There are four basic areas in which the hospice differs from the traditional hospital. All of these differences improve the psychosocial care of the patient. First, the focus of the hospice is on the person, thus counteracting the dehumanization of hospitals. Through a variety of means, patients are made to feel like people. Patients are introduced as people rather than as medical cases, acquaintanceships are built among patients and the staff, attention is paid to the patient's thoughts and feelings, and a general emphasis is placed on the patient's overall well-being.

Second, the hospice encourages rather than discourages family interaction. Spouses are recognized and welcomed, and children are permitted to visit except when it is clearly medically inadvisable. Family members are taught to help care for the patient. The family may even get to know other patients. Furthermore, it is recognized that family members also face difficulties because of the patient's illness, and therefore psychosocial support services are offered to the family.

Third, more attention is paid to the proper control of pain in hospices than in traditional acute care hospitals. Whereas hospitals are likely to view pain mechanistically, in hospices the significant psychosocial aspects of pain are recognized. Instead of administering pain medication on a strict and rigid schedule according to doctors' orders, in the hospice pain medication is administered when the patient needs it. In addition, the patient is assured that pain medication will be available when it is needed; elimination of the *fear* of pain helps to reduce the pain. With the focus on the *quality* of the patient's life, the type of pain medication used in hospices is very important. Hospice personnel endeavor to allow the patient to function normally to the greatest possible extent while pain is controlled. This hopeful emphasis in itself helps control pain. But hospices have also helped pioneer new pain control preparations. For example, St. Christopher's developed Brompton's mixture for controlling pain in terminal cancer patients. In England, this might consist of heroin, cocaine, alcohol, chloroform, and sugar. In the United States, morphine and a tranquilizer may be substituted for the heroin. The precise mixture is not as important as the emphasis on pain control medication that preserves the psychosocial functioning of the patient.

Fourth, hospices are more likely than acute care hospitals to rely on allied health professionals. Hospitals give an extraordinary range of duties and responsibilities to physicians. Hospices are more willing to rely on social workers, pharmacists, clergy, and psychologists. The full range of patient and family needs is therefore more likely to be addressed.

The hospice movement fits in well with some promising trends in America health care. Most obviously, it encourages increased sensitivity to dying and death. It is also compatible with increased emphasis on home care. Hospice staff have ties to the family and form a small community; it is easier for seriously ill patients to remain at

Box 11–3
Cost Effectiveness

Throughout this book we have pointed out the many important social psychological factors to which practitioners should pay attention in their care of patients. Some practitioners and administrators might feel, however, that these matters are impractical because they require time and effort, and therefore might render medical care too expensive. Evidence from research suggests, though, that attention to social psychological issues is *cost effective*. That is, the benefits of such attention generally outweigh its costs. For example, as we noted earlier in this chapter, patients who are given information about what they will exper-

ience before and after surgery or an uncomfortable medical procedure tend to have less anxiety about it. When they are prepared for what will happen to them, patients have a better outcome of treatment, and they may be discharged from the hospital sooner than patients who are confused and upset. Thus the extra time it takes to prepare patients often pays off in terms of reduced costs for subsequent care. Many related examples of cost-effective procedures can be found throughout this book. The use of social psychology in medicine often has economic as well as humanitarian value.

home and return to the institution only when absolutely medically necessary. (Such home care may have important implications for cost control as well.) Finally, the hospice movement fits in with the trends toward health maintenance organizations and other group practices in which teams of health professionals cooperate to produce efficient health care.

Although hospice care has been established primarily for the terminally ill, its emphases provide promising alternatives to certain types of existing hospital care. Although hospitals as they are now may be excellent places for accident or heart attack victims for a short period in the initial phase of the medical problem, many aspects of hospitalization can, upon careful scrutiny, be much improved.

CONCLUSION: A NEW ROLE FOR PATIENTS

Health care (including hospitalization and nursing homes) need not foster helplessness and dehumanization. Loss of control and of social relationships produces so many negative results that changes must be made in the care of patients. In the changes that have been suggested by various social scientists, the focus is on returning responsibility for healing into the hands of the patients [62, 77].

Human beings are motivated to achieve mastery and control over their own lives. This control involves the ability to influence the environment and to have one's responses bring expected outcomes. Perceived control involves a sense of freedom of choice and an awareness of opportunities. There is a sizeable research literature that indicates that an individual's sense of control strongly influences the ability to cope with stress and might actually decrease the effects of painful stimuli [33]. There is in fact evidence which suggests that interventions that give patients preparatory information (such as descriptions of expected reactions to medical procedures or surgery that they are about to undergo) return a sense of control to patients. Patients have better reactions to anesthesia and surgery, for example, when they are active collaborators in their care [21, 34, 35, 36, 39]. (See also Box 11-3).

In short, changes in traditional hospital and other institutional care can restore some control to patients. First, most patients can profit from detailed information about the nature of their medical care and what they are likely to experience during their illness. Second, if patients are not completely indisposed by their illnesses, they should be allowed to take a more active part in their care. Third, patients should know to whom they should turn with special problems or complaints.

To help counter the various abuses of power that may result in a total institution like a hospital, the American Hospital Association has adopted a *patient's bill of rights*. These rights are presented in Box 11-4. While recognizing the special demands of certain medical situations, these guidelines place the patient at the center of the decisionmaking process in medical care. Such an orientation can be extended to all medical care.

Box 11–4
A Patient's Bill of Rights

The American Hospital Association Board of Trustees' Committee on Health Care for the Disadvantaged, which has been a consistent advocate on behalf of consumers of health care services, developed the Statement on a Patient's Bill of Rights, which was approved by the AHA House of Delegates February 6, 1973. The statement was published in several forms, one of which was the S74 leaflet in the Association's S series. The S74 leaflet is now superseded by this reprinting of the statement.

The American Hospital Association presents a Patient's Bill of Rights with the expectation that observance of these rights will contribute to more effective patient care and greater satisfaction for the patient, his physician, and the hospital organization. Further, the Association presents these rights in the expectation that they will be supported by the hospital on behalf of its patients, as an integral part of the healing process. It is recognized that a personal relationship between the physician and the patient is essential for the provision of proper medical care. The traditional physician–patient relationship takes on a new dimension when care is rendered within an organizational structure. Legal precedent has established that the institution itself also has a responsibility to the patient. It is in recognition of these factors that these rights are affirmed.

1. The patient has the right to considerate and respectful care.

2. The patient has the right to obtain from his physician complete current information concerning his diagnosis, treatment, and prognosis in terms the patient can be reasonably expected to understand. When it is not medically advisable to give such information to the patient, the information should be made available to an appropriate person in his behalf. He has the right to know, by name, the physician responsible for coordinating his care.

3. The patient has the right to receive from his physician information necessary to give informed consent prior to the start of any procedure and/or treatment. Except in emergencies, such information for informed consent should include but not necessarily be limited to the specific procedure and/or treatment, the medically significant risks involved, and the probable duration of incapacitation. Where medically significant alternatives for care or treatment exist, or when the patient requests information concerning medical alternatives, the patient has the right to such information. The patient also has the right to know the name of the person responsible for the procedures and/or treatment.

4. The patient has the right to refuse treatment to the extent permitted by law and to be informed of the medical consequences of his action.

5. The patient has the right to every consideration of his privacy concerning his own medical care program. Case discussion, consultation, examination, and treatment are confidential and should be conducted discreetly. Those not directly involved in his care must have the permission of the patient to be present.

6. The patient has the right to expect that all communications and records pertaining to his care should be treated as confidential.

7. The patient has the right to expect that within its capacity a hospital must make reasonable response to the request of a patient for services. The hospital must provide evaluation, service, and/or referral as indicated by the urgency of the case. When medically permissable, a patient may be transferred to another facility only after he has received complete information and explanations concerning the needs for and alternatives to such a transfer. The institution to which the patient is to be transferred must first have accepted the patient for transfer.

8. The patient has the right to obtain information as to any relationship of his hospital to other health care and educational institutions insofar as his care is concerned. The patient has the right to obtain information as to the existence of any professional relationships among individuals, by name, who are treating him.

9. The patient has the right to be advised if the hospital proposes to engage in or perform human experimentation affecting his care or treatment. The patient has the right to refuse to participate in such research projects.

10. The patient has the right to expect reasonable continuity of care. He has the right to know in advance what appointment times and physicians are available and where. The patient has the right to expect that the hospital will provide a mechanism whereby he is informed by his physician or a delegate of the physician of the patient's continuing health care requirements following discharge.

11. The patient has the right to examine and receive an explanation of his bill regardless of source of payment.

12. The patient has the right to know what hospital rules and regulations apply to his conduct as a patient.

No catalog of rights can guarantee for the patient the kind of treatment he has a right to expect. A hospital has many functions to perform, including the prevention and treatment of disease, the education of both health professionals and patients, and the conduct of clinical research. All these activities must be conducted with an overriding concern for the patient, and, above all, the recognition of his dignity as a human being. Success in achieving this recognition assures success in the defense of the rights of the patient.

References

CHAPTER 1
INTRODUCTION TO SOCIAL PSYCHOLOGY
AND MEDICINE

1. Adams, J. S., and Jacobsen, P. Effects of wage inequities on work quality. *Journal of Abnormal and Social Psychology,* 1964, *69,* 19–25.
2. Adams, J. S. Inequity in social exchange. In L. Berkowitz, ed., *Advances in Experimental Social Psychology.* Vol. II. New York: Academic Press, 1965, pp. 267–299.
3. Aristotle. *The Nicomachean Ethics.* Translated by J. Welldon. London: Macmillan, 1908.
4. Berkowitz, L., ed. *Advances in Experimental Social Psychology.* Vol. 6. New York: Academic Press, 1972.
5. Bernstein, L., and Bernstein, R. S. *Interviewing: A Guide for Health Professionals.* 3rd ed. New York: Appleton-Century-Crofts, 1980.
6. Blau, P. *Exchange and Power in Social Life.* New York: John Wiley, 1964.
7. Blau, P. Social exchange. In D. Sills, ed., *International Encyclopedia of the Social Sciences.* New York: Macmillan, 1968, pp. 452–457.
8. Caplan, R. D. Patient, provider, and organization: Hypothesized determinants of adherence. In S. J. Cohen, ed., *New Directions in Patient Compliance.* Lexington, Mass.: D. C. Heath, 1979, pp. 75–100.
9. Cartwright, L. K. Sources and effects of stress in health careers. In G. C. Stone, F. Cohen, and N. E. Adler, eds., *Health Psychology.* San Francisco: Jossey-Bass, 1979, p. 419.
10. Clendening, L., ed. *Source Book of Medical History.* New York: Dover, 1942.
11. Cohen, F. Personality, stress, and the development of physical illness. In G. C. Stone, F. Cohen, and N. E. Adler, eds., *Health Psychology.* San Francisco: Jossey-Bass, 1979, p. 77.
12. Cohen, F., and Lazarus, R. S. Coping with the stresses of illness. In G. C. Stone, F. Cohen, and N. E. Adler, eds., *Health Psychology.* San Francisco: Jossey-Bass, 1979, p. 217.
13. Cooley, C. H. *Human Nature and the Social Order.* Rev. ed. New York: Scribner's, 1922. (Originally published, 1902.)
14. Cramond, W. A. Renal homotransplantation—some observations on recipients and donors. *British Journal of Psychology,* 1967, *113,* 1223–1230.
15. Davidson, P. O., and Davidson, S. M., eds. *Behavioral Medicine: Changing Health Lifestyles.* New York: Brunner/Mazel, 1980.

16. Dembroski, T. M., Weiss, S. M., Shields, J. L., Haynes, S. G., and Feinleib, M., eds. *Coronary-Prone Behavior*. New York: Springer-Verlag, 1978.

17. DiMatteo, M. R. A social-psychological analysis of physician-patient rapport: Toward a science of the art of medicine. *Journal of Social Issues*, 1979, *35*(1), 12–33.

18. DiMatteo, M. R., and Friedman, H. S., eds. Interpersonal relations in health care. *Journal of Social Issues*, 1979, *35*(1), (whole issue).

19. Elstein, A. S., and Bordage, G. Psychology of clinical reasoning. In G. C. Stone, F. Cohen, and N. E. Adler, eds., *Health Psychology*. San Francisco: Jossey-Bass, 1979, p. 333.

20. Fellner, C. H., and Marshall, J. R. Twelve kidney donors. *Journal of the American Medical Association*, 1968, *206* (16 December), 2703–2707.

21. Fidell, L. S. Sex role stereotypes and the American physician. *Psychology of Women Quarterly*, 1980, *4*, 313–330.

22. Fox, R. C., and Swazey, J. P. *The Courage to Fail*. Chicago: University of Chicago Press, 1974.

23. Frank, J. D. Mind-body relationships in illness and healing. *Journal of the International Academy of Preventive Medicine*, 1977, *2*(3).

24. Friedman, H. S. Nonverbal communication between patients and medical practitioners. *Journal of Social Issues*, 1979, *35*(1), 82–99.

25. Friedman, M., and Rosenman, R. H. *Type A Behavior and Your Heart*. New York: Alfred A. Knopf, 1974.

26. Gallup, G. G., Jr. Self-recognition in primates: A comparative approach to the bidirectional properties of consciousness. *American Psychologist*, 1977, *32*, 329–338.

27. Glass, D. *Behavior Patterns, Stress and Coronary Disease*. Hillsdale, N.J.: Lawrence Erlbaum, 1977.

28. Gouldner, A. The norm of reciprocity: A preliminary statement. *American Sociological Review*, 1960, *25*, 161–179.

29. Haynes, R. B., Taylor, D. W., and Sackett, D. L. *Compliance in Health Care*. Baltimore: Johns Hopkins University Press, 1979.

30. Henderson, T. B., Hall, S. M., and Lipton, H. L. Changing self-destructive behaviors. In G. C. Stone, F. Cohen, and N. E. Adler, eds., *Health Psychology*. San Francisco: Jossey-Bass, 1979, p. 141.

31. Hippocrates. *On Decorum and the Physician*. Vol. II. Translated by W. H. S. Jones. London: William Heinemann, Ltd., 1923.

32. James, W. *The Principles of Psychology*. Vols. 1 and 2. New York: Henry Holt, 1890.

33. Jenkins, C. D. Recent evidence supporting psychologic and social risk factors for coronary disease. *New England Journal of Medicine*, 1976, *294*, 987–994; 1033–1038.

34. Kagan, N. I. Teaching interpersonal relations for the practice of medicine. *Lakartidningen*, *1974*, *71*, 4758–4760.

35. Kastenbaum, R. *Death, Society and Human Experience*. St. Louis: C. V. Mosby, 1977.

36. Kastenbaum, R. *Humans Developing: A Lifespan Perspective*. Boston: Allyn and Bacon, 1979.

37. Kastenbaum, R., and Eisenberg, R. B. *The Psychology of Death*. New York: Springer, 1972.

38. King, S. H. *Perceptions of Illness and Medical Practice*. New York: Russell Sage Foundation, 1962.

39. Kleinman, A., Eisenberg, L., and Good, B. Culture, illness, and care. *Annals of Internal Medicine*, 1978, *88*, 251–258.

40. Knowles, J. H. The responsibility of the individual. *Daedalus*, 1977, *106*, 57–80.

41. Kubler-Ross, E. *On Death and Dying.* New York: Macmillan, 1969.
42. Lerner, M. The desire for justice and reactions to victims. In J. Macaulay and L. Berkowitz, eds., *Altruism and Helping Behavior.* New York: Academic Press, 1970.
43. Lerner, M. J., and Matthews, G. Reactions to suffering of others under conditions of indirect responsibility. *Journal of Personality and Social Psychology,* 1967, *5,* 319–325.
44. Lorber, J. Good patients and problem patients: Conformity and deviance in a general hospital. *Journal of Health and Social Behavior,* 1975, 16, 213–225.
45. Lynch, J. J. *The Broken Heart: The Medical Consequences of Loneliness.* New York: Basic Books, 1977.
46. Mauss, M. *Essai sur Le Don, Forme Archaique de L' exchange* (1925). Translated by I. Cunnison. New York: W. W. Norton, 1967.
47. McIntosh, J. Process of communication, information seeking, and control associated with cancer: A selective review of the literature. *Social Science and Medicine,* 1974, *8,* 167–187.
48. Mead, G. H. *Mind, Self and Society.* Chicago: University of Chicago Press, 1934.
49. Middlebrook, P. N. *Social Psychology and Modern Life.* 2nd ed. New York: Alfred A. Knopf, 1980.
50. Moos, R. H. Social-ecological perspectives on health. In G. C. Stone, F. Cohen, and N. E. Adler, eds., *Health Psychology.* San Francisco: Jossey-Bass, 1979, p. 523.
51. Moos, R. H., and Tsu, V.D. Overview and perspective. In R. H. Moos, ed., *Coping with Physical Illness.* New York: Plenum, 1977.
52. Rahe, R. H., and Arthur, R. H. Life change and illness studies. *Journal of Human Stress,* 1978, *4*(1), 3–15.
53. Rodin, J. Somatopsychics and attribution. *Personality and Social Psychology Bulletin,* 1978, *4,* 531–540.
54. Rodin, J., and Janis, I. L. The social power of health-care practitioners as agents of change. *Journal of Social Issues,* 1979, *35*(1), 60–81.
55. Ryan, W. *Blaming the Victim.* New York: Random House, 1971.
56. Schowalter, J. E. Multiple organ transplantation and the creation of surgical siblings. *Pediatrics,* 1970, *46*(4), 576–580.
57. Selye, H. *The Stress of Life.* Rev. ed. New York: McGraw-Hill, 1976.
58. Shem, S. *The House of God.* New York: Dell, 1978.
59. Shapiro, A. K. A contribution to a history of the placebo effect. *Behavioral Science,* 1960, *5,* 109–135.
60. Skipper, J., and Leonard, R., eds., *Social Interaction and Patient Care.* Philadelphia and Toronto: J. B. Lipincott, 1965.
61. Sontag, S. *Illness as Metaphor.* New York: Farrar, Straus, and Giroux, 1978.
62. Stone, G. C. Patient compliance and the role of the expert. *Journal of Social Issues,* 1979, *35*(1), 34–59.
63. Strauss, A. L., and Glaser, B. G. *Chronic Illness and the Quality of Life.* St. Louis: C. V. Mosby, 1975.
64. Surgeon General of the United States. *Healthy People: The Surgeon General's Report on Health Promotion and Disease Prevention, 1979.* Washington, D.C.: USDHEW Pub. 79-55071, Public Health Service.
65. Taylor, S. E. Hospital patient behavior: Reactance, helplessness, or control. *Journal of Social Issues,* 1979, *35*(1), 156–184.
66. Thompson, T. *Hearts.* New York: McCall Publishing Co., 1971.
67. Torrens, P. R. *The American Health Care System: Issues and Problems.* St. Louis: C. V. Mosby, 1978.
68. Totman, R. *Social Causes of Illness.* London: Souvenir Press, 1979.

69. Wortman, C. B., and Dunkel-Schetter, C. Interpersonal relationships and cancer: A theoretical analysis. *Journal of Social Issues,* 1979, *35*(1), 120–155.

CHAPTER 2
THE ART OF MEDICINE

1. Ajzen, I., and Fishbein, M. *Understanding Attitudes and Predicting Social Behavior.* Englewood Cliffs, N.J.: Prentice-Hall, 1980.
2. Alpert, J. J. Broken appointments. *Pediatrics,* 1964, *34,* 127–132.
3. Becker, M. H. ed. *The Health Belief Model and Personal Health Behavior.* Thorofare, N.J.: Charles B. Slack, 1974.
4. Becker, M. H., and Maiman, L. A. Strategies for enhancing patient compliance. *Journal of Community Health,* 1980, *6,* 113–135.
5. Ben-Sira, Z. The function of the professional's affective behavior in client satisfaction: A revised approach to social interaction theory. *Journal of Health and Social Behavior,* 1976, *17,* 3–11.
6. Ben-Sira, Z. Affective and instrumental components in the physician–patient relationship: An additional dimension of interaction theory. *Journal of Health and Social Behavior,* 1980, *21,* 170–180.
7. Blau, P. Social exchange. In D. Sills, ed., *International Encyclopedia of the Social Sciences.* New York: Macmillan, 1968, pp. 452–457.
8. Bloom, S. W. *The Doctor and His Patient: A Sociological Interpretation.* New York: Russell Sage Foundation, 1963.
9. Blum, R. H. *The Management of the Doctor–Patient Relationship.* New York: McGraw-Hill, 1960.
10. Caplan, E. K., and Sussman, M. B. Rank-order of important variables for patient and staff satisfaction. *Journal of Health and Human Behavior,* 1966, *7,* 133–138.
11. Cartwright, L. Sources and effects of stress in health careers. In G. C. Stone, F. Cohen, and N. E. Adler, eds., *Health Psychology.* San Francisco: Jossey-Bass, 1979.
12. Chafetz, M. E. No patient deserves to be patronized. *Medical Insight,* 1970, *2,* 68–75.
13. Cobb, B. Why do people detour to quacks? *The Psychiatric Bulletin,* 1954, *3,* 66–69.
14. Davis, M. S. Variations in patients' compliance with doctors' orders: Analyses of congruence between survey responses and results of empirical investigations. *Journal of Medicine Education,* 1966, *41,* 1037–1048.
15. Davis, M. S. Variations in patients' compliance with doctors' advice: An empirical analysis of patterns of communication. *American Journal of Public Health,* 1968, *58,* 274–288.
16. Davis, M. S. Physiological, psychological and demographic factors in patient compliance with doctors' orders. *Medical Care,* 1968, *6,* 115–122.
17. DiMatteo, M. R. A social-psychological analysis of physician–patient rapport: Toward a science of the art of medicine. *Journal of Social Issues,* 1979, *35*(1), 12–33.
18. DiMatteo, M. R., Prince, L. M., and Taranta, A. Patients' perceptions of physicians' behavior: Determinants of patient commitment to the therapeutic relationship. *Journal of Community Health,* 1979, *4,* 280–290.
19. DiNicola, D. D., and DiMatteo, M. R. Communication, interpersonal influence, and resistance to medical recommendations. In Thomas Ashby Wills, ed., *Basic Processes in Helping Relationships.* New York: Academic Press, 1982.

20. Egbert, L. D., Battit, G. E., Turndorf, H., and Beecher, H. K. The value of the pre-operative visit by an anesthetist. *Journal of the American Medical Association,* 1963, *185,* 553–555.
21. Egbert, L. D., Battit, G. E., Welch, C. E., and Bartlett, M. K. Reduction of post-operative pain by encouragement and instruction of patients: A study of doctor-patient rapport. *New England Journal of Medicine,* 1964, *270,* 825–827.
22. Engel, G. L. The need for a new medical model: A challenge for biomedicine. *Science,* 1977, *196,* 129–136.
23. Engel, G. L. The care of the patient: Art or science? *The Johns Hopkins Medical Journal,* 1977, *140,* 222–232.
24. Ford, A. B., Liske, R. E., Ort, R. S., and Denton, J. C. *The Doctor's Perspective: Physicians View Their Patients and Practice.* Cleveland: Case Western Reserve University Press, 1967.
25. Fox, R. C. *Experiment Perilous: Physicians and Patients Facing the Unknown.* Glencoe, Ill.: The Free Press, 1959.
26. Francis, V., Korsch, B. M., and Morris, M. J. Gaps in doctor–patient communications: Patients' response to medical advice. *New England Journal of Medicine,* 1969, *280,* 535–540.
27. Freidson, E. *Patients' Views of Medical Practice.* New York: Russell Sage Foundation, 1961.
28. Freidson, E. *Profession of Medicine.* New York: Dodd, Mead, 1975.
29. Gray, P. G., and Cartwright, A. Choosing and changing doctors. *The Lancet,* 1953 (19 December), 1308.
30. Headlee, R. The tacit contract between doctor and patient. *Medical Insight,* 1973, *5,* 30–37.
31. Haynes, R. B. Introduction. In R. B. Haynes, D. W. Taylor, and D. L. Sackett, eds., *Compliance in Health Care.* Baltimore: Johns Hopkins University Press, 1979, pp. 1–7.
32. Hippocrates. *On Decorum and the Physician.* Vol. II. Translated by W. H. S. Jones. London: William Heinemann, Ltd., 1923.
33. Hulka, B. S. Patient–clinician interactions and compliance. In R. B. Haynes, D. W. Taylor, and D. L. Sackett, eds., *Compliance in Health Care.* Baltimore: Johns Hopkins University Press, 1979, pp. 63–77.
34. Järvinen, K. A. J. Can ward rounds be a danger to patients with myocardial infarction? *British Medical Journal,* 1955, *1,* 318–320.
35. Kasteler, J., Kane, R. L., Olsen, D. M., and Thetford, C. Issues underlying prevalence of "doctor-shopping" behavior. *Journal of Health and Social Behavior,* 1976, *17,* 328–339.
36. King, S. H. *Perceptions of Illness and Medical Practice.* New York: Russell Sage Foundation, 1962.
37. Koos, E. "Metropolis"—what city people think of their medical services. *American Journal of Public Health,* 1955, *45,* 1551–1557.
38. Korsch, B. M., Gozzi, E. K., and Francis, V. Gaps in doctor–patient communication. I. Doctor–patient interaction and patient satisfaction. *Pediatrics,* 1968, *42,* 855–871.
39. Lederer, H. D. How the sick view their world. *Journal of Social Issues,* 1952, *8,* 4–16.
40. Lynch, J. J., Thomas, S. A., Mills, M. E., Malinow, K., and Katcher, A. H. The effects of human contact on cardiac arrhythmia in coronary care patients. *The Journal of Nervous and Mental Disease,* 1974, *158,* 88–99.
41. Mechanic, D. *Medical Sociology: A Selective View.* New York: The Free Press, 1968.
42. Milmoe, S., Rosenthal, R., Blane, H. T., Chafetz, M. L., and Wolf, I. The doctor's voice: Postdictor of successful referral of alcoholic patients. *Journal of Abnormal Psychology,* 1967, *72,* 78–84.

43. Moos, R., ed. *Coping with Physical Illness. New York: Plenum, 1977.*
44. Osler, W. The master-word in medicine. In *Aequanimitas with Other Addresses to Medical Students, Nurses, and Practitioners of Medicine.* Philadelphia: Blakiston, 1904, pp. 369–371.
45. Parsons, T. *The Social System.* Glencoe, Ill.: The Free Press, 1951, pp. 428–479.
46. Parsons, T. Definitions of health and illness in the light of American values and social structure. In E. G. Jaco, eds., *Physicians, Patients and Illness.* New York: The Free Press, 1958, pp. 165–187.
47. Parsons, T. The sick role and the role of the physician reconsidered. *Millbank Memorial Fund Quarterly,* 1975, *53,* 257–278.
48. Sackett, D. L., and Snow, J. C. The magnitude of compliance and noncompliance. In R. B. Haynes, D. W. Taylor, and D. L. Sackett, eds., *Compliance in Health Care.* Baltimore: Johns Hopkins University Press, 1979, pp. 11–22.
49. Salzman, C., Shader, R., Scott, D. A., and Binstock, W. Interviewer anger and patient dropout in a walk-in clinic. *Comprehensive Psychiatry,* 1970, *11,* 267–273.
50. Shapiro, A. K. A contribution to a history of the placebo effect. *Behavioral Science,* 1960, *5,* 109–135.
51. Shapiro, A. K. Placebo effects in medicine, psychotherapy, and psychoanalysis. In A. Bergin and S. Garfield, eds., *Handbook of Psychotherapy and Behavior Change.* New York: John Wiley, 1971, pp. 439–473.
52. Shattuck, F. C. The science and art of medicine in some of their aspects. *Boston Medical and Surgical Journal,* 1907, *157,* 63–67.
53. Skipper, J. K., and Leonard, R. C., eds. *Social Interaction and Patient Care.* Philadelphia: J. B. Lippincott, 1965.
54. Stiles, W. B., Putnam, S. M., Wolf, M. H., and James, S. A. Interaction exchange structure and patient satisfaction with medical interviews. *Medical Care,* 1979, *17,* 667–679.
55. Thurlow, R. M. Malpractice: A growing threat to doctor–patient relations. *Medical Economics,* 1969 (January 20), *46,* 212.
56. Tumulty, P. A. What is a clinician and what does he do? *New England Journal of Medicine,* 1970, *283,* 20–24.
57. Vaccarino, J. M. Malpractice: The problem in perspective. *The Journal of the American Medical Association,* 1977, *238,* 861–863.
58. Wilson, R. N., and Bloom, S. W. Patient–practitioner relationships. In H. E. Freeman, S. Levine, and L. G. Reeder, eds., *Handbook of Medical Sociology.* Englewood Cliffs, N.J.: Prentice-Hall, 1972, pp. 315–339.

CHAPTER 3
PATIENT COOPERATION WITH TREATMENT

1. Alpert, J. J. Broken appointments. *Pediatrics,* 1964, *34,* 127–132.
2. Baekeland, F., and Lundwall, L. Dropping out of treatment: A critical review. *Psychological Bulletin,* 1975, *82,* 738–783.
3. Becker, M. H., ed. *The Health Belief Model and Personal Health Behavior.* Thorofare, N.J.: Charles B. Slack, 1974.
4. Becker, M. H., and Maiman, L. A. Strategies for enhancing patient compliance. *Journal of Community Health,* 1980, *6,* 113–135.
5. Becker, M. H., Maiman, L. A., Kirscht, J. P. Haefner, D. P., Drachman, R. H., and Taylor, D. W. Patient perceptions and compliance: Recent studies of the Health Belief Model. In R. B. Haynes, D. W. Taylor, and D. L. Sackett, eds., *Compliance in Health Care.* Baltimore: Johns Hopkins University Press, 1979, pp. 78–109.

6. Bloom, S. W. *The Doctor and His Patient: A Sociological Interpretation.* New York: Russell Sage Foundation, 1963.
7. Boyd, J. R., Covington, T. R., Stanaszek, W. F., and Coussons, R. T. Drug-defaulting. II. Analysis of noncompliance patterns. *American Journal of Hospital Pharmacy,* 1974, *31,* 485–491.
8. Brehm, J. W. *A Theory of Psychological Reactance.* New York: Academic Press, 1966.
9. Caplan, R. D., Robinson, E. A. R., French, J. R. P., Jr., Caldwell, J. R., and Shinn, M. *Adhering to Medical Regimens: Pilot Experiments in Patient Education and Social Support.* Ann Arbor: Research Center for Group Dynamics, Institute for Social Research, University of Michigan, 1976.
10. Charney, E. Patient–doctor communication: Implications for the clinician. *Pediatric Clinics of North America,* 1972, *19,* 263–279.
11. Dahl, J. C. Rational management of hypertension. *Minnesota Medicine,* 1977, *60,* 311–314.
12. Davis, M. S. Variations in patients' compliance with doctors' orders: Analysis of congruence between survey responses and results of empirical investigations. *Journal of Medical Education,* 1966, *41,* 1037–1048.
13. French, J. R. P., Jr., and Raven, B. H. The bases of social power. In D. Cartwright, ed., *Studies in Social Power.* Ann Arbor: Institute for Social Research, University of Michigan, 1959, pp. 150–167.
14. Gillum, R. F., and Barsky, A. J. Diagnosis and management of patient noncompliance. *Journal of the American Medical Association,* 1974, *228,* 1563–1567.
15. Gordis, L. Methodological issues in the measurement of patient compliance. In D. L. Sackett and R. B. Haynes, eds., *Compliance with Therapeutic Regimens.* Baltimore: Johns Hopkins University Press, 1976, pp. 51–66.
16. Gordis, L. Conceptual and methodologic problems in measuring patient compliance. In R. B. Haynes, D. W. Taylor, and D. L. Sackett, eds., *Compliance in Health Care.* Baltimore: Johns Hopkins University Press, 1979, pp. 23–45.
17. Gordis, L., Markowitz, M., and Lilienfeld, A. M. Studies in the epidemiology and preventability of rheumatic fever. IV. A quantitative determination of compliance in children on oral penicillin prophylaxis. *Pediatrics,* 1969, *43,* 173–182.
18. Haynes, R. B. Introduction. In R. B. Haynes, D. W. Taylor, and D. L. Sackett, eds., *Compliance in Health Care.* Baltimore: Johns Hopkins University Press, 1979, pp. 1–7.
19. Haynes, R. B. Taking medication: Short- and long-term strategies. Paper delivered at conference, "Promoting Long-Term Health Behaviors." Institute for Advancement of Human Behavior. New York: Guilford Publications, 1980.
20. Haynes, R. B., Taylor, D. W., and Sackett, D. L., eds., *Compliance in Health Care.* Baltimore: Johns Hopkins University Press, 1979.
21. Hulka, B., Cassel, J., Kupper, L., and Burdette, J. Communication, compliance, and concordance between physicians and patients with prescribed medications. *American Journal of Public Health,* 1976, *66,* 847–853.
22. Kasl, S. V. Issues in patient adherence to health care regimens. *Journal of Human Stress,* 1975, *1,* 5–17.
23. King, S. H. *Perceptions of Illness and Medical Practice.* New York: Russell Sage Foundation, 1962.
24. Korsch, B. M., Gozzi, E. K., and Francis, V. Gaps in doctor–patient communications: I. Doctor–patient interaction and patient satisfaction. *Pediatrics,* 1968, *42,* 855–871.
25. Korsch, B. M., and Negrete, V. F. Doctor–patient communication. *Scientific American,* 1972, *227,* 66–74.

26. Ley, P., and Spelman, M. S. *Communicating with the Patient.* London: Staples Press, 1967.
27. MacDonald, M. E., Hagberg, K. L., and Grossman, B. J. Social factors in relation to participation in follow-up care of rheumatic fever. *Journal of Pediatrics,* 1963, *62,* 503–513.
28. McKinlay, J. Social networks, lay consultation, and help-seeking behavior. *Social Forces,* 1973, *51,* 275–292.
29. Nall, F., and Speilberg, J. Social and cultural factors in responses of Mexican Americans to medical treatment. *Journal of Health and Social Behavior,* 1967, *8,* 299–308.
30. Osler, Sir W. Lecture to medical students. *Albany Medical Annals,* 1899, *20,* 307.
31. Porter, A. Drug defaulting in a general practice. *British Medical Journal,* 1969, *1,* 218–222.
32. Rodin, J., and Janis, I. L. The social power of health-care practitioners as agents of change. *Journal of Social Issues,* 1979, *35*(1), 60–81.
33. Rosenstock, I. M. The health belief model and preventive health behavior. In M. H. Becker, ed., *The Health Belief Model and Personal Health Behavior.* Thorofare, N.J.: Charles B. Slack, 1974, pp. 27–59.
34. Rubel, A. J. Concepts of disease in Mexican-American culture. *American Anthropologist,* 1960, *62,* 795–814.
35. Sackett, D. L. The magnitude of compliance and noncompliance. In D. L. Sackett and R. B. Haynes, eds., *Compliance with Therapeutic Regimens.* Baltimore: Johns Hopkins University Press, 1976, pp. 9–25.
36. Sackett, D. L. A compliance practicum for the busy practitioner. In R. B. Haynes, D. W. Taylor, and D. L. Sackett, eds., *Compliance in Health Care.* Baltimore: Johns Hopkins University Press, 1979, pp. 286–294.
37. Sackett, D. L., and Snow, J. C. The magnitude of compliance and noncompliance. In R. B. Haynes, D. W. Taylor, and D. L. Sackett, eds., *Compliance in Health Care.* Baltimore: Johns Hopkins University Press, 1979, pp. 11–22.
38. Snow, L. Folk-medical beliefs and their implications for care of patients. *Annals of Internal Medicine,* 1974, *81,* 82–96.
39. Stiles, W. B., Putnam, S. M., Wolf, M. H., and James, S. A. Interaction exchange structure and patient satisfaction with medical interviews. *Medical Care,* 1979, *17,* 667–679.
40. Stone, G. C. Patient compliance and the role of the expert. *Journal of Social Issues,* 1979, *35*(1), 34–59.
41. Svarstad, B. Physician–patient communication and patient conformity with medical advice. In D. Mechanic, ed., *The Growth of Bureaucratic Medicine.* New York: John Wiley, 1976, pp. 220–238.
42. Szasz, T. S., and Hollender, M. H. A contribution to the philosophy of medicine: The basic models of the doctor–patient relationship. *Archives of Internal Medicine,* 1956, *97,* 585–592.
43. Zola, I. K. Pathways to the doctor—from person to patient. *Social Science and Medicine,* 1973, *7,* 677–689.

CHAPTER 4
THE MIND AND THE BODY

1. Adams, R. Alterations in nervous function. In K. Isselbacher, ed., *Harrison's Principles of Internal Medicine.* 9th ed. New York: McGraw-Hill, 1980, pp. 68–74.

2. Beecher, H. K. *Measurement of Subjective Responses: Quantitative Effects of Drugs.* New York: Oxford University Press, 1959.

3. Benson, H., and Epstein, M. The placebo effect: A neglected asset in the care of patients. *Journal of the American Medical Association,* 1975, *232,* 1225-1226.

4. Birbaumer, N., and Kimmel, H., eds. *Biofeedback and Self-Regulation.* Hillsdale, N.J.: L. Erlbaum, 1979.

5. Blackman, S. The effects of nonverbal expression and cognition on the perception of pain. Ph.D. dissertation, University of California, Riverside, 1980.

6. Bowsher, D., Mumford, J., Lipton, S., and Miles, J. Treatment of intractable pain by accupuncture. *Lancet,* 1973, *2,* 57-60.

7. Chaves, J., and Barber, T. X. Hypnotism and surgical pain. In M. Weisenberg, ed., *Pain: Clinical and Experimental Perspectives.* St. Louis: C. V. Mosby, 1975, pp. 225-239.

8. Cobb, B. Why do people detour to quacks? *The Psychiatric Bulletin,* 1954, *3,* 66-69.

9. Cohen, F. Personality, stress, and the development of physical illness. In G. C. Stone, F. Cohen, and N. E. Adler, eds., *Health Psychology.* San Francisco: Jossey-Bass, 1979, pp. 71-111.

10. Cousins, N. *Anatomy of an Illness as Perceived by the Patient.* New York: W. W. Norton, 1979.

11. Darwin, C. *The Expression of the Emotions in Man and Animals.* London: John Murray, 1872.

12. Degood, D. E. A behavioral pain-management program: Expanding the psychologist's role in a medical setting. *Professional Psychology,* 1979, *10,* 491-502.

13. Descartes. *Selections.* Edited by R. Eaton. New York: Scribner's, 1955.

14. Deutsch, F., Jones, A., Stokuis, B., Fryberger, H., and Stunkard, A., eds., *Advances in Psychosomatic Medicine.* New York: Hafner, 1964.

15. Dubos, R. Bolstering the body against disease. *Human Nature,* 1978, *1*(8), 68-72.

16. Earthquake in Chicago. *Time,* April 9, 1951.

17. Frank, J. D. Emotional reactions of American soldiers to an unfamiliar disease. *American Journal of Psychiatry,* 1946, *102,* 631-640.

18. Frank, J. D. Mind-body relationships in illness and healing. *Journal of the International Academy of Preventive Medicine,* 1977, *2*(3).

19. Friedman, H. S., and DiMatteo, M. R. Health care as an interpersonal process. *Journal of Social Issues,* 1979, *35*(1), 1-11.

20. Gurin, J. The science watch: Homeopathy. *Harvard Magazine,* May-June and November-December 1979.

21. Herrick, J. W. Placebos, psychosomatic, and psychogenic illness and psychotherapy. *The Psychological Record,* 1976, *26,* 327-342.

22. James, W. *The Principles of Psychology.* New York: Henry Holt, 1910.

23. Johnson, J. Effects of accurate expectations about sensations on the sensory and distress components of pain. *Journal of Personality and Social Psychology,* 1973, *27,* 261-275.

24. Jones, R. A. *Self-fulfilling prophecies.* Hillsdale, N.J.: L. Erlbaum, 1977.

25. Jones, R. Expectations and illness. In H. S. Friedman and M. R. DiMatteo, eds., *Interpersonal Issues in Health Care.* New York: Academic Press, 1982.

26. Jospe, M. *The Placebo Effect.* Lexington, Mass.: Lexington Books, 1978.

27. Kaplan, R. Coping with stressful medical examinations. In H. S. Friedman and M. R. DiMatteo, eds., *Interpersonal Issues in Health Care.* New York: Academic Press, 1982.

28. Leigh, H., and Reiser, M. *The Patient: Biological, Psychological and Social Dimensions of Medical Practice.* New York: Plenum, 1980.

29. Levine, J. D., Gordon, N., and Fields, H. The mechanism of placebo analgesia. *Lancet,* 1978, *2,* 654-657.

30. Loesser, J. D. Low back pain. In J. Bonica, ed., *Pain*. New York: Raven Press, 1980, pp. 363–377.
31. Marsland, D. W., Wood, M. B., and Mayo, F. The databank for patient care, curriculum, and research in family practice: 526,196 patient problems. *Journal of Family Practice*, 1976, *3*, 25–28.
32. Meichenbaum, D. H., and Turk, D. The cognitive-behavioral management of anxiety, anger, and pain. In P. Davidson, ed., *The Behavioral Management of Anxiety, Depression and Pain*. New York: Brunner/Mazel, 1976.
33. Melzack, R. *The Puzzle of Pain*. New York: Basic Books, 1973.
34. Melzack, R., and Wall, P. D. Pain mechanisms: A new theory. *Science*, 1965, *150*, 971.
35. *Newsweek*. Medicine. December 8, 1952.
36. *Newsweek*. Medicine. June 27, 1977.
37. Pfungst, O. *Clever Hans: The Horse of Mr. Von Osten*. New York: Holt, Rinehart, and Winston, 1965.
38. Richman, J., and Goldthorp, W. O. Fatherhood: The social construction of pregnancy and birth. In S. Kitzinger and J. A. Davis, eds., *The Place of Birth*. Oxford: Oxford University Press, 1978.
39. Roethlisberger, F. J., and Dickson, W. *Management and the Worker*. Cambridge, Mass.: Harvard University Press, 1939.
40. Rosenthal, R. *Experimenter Effects in Behavioral Research*. New York, Appleton-Century-Crofts, 1966.
41. Shapiro, A. K. A contribution to a history of the placebo effect. *Behavioral Science*, 1960, *5*, 109–135.
42. Shapiro, A. K. Factors contributing to the placebo effect. *American Journal of Psychotherapy*, 1964, *18*, 73–88.
43. Shapiro, A. K. Placebo effects in medicine, psychotherapy, and psychoanalysis. In A. E. Bergin and S. L. Garfield, eds., *Handbook of Psychotherapy and Behavior Change*. New York: John Wiley, 1971, pp. 439–473.
44. Sternbach, R. A. *Pain Patients: Traits and Treatments*. New York: Academic Press, 1974.
45. Szasz, T. S. *Pain and Pleasure*. New York: Basic Books, 1957.
46. *Time*. Medicine. July 26, 1963.
47. *Time*. Medicine. June 20, 1977.
48. Weisenberg, M., ed. *Pain: Clinical and Experimental Perspectives*. St. Louis: C. V. Mosby, 1975.
49. Weisenberg, M. Pain and pain control. *Psychological Bulletin*, 1977, *84*, 1008–1044.
50. Weitz, S. Sex differences in nonverbal communication. *Sex Roles*, 1976, *2*, 175–184.
51. Wolf, S. The Pharmacology of placebos. *Pharmacology Review*, 1959, *11*, 698.
52. Wortman, C. B., and Dunkel-Schetter, C. Interpersonal relationships and cancer: A theoretical analysis. *Journal of Social Issues*, 1979, *35*(1), 120–155.
53. Zborowski, M. *People in Pain*. San Francisco: Jossey-Bass, 1969.

CHAPTER 5
COMMUNICATION WITH PATIENTS: VERBAL AND NONVERBAL

1. Allport, G. W. *The Nature of Prejudice*. Garden City, N.Y.: Addison-Wesley, 1954.
2. Altman, I. The communication of interpersonal attitudes: An ecological approach.

In T. L. Huston, ed., *Foundations of Interpersonal Attraction.* New York: Academic Press, 1974.

3. Argyle, M. *Bodily Communication.* New York: International Universities Press, 1975.

4. Barnlund, D. C. The mystification of meaning: Doctor-patient encounters. *Journal of Medical Education,* 1976, *51,* 716-725.

5. Becker, M. H., and Maiman, L. A. Strategies for enhancing patient compliance. *Journal of Community Health,* 1980, *6*(2), 113-135.

6. Ben-Sira, Z. The function of the professional's affective behavior in client satisfaction: A revised approach to social interaction theory. *Journal of Health and Social Behavior,* 1976, *17,* 3-11.

7. Ben-Sira, Z. Affective and instrumental components in the physician-patient relationship. An additional dimension of interaction theory. *Journal of Health and Social Behavior,* 1980, *21,* 170-180.

8. Bernstein, L., and Bernstein, R. S. *Interviewing: A Guide for Health Professionals.* 3rd ed. New York: Appleton-Century-Crofts, 1980.

9. Blackman, S. L. The effects of nonverbal expression and cognition on the perception of pain. Ph.D. dissertation, University of California, Riverside, 1980.

10. Bloch, M. *The Royal Touch.* Translated by F. E. Anderson. Montreal: McGill-Queen's University Press, 1973. (Originally published, 1961.)

11. Blondis, M. N., and Jackson, B. E. *Nonverbal Communication with Patients.* New York: John Wiley, 1977.

12. Bloom, S. W. *The Doctor and His Patient: A Sociological Interpretation.* New York: Russell Sage Foundation, 1963.

13. Cannell, C. F., Oksenberg, L., and Converse, J. M., eds., *Experiments in Interviewing Techniques: Field Experiments in Health Reporting, 1971-1977.* Ann Arbor: Survey Research Center Institute for Social Research, 1977.

14. Christy, N. P. English is our second language. *New England Journal of Medicine,* 1979, *300*(17), 979-981.

15. Daubenmire, M. J. Nurse-patient-physician communicative interaction process. In H. Werley, A. Zuzich, M. Zajkowski, and A. Zngornik, eds., *Health Research: The Systems Approach.* New York: Springer, 1976.

16. Davis, F. Uncertainty in medical prognosis: Clinical and functional. *American Journal of Sociology,* 1960, *66,* 41-47.

17. Davitz, J. R. *The Communication of Emotional Meaning.* New York: McGraw-Hill, 1964.

18. DiMatteo, M. R., Friedman, H. S., and Taranta, A. Sensitivity to bodily nonverbal communication as a factor in practitioner-patient rapport. *Journal of Nonverbal Behavior,* 1979, *4,* 18-26.

19. DiMatteo, M. R., Taranta, A., Friedman, H. S., and Prince, L. M. Predicting patient satisfaction from physicians' nonverbal communication skills. *Medical Care,* 1980, *18,* 376-387.

20. Duncan, D. S., Jr., and Rosenthal, R. Vocal emphasis in experimenters' introduction reading as unintended determinant of subjects' responses. *Language and Speech,* 1968, *11,* 20-26.

21. Ekman, P., and Friesen, W. Nonverbal leakage and clues to deception. *Psychiatry,* 1969, *32,* 88-105.

22. Ekman, P., and Friesen, W. *Unmasking the Face.* Englewood Cliffs, N.J.: Prentice-Hall, 1975.

23. Ekman, P., Friesen, W., and Ellsworth, P. *Emotion in the Human Face.* New York: Pergamon Press, 1972.

24. Ellsworth, P. Direct gaze as a social stimulus: The example of aggression. In P.

Pliner, L. Krames, and T. Alloway, eds., *Nonverbal Communication of Aggression.* New York: Plenum, 1975.

25. Ellsworth, P., Friedman, H., Perlick, D., and Hoyt, M. Some effects of gaze on subjects motivated to seek or to avoid social comparison. *Journal of Experimental Social Psychology,* 1978, *14,* 69–87.
26. Engel, G. L. The care of the patient: Art of science? *The Johns Hopkins Medical Journal,* 1977, *140,* 222–232.
27. Exline, R. V. Visual interaction: The glance of power and preference. In J. Cole, ed., *Nebraska Symposium on Motivation 1971.* Lincoln: University of Nebraska Press, 1972.
28. Francis, V., Korsch, B., and Morris, M. Gaps in doctor–patient communication: Patients' response to medical advice. *New England Journal of Medicine,* 1969, *280*(10), 535–540.
29. Freemon, B., Negrete, V. F., Davis, M., and Korsch, B. M. Gaps in doctor–patient communication: Doctor–patient interaction analysis. *Pediatric Research,* 1971, *5,* 298–311.
30. Freidson, E. *Profession of Medicine.* New York: Dodd, Mead, 1970.
31. Friedman, H. S. The interactive effects of facial expressions of emotion and verbal messages on perceptions of affective meaning. *Journal of Experimental Social Psychology,* 1979, *15,* 453–469.
32. Friedman, H. S. Nonverbal communication between patients and medical practitioners. *Journal of Social Issues,* 1979, *35*(1), 82–99.
33. Friedman, H. S. Nonverbal communication in medical interaction. In H. S. Friedman and M. R. DiMatteo, eds., *Interpersonal Issues in Health Care.* New York: Academic Press, 1982.
34. Friedman, H. S., DiMatteo, M. R., and Taranta, A. A study of the relationship between individual differences in nonverbal expressiveness and factors of personality and social interaction. *Journal of Research in Personality,* 1980, *14,* 351–364.
35. Goffman, E. *Stigma.* Englewood Cliffs, N.J.: Prentice-Hall, 1963.
36. Golden, J. S., and Johnston, G. D. Problems of distortion in doctor–patient communications. *Psychiatry in Medicine,* 1970, *1,* 127–149.
37. Gordon, R. L. *Interviewing, Strategy, Techniques, and Tactics.* Homewood, Ill.: Dorsey Press, 1980.
38. Goodman, R., and Gorlin, R. *The Face in Genetic Disorders.* St. Louis: C. V. Mosby, 1970.
39. Hall, E. T. *The Hidden Dimension.* Garden City, N.Y.: Doubleday, 1966.
40. Harlow, H. F., and Zimmermann, R. R. Affectional responses in the infant monkey. *Science,* 1959, *130,* 421–432.
41. Henley, N. M. *Body Politics.* Englewood Cliffs, N.J.: Prentice-Hall, 1977.
42. Hippocrates. *The Medical Works of Hippocrates.* Translated by J. Chadwick and W. N. Mann. Oxford: Blackwell Scientific Publications, 1950.
43. Johnson, B. S. The meaning of touch in nursing. *Nursing Outlook,* 1965, *13,* 59–60.
44. Jourard, S. M. An exploratory study of body-accessibility. *British Journal of Social and Clinical Psychology,* 1966, *5,* 221–231.
45. Kleck, R. Physical stigma and nonverbal cues emitted in face-to-face interaction. *Human Relations,* 1968, *21,* 119–128.
46. Knapp, M. L. *Nonverbal Communication in Human Interaction.* New York: Holt, Rinehart and Winston, 1978.
47. Knapp, M. L., Hart, R. P., and Dennis, H. S. An exploration of deception as a communication construct. *Human Communication Research,* 1974, *1,* 15–29.

48. Koos, E. *The Health of Regionville*. New York: Columbia University Press, 1954, p. 77.
49. Korsch, B. M., Gozzi, E. K., and Francis, V. Gaps in doctor-patient communication. I. Doctor-patient interaction and patient satisfaction. *Pediatrics*, 1968, *42*, 855–871.
50. Lanzetta, J. T., Cartwright-Smith, J., and Kleck, R. Effects of nonverbal dissimulation on emotional experience and autonomic arousal. *Journal of Personality and Social Psychology*, 1976, *33*, 354–370.
51. Largey, G. P., and Watson, D. R. The sociology of odors. *American Journal of Sociology*, 1972, *77*, 1021–1033.
52. Lederer, H.D. How the sick view their world. *Journal of Social Issues*, 1952, *8*, 4–16.
53. Leventhal, H., and Sharp, E. Facial expressions as indicators of distress. In S. S. Tomkins and C. E. Izard, eds., *Affect, Cognition and Personality: Empirical Studies*. New York: Springer, 1965.
54. Ley, P., and Spelman, M. S. Communication in an outpatient setting. *British Journal of Social and Clinical Psychology*, 1965, *4*, 114–116.
55. Liggett, J. *The Human Face*. New York: Stein and Day, 1974.
56. Lorber, J. Good patients and problem patients: Conformity and deviance in a general hospital. *Journal of Health and Social Behavior*, 1975, *16*, 213–225.
57. Marquis, K. H. Effects of social reinforcement on health reporting in the household interview. *Sociometry*, 1970, *33*(2), 203–215.
58. Mazullo, J. M., Lasagna, L., and Griner, P. F. Variations in interpretation of prescription instructions. *Journal of the American Medical Association*, 1974, *227*(8), 929–930.
59. McIntosh, J. Processes of communication, information seeking and control associated with cancer: A selective review of the literature. *Social Science and Medicine*, 1974, *8*, 167–187.
60. McKinlay, J. Who is really ignorant? *Journal of Health and Social Behavior*, 1975, *16*, 3–12.
61. Meerloo, J. A. M. *Unobtrusive Communication*. Assen, The Netherlands: Koninklijke Van Gorcum and Comp. N. V., 1964.
62. Mehrabian, A. *Nonverbal Communication*. Chicago: Aldine-Atherton, 1972.
63. Milmoe, S., Rosenthal, R., Blane, H. T., Chafetz, M. E., and Wolf, I. The doctor's voice: Postdictor of successful referral of alcoholic patients. *Journal of Abnormal Psychology*, 1967, *72*, 78–84.
64. Montague, A. *Touching*. New York: Harper and Row, 1978.
65. O'Brien, M. J. *Communications and Relationships in Nursing*. St. Louis: C. V. Mosby, 1974.
66. Orwell, G. *1984*. New York: Harcourt, Brace, 1949.
67. Pomeroy, W. B. *Dr. Kinsey and the Institute for Sex Research*. New York: Harper and Row, 1972.
68. Pratt, L., Seligmann, A., and Reader, G. Physicians' views on the level of medical information among patients. *American Journal of Public Health*, 1957, *47*, 1277–1283.
69. Riscalla, L. Healing by laying on of hands: Myth or fact. *Ethics in Science and Medicine*, 1975, *2*, 167–171.
70. Rodin, J., and Janis, I. L. The social power of health-care practitioners as agents of change. *Journal of Social Issues*, 1979, *35*(1), 60–81.
71. Rosenthal, R., Hall, J. H., DiMatteo, M. R., Rogers, P. L., and Archer, D. *Sensitivity to Nonverbal Communication: The PONS Test*. Baltimore: Johns Hopkins University Press, 1979.

72. Samora, J., Saunders, L., and Larson, R. F. Medical vocabulary knowledge among hospital patients. *Journal of Health and Human Behavior,* 1961, *2,* 83–89.
73. Schachter, S. *The Psychology of Affiliation.* Palo Alto, Calif.: Stanford University Press, 1959.
74. Segall, A., and Roberts, L. W. A comparative analysis of physician estimates and levels of medical knowledge among patients. *Sociology of Health and Illness,* 1980, *2*(3), 317–334.
75. Slack, W. V. A computer-based medical history system. *New England Journal of Medicine,* 1966, 274(4), 194–198.
76. Slack, W. V. Computer-based interviewing system dealing with nonverbal behavior as well as keyboard responses. *Science,* 1971, *171,* 84–87.
77. Slack, W. V. Patient-computer dialogue. *New England Journal of Medicine,* 1972, *286*(24), 1304–1309.
78. Szasz, T. S. *Pain and Pleasure: A Study of Bodily Feelings.* New York: Basic Books, 1957.
79. Thompson, T. *Hearts.* New York: McCall Publishing Co., 1971.
80. Vine, I. Communication by facial-visual signals. In J. H. Crook, ed., *Social Behavior in Birds and Mammals.* London and New York: Academic Press, 1970, pp. 279–354.
81. Waitzkin, H., and Stoeckle, J. D. The communication of information about illness: Clinical, sociological and methodological considerations. *Advances in Psychosomatic Medicine,* 1972, *8,* 180–215.
82. Waitzkin, H., and Waterman, B. *The Exploitation of Illness in Capitalist Society.* Indianapolis, Ind.: Bobbs-Merrill, 1974.
83. Whitcher, S., and Fisher, J. Multidimensional reaction to therapeutic touch in a hospital setting. *Journal of Personality and Social Psychology,* 1979, *37,* 87–96.
84. Whorf, B. L. *Language, Thought, and Reality: Selected Writings of Benjamin Lee Whorf,* edited by J. Carroll. Cambridge, Mass.: M.I.T. Press, 1956.

CHAPTER 6
THE NATURE OF ILLNESS

1. Asch, S. E. Effects of group pressure upon the modification and distortion of judgements. In H. Gretzkow, ed., *Groups, Leadership and Men.* Pittsburgh: Carnegie Press, 1951, pp. 177–190.
2. Balint, M. *The Doctor, His Patient and the Illness.* New York: International Universities Press, 1957.
3. Berkanovic, E. Lay conceptions of the sick role. *Social Forces,* 1972, *51,* 53–64.
4. Clark, M. *Health in the Mexican-American Culture,* 2nd ed. Berkeley: University of California Press, 1970.
5. Davitz, L. J., Sameshima, Y., and Davitz, J. Suffering as viewed in six different cultures. *American Journal of Nursing,* (August) 1976, *76*(8), 1296–1297.
6. Duff, R. S., and Hollingshead, A. B. *Sickness and Society.* New York: Harper and Row, 1968.
7. Field, M. G. *Doctor and Patient in Soviet Russia.* Cambridge, Mass.: Harvard University Press, 1957.
8. Gentry, W. D. Preadmission behavior. In W. D. Gentry and R. B. Williams, eds., *Psychological Aspects of Myocardial Infarction and Coronary Care.* 2nd ed. St. Louis: C. V. Mosby, 1979, pp. 67–77.
9. Gentry, W. D., and Haney, T. Emotional and behavioral reaction to acute myocardial infarction. *Heart and Lung,* 1975, *4,* 738.

10. Goffman, E. L. *Stigma*. Englewood Cliffs, N.J.: Prentice-Hall, 1963.
11. Jones, E. E., Kanouse, D., Kelley, H., Nisbett, R., Valins, S., and Weiner, B. *Attribution: Perceiving the Causes of Behavior*. Morristown, N.J.: General Learning Press, 1972.
12. Jones, E. E., and Nisbett, R. E. The actor and the observer: Divergent perceptions of the causes of behavior. In E. E. Jones, ed., *Attribution: Perceiving the Causes of Behavior*. Morristown, N.J.: General Learning Press, 1972, pp. 79-94.
13. Kasl, S. V., and Cobb, S. Health behavior, illness behavior, and sick role behavior. I., *Archives of Environmental Health*, 1966, *12*, 246-266 (February 1966); II., 1966, *12*, 534-541 (April 1966).
14. Kelley, H. H. Attribution theory in social psychology. In D. Levine, ed., *Nebraska Symposium on Motivation*, 1967 (Vol. 15). Lincoln: University of Nebraska Press, 1967, pp. 192-238.
15. Kiev, A. *Curanderismo: Mexican-American Folk Psychiatry*. New York: The Free Press, 1968.
16. Koos, E. *The Health of Regionville*. New York: Columbia University Press, 1954.
17. Lurie, H. J., and Lawrence, G. L. Communication problems between rural Mexican-American patients and their physicians: Description of a solution. *American Journal of Orthopsychiatry*, 1972, *49*(5), 777-783.
18. Mathis, J. L. A sophisticated version of voodoo death. *Psychosomatic Medicine*, 1964, *26*(2), 104-107.
19. Mechanic, D. Illness and social disability: Some problems in analysis. *Pacific Sociological Review*, 1959, *2*, 37-41.
20. Mechanic, D. The concept of illness behavior. *Journal of Chronic Disease*, 1962, *15*, 189-194.
21. Mechanic, D. Response factors in illness: The study of illness behavior. *Social Psychiatry*, 1966, *1*, 11-20.
22. Mechanic, D., and Volkart, E. H. Illness behavior and medical diagnoses. *Journal of Health and Human Behavior*, 1960, *1*, 86-94.
23. Mechanic, D., and Volkart, E. H. Stress, illness behavior and the sick role. *American Sociological Review*, 1961, *26*, 51-58.
24. Minuchin, S., Montalvo, B., Guerney, B., Jr., Rosman, B., and Schumer, K. *Families of the Slums*. New York: Basic Books, 1967.
25. Moss, A. J., and Goldstein, S. The pre-hospital phase of acute myocardial infarction. *Circulation*, 1970, *41*, 737.
26. Nall, F. C., and Speilberg, J. Social and cultural factors in the responses of Mexican-Americans to medical treatment. *Journal of Health and Social Behavior*, 1967, 8(4), 299-308.
27. Norman, J. C., ed. *Medicine in the Ghetto*. New York: Appleton-Century-Crofts, 1969.
28. Olin, H. S., and Hackett, T. P. The denial of chest pain in 32 patients with acute myocardial infarction. *Journal of the American Medical Association*, 1964, *190*, 977.
29. Padilla, A., and Ruiz, R. A. *Latino Mental Health*. Rockville, Md.: National Institute of Mental Health, 1973.
30. Paige, K. Women learn to sing the menstrual blues. *Psychology Today*, 1973, *7*, 41-46.
31. Parsons, T. Definitions of health and illness in the light of American values and social structure. In E. G. Jaco, ed., *Patients, Physicians and Illness*. New York: The Free Press, 1958, pp. 165-187.
32. Phillips, D. L. Self-reliance and the inclination to adopt the sick role. *Social Forces*, 1965, *43*, 555-563.

33. Pilowsky, I., and Spence, N. D. Ethnicity and illness behaviors. *Psychological Medicine,* 1977, *7,* 447–452.
34. Quesada, G. M. Language and communication barriers for health delivery to a minority group. *Social Science and Medicine,* 1976, *10,* 323–327.
35. Rubel, A. J. Concepts of disease in Mexican-American culture. *American Anthropologist,* 1960, *62*(5), 795–814.
36. Saunders, L. *Cultural Differences and Medical Care.* New York: Russell Sage Foundation, 1954.
37. Schachter, S. *The Psychology of Affiliation.* Palo Alto, Calif.: Stanford University Press, 1959.
38. Schachter, S., and Singer, J. E. Cognitive, social and physiological determinants of emotional state. *Psychological Review,* 1962, *69,* 379–399.
39. Segall, A. The sick role concept: Understanding illness behavior. *Journal of Health and Social Behavior,* 1972 (June), *17,* 163–170.
40. Segall, A. Sociocultural variation in sick role behavioral expectations. *Social Science and Medicine,* 1976, *10,* 47–51.
41. Smelser, N. J. *Theory of Collective Behavior.* New York: The Free Press, 1963.
42. Sternbach, R. A., and Tursky, B. Ethnic differences among housewives in psychological and skin potential responses to electric shock. *Psychophysiology,* 1965, *1,* 241–246.
43. Storms, M. D., and Nisbett, R. E. Insomnia and the attribution process. *Journal of Personality and Social Psychology,* 1970, *16,* 319–328.
44. Tjoe, S. L., and Luria, M. H. Delays in reaching the cardiac care unit: An analysis. *Chest,* 1972, *61,* 617.
45. Whorf, B. L. *Language, Thought and Reality.* Cambridge, Mass.: MIT press, 1957.
46. Zborowski, M. Cultural components in responses to pain. *Journal of Social Issues,* 1952, *8,* 16–30.
47. Zborowski, M. *People in Pain.* San Francisco: Jossey-Bass, 1969.
48. Zola, I. Problems of communication, diagnosis and patient care. *Journal of Medical Education,* 1963, *10,* 829–838.
49. Zola, I. K. Illness behavior of the working class. In A. Shostak and W. Gomberg, eds., *Studies of the American Worker.* Englewood Cliffs, N.J.: Prentice-Hall, 1964.
50. Zola, I. K. Culture and symptoms: An analysis of patients presenting complaints. *American Sociological Review,* 1966, *31,* 615.
51. Zola, I. K. Studying the decisions to see a doctor. *Advances in Psychosomatic Medicine,* 1972, *8,* 226–227.

CHAPTER 7
PSYCHOLOGICAL FACTORS IN THE ETIOLOGY OF ILLNESS

1. Alexander, F. *Psychosomatic Medicine: Its Principles and Applications.* New York: W. W. Norton, 1950.
2. Antonovsky, A. *Health, Stress and Coping.* San Francisco: Jossey-Bass, 1979.
3. Beck, A. T. *Cognitive Therapy and the Emotional Disorders.* New York: International Universities Press, 1976.
4. Benson, M. *The Relaxation Response.* New York: Wm. Morrow, 1975.
5. Brown, G. W. Meaning, measurement, and stress of life events. In B. S. Dohrenwend and B. P. Dohrenwend, eds., *Stressful Life Events: Their Nature and Effects.* New York: John Wiley, 1974, pp. 217–244.

6. Cannon, W. B. *Wisdom of the Body.* New York: W. M. Norton, 1932.
7. Cannon, W. B. Voodoo death. *American Anthropologist,* 1942, *44,* 169–181.
8. Canter, A., Imboden, J. B., and Cluff, L. E. The frequency of physical illness as a function of prior psychological vulnerability and contemporary stress. *Psychosomatic Medicine,* 1966, *28,* 344–350.
9. Clayton, P. J. Mortality and morbidity in the first year of widowhood. *Archives of General Psychiatry,* 1974, *30,* 747–750.
10. Cohen, F. Personality, stress, and the development of physical illness. In G. C. Stone, F. Cohen, and N. E. Adler, eds., *Health Psychology.* San Francisco: Jossey-Bass, 1979, pp. 77–111.
11. Cousins, N. *Anatomy of an Illness as Perceived by the Patient.* New York: W. W. Norton, 1979.
12. Dembroski, T. M., Weiss, S. M., Shields, J. L., Haynes, S. G., and Feinlieb, M., eds. *Coronary-Prone Behavior.* New York: Springer-Verlag, 1978.
13. Donald, C. A., Ware, J. E., Jr., Brook, R. H., and Davies-Avery, A. Conceptualization and measurement of health for adults in the health insurance study. Vol. 4. *Social health.* Santa Monica: The Rand Corporation R-4-HEW, 1978.
14. Engel, G. L. A life setting conducive to illness: The giving up–given up complex. *Bulletin of the Menninger Clinic,* 1968, *32,* 355–365.
15. Engel, G. L. Sudden and rapid death during psychological stress: Folklore or folk wisdom? *Annals of Internal Medicine,* 1971, *74,* 771–782.
16. Engel, G. L., and Schmale, A. H. Psychoanalytic theory of somatic disorder. *Journal of the American Psychoanalytic Association,* 1967, *15,* 344–363.
17. Erikson, K. *Everything in Its Path.* New York: Simon and Schuster, 1977.
18. Friedman, M., and Rosenman, R. H. *Type A Behavior and Your Heart.* New York: Alfred A. Knopf, 1974.
19. Gersten, J. C., Langer, T. S., Eisenberg, J. G., and Orzeck, L. Child behavior and life events: Undesirable change or change per se? In B. S. Dohrenwend and B. P. Dohrenwend, eds., *Stressful Life Events: Their Nature and Effects.* New York: John Wiley, 1974, pp. 159–170.
20. Glass, D. C. *Behavior Patterns, Stress and Coronary Disease.* Hillsdale, N.J.: L. Erlbaum, 1977.
21. Glass, D. C. Stress, behavior patterns, and coronary disease. *American Scientist,* 1977, *65,* 177.
22. Gore, S. The effect of social support in moderating the health consequences of unemployment. *Journal of Health and Social Behavior,* 1978, 19(2), 157–165.
23. Graham, S. The sociological approach to epidemiology. *American Journal of Public Health,* 1974, *64,* 1046–1049.
24. Holmes, T. H., and Masuda, M. Life change and illness susceptibility. In B. S. Dohrenwend and B. P. Dohrenwend, eds., *Stressful Life Events: Their Nature and Effects.* New York: John Wiley, 1974, pp. 45–72.
25. Holmes, T. H., and Rahe, R. H. *Schedule of Recent Experiences.* Seattle: School of Medicine, University of Washington, 1967.
26. Holmes, T. H., and Rahe, R. H. The social readjustment rating scale. *Journal of Psychosomatic Research,* 1967, *11,* 213–218.
27. Ireton, H., and Cassata, D. A psychological systems review. *The Journal of Family Practice,* 1976, 3(2), 155–159.
28. Jacobs, S., and Ostfeld, A. M. An epidemiological review of the mortality of bereavement. *Psychosomatic Medicine,* 1977, *39,* 344–357.
29. Janis, I. L. *Psychological Stress: Psychoanalytic and Behavioral Studies of Surgical Patients.* New York: John Wiley, 1958.
30. Jenkins, C. D. The coronary-prone personality. In W. D. Gentry, and R. B. Wil-

liams, Jr., eds., *Psychological Aspects of Myocardial Infarction and Coronary Care.* 2nd ed. St. Louis: C. V. Mosby, 1979, pp. 5–30.

31. Jenkins, C. D., Rosenman, R. H., and Friedman, M. Development of an objective psychological test for the determination of the coronary-prone behavior pattern in employed men. *Journal of Chronic Disease,* 1967, *20,* 371.

32. Jenkins, C. D., Rosenman, R. H., and Zyzanski, S. J. Prediction of clinical coronary heart disease by a test for the coronary-prone behavior pattern. *New England Journal of Medicine,* 1974, *290,* 1271.

33. Jenkins, C. D., Zyzanski, S. J., and Rosenman, R. H. *Manual for the Jenkins Activity Survey.* New York: Psychological Corporation, 1978.

34. Kaplan, R. Coping with stressful medical examinations. In H. S. Friedman, and M. R. DiMatteo, eds., *Interpersonal Issues in Health Care.* New York: Academic Press, 1982.

35. Knowles, J. H. The responsibility of the individual. *Daedalus,* 1977, *106,* 57–80.

36. Kobasa, S. Stressful life events, personality and health: An inquiry into hardiness. *Journal of Personality and Social Psychology,* 1979, *37*(1), 1–11.

37. Kostrubala, T. *The Joy of Running.* New York: Simon and Schuster, 1976.

38. Leibowitz, J. O. *The History of Coronary Heart Disease.* Berkeley: University of California Press, 1970.

39. Levy, L., and Herzog, A. Effects of population density and crowding on health and social adaptation in the Netherlands. *Journal of Health and Social Behavior,* 1974, *15,* 228–240.

40. Liem, J. H., and Liem, R. Life events, social supports and physical and psychological well-being. Paper presented at annual meetings of the American Psychological Association, Washington, D.C., 1976.

41. Lin, N., Simeone, R. S., Ensel, W. M., and Kuo, W. Social support, stressful life events, and illness: A model and an empirical test. *Journal of Health and Social Behavior,* 1979, *20*(2), 108–119.

42. Lynch, J. J. *The Broken Heart: The Medical Consequences of Loneliness.* New York: Basic Books, 1977.

43. Mason, J. W. Specificity in the organization of neuroendocrine response profiles. In P. Seeman and G. M. Brown, eds., *Frontiers in Neurology and Neuroscience Research.* First International Symposium of the Neuroscience Institute. Toronto: University of Toronto, 1974.

44. Mason, J. W. A historical view of the stress field: Part I. *Journal of Human Stress,* 1975, *1*(1), 6–12.

45. Mechanic, D. *Medical Sociology.* New York: The Free Press, 1968.

46. Mechanic, D. Social psychological factors affecting the presentation of bodily complaints. *New England Journal of Medicine,* 1972, *286,* 1132–1139.

47. Mechanic, D., and Volkart, E. H. Stress, illness behavior, and the sick role. *American Sociological Review,* 1961, *26,* 51–58.

48. Menninger, K. A., and Menninger, W. C. Psychoanalytic observations in cardiac disorders. *American Heart Journal,* 1936, 11(10).

49. Meyer, A. Cited in A. Lief, ed., *The Commonsense Psychiatry of Dr. Adolf Meyer.* New York: McGraw-Hill, 1948.

50. Moss, G. E. *Illness, Immunity and Social Interaction: The Dynamics of Biosocial Resonation.* New York: John Wiley, 1973.

51. Pearlin, L. I., and Schooler, C. The structure of coping. *Journal of Health and Social Behavior,* 1978, *19*(1), 2–21.

52. Pelletier, K. *Mind as Healer, Mind as Slayer.* New York: Dell, 1977.

53. Pennebaker, J. W., Burnan, M. A., Schaeffer, M. A., and Harper, D. C. Lack of control as a determinant of perceived physical symptoms. *Journal of Personality*

and Social Psychology, 1977, 35, 167–174.

54. Pennebaker, J., and Skelton, J. Psychological parameters of physical symptoms. *Personality and Social Psychology Bulletin*, 1978, 4, 524–530.

55. Phillips, D. L. Rejection: A possible consequence of seeking help for mental disorders. *American Sociological Review*, 1963, 28, 963–972.

56. Rabkin, J. G., and Struening, E. L. Life events, stress, and illness. *Science*, 1976, 194, 1013–1020.

57. Rahe, R. H. Subjects' recent changes and their near-future illness susceptibility. *Advances in Psychosomatic Medicine, 1972, 8*, 2–19.

58. Rahe, R. H. The pathway between subjects' recent life changes and their near-future illness reports: Representative results and methodological issues. In B. S. Dohrenwend and B. P. Dohrenwend, eds., *Stressful Life Events: Their Nature and Effects*. New York: John Wiley, 1974, pp. 73–86.

59. Rahe, R. H., and Arthur, R. H. Life change and illness studies. *Journal of Human Stress*, 1978, 4(1), 3–15.

60. Rahe, R. W., McKean, J. D., and Arthur, R. J. A longitudinal study of life change and illness patterns. *Journal of Psychosomatic Research*, 1967, 10, 355–366.

61. Richter, C. P. On the phenomenon of sudden death in animals and man. *Psychosomatic Medicine*, 1957, 19, 191–198.

62. Rosenman, R. H., Friedman, M. Straus, R., Wurm, M., Kositcheck, R. Hahn, W., and Werthesson, N. A predictive study of coronary heart disease. The western collaborative group study. *Journal of the American Medical Association*, 1964, 189, 15.

63. Rosenman, R. H., Friedman, M., Straus, R., Jenkins, D., Zyzanski, S., and Wurm, M. Coronary heart disease in the western collaborative group study: A follow-up experience of 4½ years. *Journal of Chronic Disease*, 1970, 23, 173.

64. Rotter, J. B. Generalized expectancies for internal versus external control of reinforcement. *Psychological Monographs*, 1966, 80(1), No. 609.

65. Rowland, K. R. Environmental events predicting death for the elderly. *Psychological Bulletin*, 1977, 84, 349–372.

66. Schmale, A. H., Jr. Giving up as a final common pathway to changes in health. *Advances in Psychosomatic Medicine, 1972, 8*, 20–40.

67. Schmale, A. H., Jr., and Engel, G. L. The giving up–given up complex illustrated on film. *Archives of General Psychiatry*, 1967, 17, 135–145.

68. Schmale, A. H., Jr., and Iker, H. P. The affect of hopelessness and the development of cancer. I. Identification of uterine cervical cancer in women with atypical cytology. *Psychosomatic Medicine*, 1966, 28, 714–721.

69. Schmale, A. H., Jr., and Iker, H. P. Hopelessness as a predictor of cervical cancer. *Social Science and Medicine*, 1971, 5, 95–100.

70. Schultz, D. *Growth Psychology*. New York: D. Van Nostrand, 1977.

71. Seligman, M. E. *Helplessness*. San Francisco: W. H. Freeman, 1975.

72. Selye, H. *The Stress of Life*. New York: McGraw-Hill, 1956.

73. Sheehan, G. *Dr. Sheehan: On Running*. Mt. View, Calif.: World Publications, 1975.

74. Surgeon General of the United States. *Healthy People: The Surgeon General's Report on Health Promotion and Disease Prevention, 1979*. Washington, D.C.: USDHEW Pub. 79-55071. Public Health Service.

75. Toffler, A. *Future Shock*, New York: Bantum Books, 1971.

76. Torrens, P. R. *The American Health Care System: Issues and Problems*. St. Louis: C. V. Mosby, 1978.

77. Wolff, H., and Goodell, H. *Stress and Disease*. 2nd ed. Springfield, Ill.: Charles C. Thomas, 1968.

CHAPTER 8
CHRONIC ILLNESS: PSYCHOSOCIAL
ASPECTS OF DISABILITY

1. Abram, H. S. Survival by machine: The psychological stress of chronic hemo-dialysis. *Psychiatry in Medicine,* 1970, *1,* 37–51.
2. ACS 1979 Survey. Report on the social, economic and psychological needs of cancer patients in California. San Francisco: American Cancer Society, 1974.
3. Adler, A. Neuropsychiatric complications in victims of Boston's Cocoanut Grove disaster. *Journal of the American Medical Association,* 1943, *123,* 1098–1101.
4. Adler, M. L. Kidney transplantation and coping mechanisms. *Psychosomatics,* 1972, *13,* 337–341.
5. Andreasen, N. J. C., and Norris, A. S. Long-term adjustment and adaptation mechanisms in severely burned adults. *Journal of Nervous and Mental Disease,* 1972, *154*(5), 352–362.
6. Benoliel, J. Q. Childhood diabetes: The commonplace in living becomes uncom-mon. In A. L. Strauss, ed., *Chronic Illness and the Quality of Life.* St. Louis: C. V. Mosby, 1975, pp. 89–98.
7. Brodland, G. A., and Andreasen, N. J. C. Adjustment problems of the family of the burned patient. *Social Casework,* 1974, *55,* 13–18.
8. Cantor, R. C. *And a Time to Live: Toward Emotional Well-Being During the Crisis of Cancer.* New York: Harper and Row, 1978.
9. Caplan, R. Patient, provider, and organization: Hypothesized determinants of adherence. In S. J. Cohen, ed., *New Directions in Patient Compliance.* Lexington, Mass.: D. C. Heath, 1979, pp. 75–100.
10. Cassem, N. H., and Hackett, T. P. Psychological rehabilitation of myocardial infarction patients in the acute phase. *Heart and Lung,* 1973, *2,* 382.
11. Cobb, S. Social support as a moderator of life stresses. *Psychosomatic Medicine,* 1976, *38*(5), 300–314.
12. Cobb, S., and Erbe, C. Social support for the cancer patient. *Forum on Medicine,* 1978, *1*(8), 24–29.
13. Cohen, F., and Lazarus, R. S. Coping with the stresses of illness. In G. C. Stone, F. Cohen, and N. E. Adler, eds., *Health Psychology.* San Francisco: Jossey-Bass, 1979.
14. Croog, S. H., and Levine, S. After the heart attack: Social aspects of rehabilita-tion. *Medical Insight,* 1973, *5,* 10.
15. Davis, F. *Passage Through Crisis.* Indianapolis: Bobbs Merrill, 1963.
16. DiMatteo, M. R., and Friedman, H. S. *A New Undergraduate Science Course in Social Psychology and Health.* Report to the National Science Foundation, Local Course Improvement Grant. Riverside, Calif., January 1981.
17. Donavan, M., and Pierce, S. *Cancer Care Nursing.* New York: Appleton-Century-Crofts, 1976.
18. Glaser, H. H., Harrison, G. S., and Lynn, D. B. Emotional implications of con-genital heart disease in children. *Pediatrics,* 1964, *33,* 367.
19. Goffman, E. *Stigma.* Englewood Cliffs, N.J.: Prentice-Hall, 1963.
20. Green, M. Care of the child with a long-term life-threatening illness: Some prin-ciples of management. *Pediatrics,* 1967, *39,* 441.
21. Greenfield, N. S., Roessler, R., and Crosley, A. P. Ego strength and length of re-covery from infectious mononucleosis. *Journal of Nervous and Mental Disease,* 1959, *128,* 125–128.

22. Gulledge, A. D. Psychological aftermaths of myocardial infarction. In W. D. Gentry, and R. B. Williams, Jr., eds., *Psychological Aspects of Myocardial Infarction and Coronary Care.* St. Louis: C. V. Mosby, 1979, pp. 113–130.
23. Haan, N. *Coping and Defending.* New York: Academic Press, 1977.
24. Janis, I. L. *Psychological Stress: Psychoanalytic and Behavioral Studies of Surgical Patients.* New York: John Wiley, 1958.
25. Kahana, R. J., and Bibring, G. L. Personality types in medical management. In N. E. Zinberg, ed., *Psychiatry and Medical Practice in a General Hospital.* New York: International Universities Press, 1964.
26. Kelly, O. E. *Make Today Count.* New York: Delacorte Press, 1975.
27. Lasagna, L. Physicians' behavior toward the dying patient. In O. Brim, H. Freeman, S. Levine, and N. Scotch, eds., *The Dying Patient.* New York: Russell Sage Foundation, 1970.
28. Lasser, T. *Reach to Recovery.* New York: American Cancer Society, 1974.
29. Lerner, M. The desire for justice and reactions to victims. In J. Macaulay and L. L. Berkowitz, eds., *Altruism and Helping Behavior.* New York: Academic Press, 1970, pp. 205–229.
30. Lieberman, M. A. *Self-help Groups for Coping with Crisis.* San Francisco: Jossey-Bass, 1979.
31. Lipowski, Z. J. Psychosocial aspects of disease. *Annals of Internal Medicine,* 1969, *71,* 1197–1206.
32. Mattsson, A. The crisis of illness: Chronic conditions. *Pediatrics,* 1972, *50,* 801–811.
33. Moos, R. H., and Tsu, V. D. Overview and perspective. In R. H. Moos, ed., *Coping with Physical Illness.* New York: Plenum, 1977.
34. Reichsman, F., and Levy, N. B. Problems in adaptation to maintenance. *Archives of Internal Medicine,* 1972, *130,* 859–865.
35. Ryan, W. *Blaming the Victim.* New York: Random House, 1971.
36. Schulman, B. A. Active patient orientation and outcomes in hypertensive treatment: Application of a socio-organizational perspective. *Medical Care,* 1979, *17*(3), 267–280.
37. Simonton, C., Matthews-Simonton, S., and Creighton, J. *Getting Well Again: A Step-by-Step Self Help Guide to Overcoming Cancer for Patients and Their Families.* New York: St. Martin's Press, 1978.
38. Sontag, S. *Illness as Metaphor.* New York: Farrar, Straus, and Giroux, 1978.
39. Strauss, A. L., and Glaser, B. *Chronic Illness and the Quality of Life.* St. Louis: C. V. Mosby, 1975.
40. Tisza, V. B. Management of the parents of the chronically ill child. *American Journal of Orthopsychiatry,* 1962, *32,* 53–59.
41. U.S. Public Health. *Chronic Conditions and Limitations of Activity and Mobility: July 1965–June 1967.* Public Health Service Publication: No. 1000, Series 10-61. USDHEW, PHS, Mental Health Administration, Washington, D.C., January 1971.
42. Vernon, D., Foley, J., Sipowicz, R., and Schulman, J. *The Psychological Responses of Children to Hospitalization and Illness: A Review of the Literature.* Springfield, Ill.: Charles C Thomas, 1965.
43. Wishnie, H. A., Hackett, T. P., and Cassem, N. H. Psychological hazards of convalescence following myocardial infarction. *Journal of the American Medical Association,* 1971, *215,* 1292–1296.
44. Wortman, C. B., and Dunkel-Schetter, C. Interpersonal relationships and cancer: A theoretical analysis. *Journal of Social Issues,* 1979, *35*(1), pp. 120–155.

CHAPTER 9
DYING AND DEATH

1. Anthony, S. *The Discovery of Death in Childhood and After.* New York: Basic Books, 1972. (Revision of *The Child's Discovery of Death.* New York: Harcourt, Brace and World, 1940.)
2. Barton, D. The need for including instruction on death and dying in the medical curriculum. *Journal of Medical Education,* 1972, *47,* 169–175.
3. Becker, E. *The Denial of Death.* New York: The Free Press, 1973.
4. Brown, F. Depression and childhood bereavement. *Journal of Mental Science,* 1961, *107,* 754–777.
5. Bryer, K. The Amish way of death. *American Psychologist,* 1979, *34,* 255–261.
6. Bugen, L. A. Emotions: Their presence and impact upon the helping role. In Charles A. Garfield, ed., *Stress and Survival.* St. Louis: C. V. Mosby, 1979, pp. 138–145.
7. Caine, L. *Widow.* New York: Bantam Books, 1974.
8. Caine, L. *Lifelines.* New York: Dell, 1978.
9. Caughill, R. E., ed. *The Dying Patient.* Boston: Little, Brown, 1976.
10. Clayton, P., Desmarais, L., and Winokur, G. A study of normal bereavement. *American Journal of Psychiatry,* 1968, *125,* 168–178.
11. Curtin, S. R. *Nobody Ever Died of Old Age: In Praise of Old People in Outrage at Their Loneliness.* Boston: Little, Brown, 1972.
12. Dempsey, D. *The Way We Die: An Investigation of Death and Dying in America Today.* New York: McGraw-Hill, 1975.
13. Douglas, J. D. *The Social Meaning of Suicide.* Princeton: Princeton University Press, 1967.
14. Erickson, R. C., and Hyerstay, B. J. The dying patient and the double-bind hypothesis. In Charles A. Garfield, ed., *Stress and Survival.* St. Louis: C. V. Mosby, 1979, pp. 298–306.
15. Farberow, N. L., and Shneidman, E. S., eds. *The Cry for Help.* New York: McGraw-Hill, 1965.
16. Feifel, H., ed. *The Meaning of Death.* New York: McGraw-Hill, 1959.
17. Feifel, H. The function of attitudes toward death. In *Death and Dying: Attitudes of Patient and Doctor.* Vol. 5, Symposium 11. New York: Group for the Advancement of Psychiatry, 1965.
18. Fishoff, J., and O'Brien, N. After a child dies. *Pediatrics,* 1976, *88,* 140–146.
19. Furman, E. F. *A Child's Parent Dies.* New Haven: Yale University Press, 1974.
20. Futterman, E. H., Hoffman, I., and Sabshin, M. Parental anticipatory mourning. In B. Schoenberg, A. C. Carr, D. Peretz, and A. H. Kutscher, eds., *Psychosocial Aspects of Terminal Care.* New York: Columbia University Press, 1972.
21. Garfield, C. A., ed. *Stress and Survival: The Emotional Realities of Life Threatening Illness.* St. Louis: C. V. Mosby, 1979.
22. Glick, I. O., Weiss, R. S., and Parkes, C. M. *The First Year of Bereavement.* New York: Wiley-Interscience, 1974.
23. Gorer, G. D. *Grief and Mourning.* Garden City, N.Y.: Doubleday, 1965. (Reprinted by Arno Press, 1977.)
24. Kalish, R. A. Social distance and the dying. *Community Mental Health Journal,* 1966, *2,* 152–155.
25. Kastenbaum, R. J. *Death, Society and Human Experience.* St. Louis: C. V. Mosby, 1977.
26. Kastenbaum, R. "Healthy dying": A paradoxical quest continues. *Journal of Social Issues,* 1979, *35*(1), 185–206.

27. Kastenbaum, R. Dying is healthy and death a bureaucrat: Our fantasy machine is alive and well. In H. S. Friedman, and M. R. DiMatteo, eds., *Interpersonal Issues in Health Care*. New York: Academic Press, 1982.
28. Kastenbaum, R., and Aisenberg, R. B. *The Psychology of Death*. New York: Springer, 1972.
29. Kastenbaum, R., and Costa, P. T., Jr. Psychological perspectives on death. In M. R. Rosenzweig and L. W. Porter, eds., *Annual Review of Psychology*. Palo Alto, Calif.: Annual Reviews, Inc., 1977, Vol. 28, pp. 225-250.
30. Kennell, J. H., and Klaus, M. H. Caring for parents of an infant who dies. In M. H. Klaus and J. H. Kennell, eds., *Maternal-Infant Bonding*. St. Louis: C. V. Mosby, 1976.
31. Kübler-Ross, E. *On Death and Dying*. New York: Macmillan, 1969.
32. Ladurie, E. *Montaillou: The Promised Land of Error*. New York: G. Braziller, 1978.
33. Lewis, S., and Armstrong, S. H. Children with terminal illness: A selected review. *International Journal of Psychiatry in Medicine*, 1977, *8*(1), 73-82.
34. Lindemann, E. The symptomatology and management of acute grief. *American Journal of Psychiatry*, 1944, *101*, 141-148.
35. Maslach, C. The burn-out syndrome and patient care. In Charles A. Garfield, ed., *Stress and Survival*. St. Louis: C. V. Mosby, 1979, pp. 111-120.
36. Miller, M. *Suicide After Sixty: The Final Alternative*. New York: Springer, 1979.
37. Moriarty, D. M., ed. *The Loss of Loved Ones*. Springfield, Ill.: Charles C Thomas, 1967.
38. Nagy, M. The child's theories concerning death. *Journal of Genetic Psychology*, 1948, *73*, 3-27.
39. Parkes, C. M. *Bereavement*. New York: International Universities Press, 1972.
40. Piaget, J. *The Child's Conception of the World*. Patterson, N.J.: Littlefield, Adams, 1960.
41. Pincus, L. *Death and the Family*. New·York: Vintage Books, 1974.
42. Rochlin, G. How younger children view death and themselves. In E. A. Grollman, ed., *Explaining Death to Children*. Boston: Beacon Press, 1967, pp. 51-88.
43. Rothenberg, M. Reactions of those who treat children with cancer. *Pediatrics*, 1967, *40*, 507.
44. Seligmann, J., and Agrest, S. A right to die. *Newsweek*, April 12, 1976.
45. Shephard, M. *Someone You Love Is Dying: A Guide for Helping and Coping*. New York: Charter, 1975.
46. Vernick, J., and Karon, M. Who's afraid of death on a leukemia ward? *American Journal of Diseases of Children*, 1965, *109*, 393-397.
47. Weisman, A. D., and Worden, J. W. Psychosocial analysis of cancer deaths. *Omega*, 1975, *6*, 61-65.
48. Wiener, J. M. Response of medical personnel to the fatal illness of a child. In B. Schoenberg, G. C. Carr, S. Peretz, and A. H. Kutscher, eds., *Loss and Grief: Psychological Management in Medical Practice*. New York: Columbia University Press, 1970.

CHAPTER 10
THE HEALTH CARE PROFESSIONAL

1. Adler, N. E. Abortion: A social-psychological perspective. *Journal of Social Issues*, 1979, *35*(1), 100-119.
2. Barron-McBride, A. *Living with Contradictions*. New York: Harper-Colophon, 1976.

3. Becker, H. S., and Geer, B. The fate of idealism in medical school. *American Sociological Review*, 1958, *23*, 50–56.
4. Becker, H. S., Geer, B., Hughes, E. C., and Strauss, A. M. *Boys in White: Student Culture in Medical School*. Chicago: University of Chicago Press, 1961.
5. Blachly, P. H., Disher, W., and Roduner, G. Suicide by physicians. *Bulletin of Suicidology*, December 1968, 1–18.
6. California Medical Association. What you need to know about impairment in physicians. CMA *Newsletter*—division of scientific and educational activities, 731 Market St., San Francisco, 94103.
7. Campbell, M. A. *Why Would a Girl Go into Medicine?* Westbury, N.Y.: The Feminist Press, 1973.
8. Cartwright, L. K. Personality changes in a sample of young women physicians. *Journal of Medical Education*, 1977, *52*, 467–474.
9. Cartwright, L. K. Career satisfaction and role harmony in a sample of young women physicians. *Journal of Vocational Behavior*, 1978, *12*, 184–196.
10. Cartwright, L. K. Sources and effects of stress in health careers. G. C. Stone, F. Cohen, and N. E. Adler, eds., *Health Psychology*. San Francisco: Jossey-Bass, 1979.
11. Char, W. F., and McDermott, J. F. Abortions and acute identity crisis in nurses. *American Journal of Psychiatry*, 1972, *128*, 66–71.
12. Christie, R., and Merton, R. K. Procedures for the sociological study of the value climate in medical schools. *Journal of Medical Education*, 1958, *33*, 125–133 (part 2).
13. Council on mental health: The sick physician. *Journal of the American Medical Association*, 1973, *223*(6), 684–687.
14. Craig, A. G., and Pitts, F. N. Suicide by physicians. *Diseases of the Nervous System*, 1968, *29*, 763–772.
15. Dawes, R. M. Case by case versus rule-generated procedures for the allocation of scarce resources. In M. F. Kaplan and S. Schwartz, eds., *Human Judgment and Decision Processes in Applied Settings*. New York: Academic Press, 1977.
16. Djerassi, E. Some problems of occupational diseases of dentists. *International Dental Journal*, 1971, *21*, 252–269.
17. Elstein, A. S. Clinical judgment: Psychological research and medical practice. *Science*, 1976, *194*, 696–700.
18. Elstein, A. S., and Bordage, G. Psychology of clinical reasoning. In G. C. Stone, F. Cohen, and N. E. Adler, eds., *Health Psychology*. San Francisco: Jossey-Bass, 1979.
19. Engel, G. L. The need for a new medical model: A challenge for biomedicine. *Science*, 1977, *196*, 129–136.
20. Everson, R. B., and Fraumeni, J. F. Mortality among medical students and young physicians. *Journal of Medical Education*, 1975, *50*, 809–811.
21. Fox, R. *Experiment Perilous*. Philadelphia: University of Pennsylvania Press, 1959.
22. Funkenstein, D. *Medical Students, Medical Schools, and Society During Five Eras*. Cambridge, Mass.: Ballinger, 1978.
23. Goldberg, L. R. Man versus model of man: A rationale, plus some evidence for a method of improving on clinical inferences. *Psychological Bulletin*, 1970, *73*, 422–432.
24. Gough, H. G. A factorial study of medical specialty preference. *British Journal of Medical Education*, 1975, *9*, 78–85.
25. Gough, H. G., and Hall, W. B. Physicians' retrospective evaluations of their medical education. *Research in Higher Education*, 1977, *7*, 29–42.
26. Gray, R. M., Newman, W. R. E., and Reinhardt, A. M. The effect of medical spe-

cialization on physicians' attitudes. *Journal of Health and Human Behavior,* 1966, *7,* 128–133.

27. Haan, N. G. Psychosocial meanings of unfavorable medical forecasts. In G. C. Stone, F. Cohen, and N. E. Adler, eds., *Health Psychology.* San Francisco: Jossey-Bass, 1979.

28. Janis, I. L. *Victims of Groupthink.* Boston: Houghton Mifflin, 1972.

29. Johnson, C. A., Hammel, R. J., and Heinen, J. S. Levels of satisfaction among hospital pharmacists. *American Journal of Hospital Pharmacy,* 1977, *34,* 241–247.

30. Kahneman, D., and Tversky, A. Subjective probability: A judgment of representativeness. *Cognitive Psychology,* 1972, *3,* 430–454.

31. Kahneman, D., and Tversky, A. On the psychology of prediction. *Psychological Review,* 1973, *80,* 237–251.

32. Kane, F. J., Feldman, M., Jain, S., and Lipton, M. A. Emotional reactions of abortion services personnel. *Archives of General Psychiatry,* 1973, *28,* 409–411.

33. King, H. Health in the medical and other learned professions. *Journal of Chronic Diseases,* 1970, *23,* 257–281.

34. Kramer, M. *Reality Shock: Why Nurses Leave Nursing.* St. Louis: C. V. Mosby, 1974.

35. Lief, H. I., and Fox, R. C. Training for "detached concern" in medical students. In H. I. Lief, V. P. Lief, and N. L. Lief, eds., *The Psychological Basis of Medical Practice.* New York: Harper and Row, Hoeber Medical Books, 1963, pp. 12–35.

36. Lowenstein, L. M. The structure and function of graduate medical education. In E. C. Shapiro, and L. M. Lowenstein, eds., *Becoming a Physician.* Cambridge, Mass.: Ballinger, 1979, pp. 93–111.

37. Maslach, C. Burned-out. *Human Behavior,* 1976, *5*(9), 16–22.

38. Modlin, H. C., and Montes, A. Narcotics addiction in physicians. *American Journal of Psychiatry,* 1964, *121,* 358–369.

39. Mumford, E. *Interns: From Students to Physicians.* Cambridge, Mass.: Harvard University Press, 1970.

40. Newsom, J. A. Help for the alcoholic physician in California. *Alcoholism: Clinical and Experimental Research,* 1977, *1*(2), 135–137.

41. Robinson, V. M. *Humor and the Health Professions.* Thorofare, N.J.: Charles B. Slack, 1977.

42. Rogoff, N. The decision to study medicine. In R. K. Merton, G. G. Reader, and P. L. Kendall, eds., *The Student Physician.* Cambridge, Mass.: Harvard University Press, 1957, pp. 109–129.

43. Rose, K. D., and Rosow, I. Physicians who kill themselves. *Archives of General Psychiatry,* 1973, *29,* 800–805.

44. Rosen, R. A., Werley, H. A., Ager, J. W., and Shea, F. P. Health professionals' attitudes toward abortion. *Public Opinion Quarterly,* 1974, *38,* 158–173.

45. Rosenberg, P. P. Catch 22—the medical model. In E. C. Shapiro, and L. M. Lowenstein, eds., *Becoming a Physician.* Cambridge, Mass.: Ballinger, 1979, pp. 81–92.

46. Roth, J. A. Some contingencies of the moral evaluation and control of clientele: The case of the hospital emergency service. *American Journal of Sociology,* 1972, *77,* 839–856.

47. Sawyer, T. Measurement and prediction: Clinical and statistical. *Psychological Bulletin,* 1966, *66,* 178–200.

48. Schumacher, C. F. Personal characteristics of students choosing different types of medical careers. *Journal of Medical Education,* 1964, *39,* 278–288.

49. Spence, T. T., Helmreich, R. L., and Deaux, K. Sex roles and sex differences. In G. Lindzey and E. Aronson, eds., *Handbook of Social Psychology.* Reading, Mass.: Addison-Wesley, in press.

50. Steppacher, R. C., and Mausner, J. S. Suicide in male and female physicians. *Journal of the American Medical Association,* 1974, *228*(3), 323–328.
51. Tesser, A., and Rosen, S. The reluctance to transmit bad news. In L. Berkowitz, ed., *Advances in Experimental Social Psychology.* New York: Academic Press, 1975.
52. Tversky, A., and Kahneman, D. Judgment under uncertainty: Heuristics and biases. *Science,* 1974, *185,* 1124–1131.
53. Vaillant, G. E. *Adaptation to Life.* Boston: Little, Brown, 1977.
54. Vaillant, G. E., Sobowale, N. C., and McArthur, C. Some psychologic vulnerabilities of physicians. *New England Journal of Medicine,* 1972, *287,* 372–375.
55. Waitzkin, H., and Waterman, B. *The Exploitation of Illness in Capitalist Society.* Indianapolis: Bobbs Merrill, 1974.

CHAPTER 11
THE HEALTH CARE ENVIRONMENT

1. American Hospital Association. *Hospital Statistics.* Chicago: American Hospital Association, 1977.
2. Amir, M. *Patterns in Forcible Rape.* Chicago: University of Chicago Press, 1971, p. 314.
3. Antonovsky, A. *Health, Stress, and Coping.* San Francisco: Jossey-Bass, 1979.
4. Beck, N. C., Geden, E. A., and Brouder, G. T. Preparation for labor: A historical perspective. *Psychosomatic Medicine,* 1979, *41,* 243–258.
5. Bemis, K. M. Current approaches to the etiology and treatment of anorexia nervosa. *Psychological Bulletin,* 1978, *85,* 593–617.
6. Bernard, V. W., Ottenberg, P., and Redl, F. Dehumanization. In N. Sanford, and C. Comstock, eds., *Sanctions for Evil.* Boston: Beacon Press, 1971, pp. 102–124.
7. Birren, J. E., and Schaie, K. W., eds., *Handbook of the Psychology of Aging.* New York: Van Nostrand Reinhold, 1977.
8. Brehm, J. W. *A Theory of Psychological Reactance.* New York: Academic Press, 1966.
9. Brown, W. A. *Psychological Care During Pregnancy and the Postpartum.* New York: Raven Press, 1979.
10. Butler, R. *Why Survive? Being Old in America.* New York: Harper and Row, 1975.
11. Butler, R. N., and Lewis, M. I. *Love and Sex After Sixty.* New York: Harper and Row, 1976.
12. Cartwright, A. *Human Relations and Hospital Care.* London: Routledge and Kegan Paul, 1964.
13. Carveth, W. B., and Gottlieb, B. H. The measurement of social support and its relation to stress. *Canadian Journal of Behavioral Science,* 1979, *11*(3), 179–188.
14. Cooperstock, R. Sex differences in the use of mood-modifying drugs: An explanatory model. *Journal of Health and Social Behavior,* 1971,. *12,* 238–244.
15. Coser, R. L. *Life in the Ward.* East Lansing: Michigan State University Press, 1962.
16. Cundy, K. R., and Ball, W., eds. *Infection Control in Health Care Facilities.* Baltimore: University Park Press, 1977.
17. Curtin, S. *Nobody Ever Died of Old Age: In Praise of Old People in Outrage at Their Loneliness.* Boston: Little, Brown, 1972.
18. Dangott, L. R., and Kalish, R. A. *A Time to Enjoy: The Pleasures of Aging.* Englewood Cliffs, N.J.: Prentice-Hall, 1979.

19. Diamond, M., and Karlen, A. *Sexual Decisions*. Boston: Little, Brown, 1980.
20. Dubos, R. J. *Man, Medicine and Environment*. New York: Praeger, 1968.
21. Egbert, L. D., Battit, G. E., Welch, C. E., and Bartlett, M. K. Reductions of postoperative pain by encouragement and instruction of patients: A study of doctor-patient rapport. *New England Journal of Medicine*, 1964, *270*, 825–827.
22. Fidell, L. S. Sex role stereotypes and the American physician. *Psychology of Women Quarterly*, 1980, *4*, 313–330.
23. Glass, D. C. *Behavior Patterns, Stress, and Coronary Disease*. Hillsdale, N.J.: Laurence Erlbaum, 1977.
24. Goffman, E. *Asylums*. Garden City, N.Y.: Doubleday, 1961.
25. Gorsuch, R., and Butler, M. Initial drug abuse: A review of predisposing social psychological factors. *Psychological Bulletin*, 1976, *83*, 120–137.
26. Gumbiner, J. Psychotherapeutic drug use: Personality, health, and demographic factors. Ph.D. dissertation, University of California, Riverside, 1981.
27. Haller, J. A., Talbert, J. L., and Dombro, R. H. *The Hospitalized Child and His Family*. Baltimore: Johns Hopkins University Press, 1967.
28. Herman, D. The rape culture. In Jo Freeman, ed., *Women: A Feminist Perspective*. 2nd ed. Palo Alto, Calif.: Mayfield Co., 1979.
29. Herzberger, S. D., and Potts, D. A. Interpersonal relations during the childbearing year. In H. S. Friedman and M. R. DiMatteo, eds., *Interpersonal Issues in Health Care*. New York: Academic Press, 1982.
30. Hofling, C. K., Brotzman, S. D., Graves, N., and Pierce, C. M. An experimental study in nurse–physician relationships. *Journal of Nervous and Mental Disease*, 1966, *143*, 171–180.
31. Hunt, M. *Sexual Behavior in the 1970's*. Chicago: Playboy Press, 1974.
32. James, W. H., Woodruff, A. B., and Werner, W. Effect of internal and external control upon changes in smoking behavior. *Journal of Consulting Psychology*, 1965, *29*, 184–186.
33. Janis, I. L. *Psychological Stress*. New York: John Wiley, 1958.
34. Johnson, J. E. Stress reduction through sensation information. In I. G. Sarason and C. D. Spielberger, eds., *Stress and Anxiety*. Vol. 2. New York: John Wiley, 1975.
35. Johnson, J. E., and Leventhal, H. Effects of accurate expectations and behavioral instructions on reactions during a noxious medical examination. *Journal of Personality and Social Psychology*, 1974, *29*, 710–718.
36. Johnson, J. E., Leventhal, H., and Dabbs, J. Contribution of emotional and instrumental response processes in adaptation to surgery. *Journal of Personality and Social Psychology*, 1971, *20*, 55–64.
37. Kanfer, F. H. Self-management methods. In F. H. Kanfer and A. P. Goldstein, eds., *Helping People Change*. 2nd ed. New York: Pergamon Press, 1980, pp. 334–389.
38. Kaplan, H. S. *The New Sex Therapy*. New York: Brunner/Mazel, 1974.
39. Kaplan, R. M. Coping with stressful medical examinations. In H. S. Friedman and M. R. DiMatteo, eds., *Interpersonal Issues in Health Care*. New York: Academic Press, 1982.
40. Karoly, P. Operant methods. In F. H. Kanfer and A. P. Goldstein, eds., *Helping People Change*. 2nd ed. New York: Pergamon Press, 1980, pp. 210–247.
41. Katz, J. L., Weiner, H., Gallagher, T. F., and Hellman, L. Stress, distress, and ego defenses. Psychoendocrine response to impending breast tumor biopsy. *Archives of General Psychiatry*, 1970, *23*, 131–142.
42. Kinsey, A. C., Pomeroy, W. B., and Martin, C. E. *Sexual Behavior in the Human Male*. Philadelphia: W. B. Saunders, 1948.

43. Kinsey, A. C., Pomeroy, W. B., Martin, C. E., and Gebhard, P. H. *Sexual Behavior in the Human Female.* Philadelphia: W. B. Saunders, 1953.
44. Kirkham, G. L. Homosexuality in prison. In J. M. Henslin, ed., *Studies in the Sociology of Sex.* New York: Appleton-Century-Crofts, 1971, p. 340.
45. Lief, H., and Karlen, A., eds. *Sex Education in Medicine.* New York: Spectrum, 1976.
46. Linn, L. Physician characteristics and attitudes toward legitimate use of psychotherapeutic drugs. *Journal of Health and Social Behavior,* 1971, *12,* 132-140.
47. LoPiccolo, J., and LoPiccolo, L., eds. *Handbook of Sex Therapy.* New York: Plenum, 1978.
48. Lorber, J. Good patients and problem patients: Conformity and deviance in a general hospital. *Journal of Health and Social Behavior,* 1975, *16,* 213-225.
49. MacDonald, A. P., Jr. Internal-external locus of control and the practice of birth control. *Psychological Reports,* 1970, *27,* 206.
50. MacFarlane, A. *The Psychology of Childbirth.* Cambridge, Mass.: Harvard University Press, 1977.
51. Mahoney, M. J. Self-reward and self-monitoring techniques for weight control. *Behavior Therapy,* 1974, *45,* 48-57.
52. Mahoney, M. J., and Mahoney, K. *Permanent Weight Control.* New York: W. W. Norton, 1976.
53. Masters, W. H., and Johnson, V. E. *Human Sexual Response.* Boston: Little, Brown, 1966.
54. Masters, W. H., and Johnson, V. E. *Human Sexual Inadequacy.* Boston: Little, Brown, 1970.
55. McGuire, J. C., and Gottlieb, B. H. Social support groups among new parents: An experimental study in primary prevention. *Journal of Clinical Child Psychology,* 1979, *8,* 111-116.
56. Mendelson, M. A. *Tender Loving Greed.* New York: Vintage Books, 1975.
57. Milgram, S. *Obedience to Authority.* New York: Harper and Row, 1974.
58. Minuchin, S., Rosman, B. L., and Baker, L. *Psychosomatic Families: Anorexia Nervosa in Context.* Cambridge, Mass.: Harvard University Press, 1978.
59. National Hospice Organization. Hospice in America, 765 Prospect Street, New Haven, CT, 06511.
60. Neugarten, B. L., ed. *Middle Age and Aging: A Reader in Social Psychology.* Chicago: University of Chicago Press, 1968.
61. *Newsweek,* November 15, 1976.
62. Pelletier, K. R. *Holistic Medicine.* New York: Delacorte Press, 1979.
63. Rank, S. G., and Jacobson, C. K. Hospital nurses' compliance with medication overdose orders: A failure to replicate. *Journal of Health and Social Behavior,* 1977, *18,* 188-193.
64. Raven, B. H., and Haley, R. W. Social influence processes and infection risk in hospitals. Los Angeles: Institute for Social Science Research, University of California Los Angeles.
65. Rodin, J. Research on eating behavior and obesity. Where does it fit in personality and social psychology. *Personality and Social Psychology Bulletin,* 1977, *3,* 333-355.
66. Rodin, J., and Janis, I. L. The social power of health-care practitioners as agents of change. *Journal of Social Issues,* 1979, 35(1), 60-81.
67. Rotter, J. B. *Social Learning and Clinical Psychology.* Englewood Cliffs, N.J.: Prentice-Hall, 1954.
68. Rotter, J. B. Generalized expectancies for internal versus external control of reinforcement. *Psychological Monographs,* 1966, *80*(1), No. 609.

69. Sanford, N., and Comstock, C., eds. *Sanctions for Evil.* Boston: Beacon Press, 1971.
70. Seeman, M., and Evans, J. W. Alienation and learning in a hospital setting. *American Sociological Review,* 1962, *27,* 772–783.
71. Seligman, M. E. *Helplessness.* San Francisco: W. H. Freeman, 1975.
72. Skipper, J. K., Tagliacozzo, D., and Mauksch, H. Some possible consequences of limited communication between patients and hospital functionaries. *Journal of Health and Human Behavior,* 1964, *5,* 34–39.
73. Sobel, D. The hospital fever. *Harvard Magazine,* 1978, *80*(5), May–June.
74. Strauss, D. Aging and old age. In R. C. Simons and H. Pardes, eds., *Understanding Human Behavior in Health and Illness.* Baltimore: Williams and Wilkins, 1977, pp. 370–378.
75. Stoddard, S. *The Hospice Movement: A Better Way of Caring for the Dying.* New York: Vintage Books, 1978.
76. Tagliacozzo, D. L., and Mauksch, H. O. The patient's view of the patient's role. In E. G. Jaco, ed., *Patients, Physicians and Illness.* 2nd ed. New York: The Free Press, 1972, pp. 162–175.
77. Taylor, S. E. Hospital patient behavior: Reactance, helplessness or control? *Journal of Social Issues,* 1979, *35*(1), 156–184.
78. U.S. Public Health Service. *Healthy People: The Surgeon General's Report on Health Promotion and Disease Prevention.* Washington, D.C.: U.S. Government Printing Office, 1979.
79. Wallston, B. S., and Wallston, K. A. Locus of control and health: A review of the literature. *Health Education Monographs,* 1978, Spring, *6*(2), 107–117.
80. Wallston, K. A., and Wallston, B. S., eds. Health locus of control. *Health Education Monographs,* 1978, *6*(2) (whole issue).
81. Wallston, B. S., Wallston, K. A., Kaplan, G. D., and Maides, S. A. Development and validation of the health locus of control (HLC) scale. *Journal of Consulting and Clinical Psychology,* 1976, *44,* 580–585.
82. Weis, K., and Borges, S. S. Victimology and rape: The case of the legitimate victim. *Issues in Criminology,* 1973, *8*(2), 105.
83. Wilson, R. The social structure of a general hospital. *Annals of the American Academy of Political and Social Science,* 1963, *346,* 67–76.
84. Zilbergeld, B. *Male Sexuality.* Boston: Little, Brown, 1978.

Index of Names

Adams, J. S., 4
Adler, N. E., 259
Andreasen, N. J. C., 206
Antonovsky, A., 165
Aristotle, 4

Barnard, C., 12
Barsky, A. J., 43
Beck, A. T., 175
Beecher, H., 69
Benson, H., 172–173
Blackman, S. L., 73
Blau, P., 3
Bloom, S. W., 84
Bourne, P., 279
Bryer, K., 224

Cannell, C., 107, 108
Cannon, W. B., 152–153
Caplan, R. D., 46–47
Carter, J., 63, 279
Cartwright, L., 271
Christy, N., 88
Cloquet, J. G., 72
Cobb, B., 28
Cohen, F., 150
Cooley, C., 8
Cooley, D., 13
Cousins, N., 59, 174

Darwin, C., 73
DeBakey, M., 13
Descartes, R., 60
Donne, J., 11–12
Duff, R., 140

Engel, G. L., 157, 248
Erikson, K. 173

Fiefel, H., 214
Fox, R. C., 19, 260–261
Frank, J. D., 60, 69
Freud, S., 72
Friedman, M., 155, 166

Gallup, G., 8
Gillum, R. F., 43
Glaser, B. G., 185, 190, 198
Glick, I. O., 221–223
Goffman, E., 136, 192
Groves, J., 42

Hall, E. T., 101
Hamlet, 211
Harlow, H. F., 97
Hippocrates, 20, 21, 22, 34, 93, 271
Hofling, C., 295
Hollender, M. I., 51–52
Hollingshead, A., 140

Note: Authors whose research is described but who are not mentioned by name in the text are not included in this index. They are included in the References (pp. 311–339).

Index of Subjects

About the Authors

M. Robin DiMatteo is Associate Professor of Psychology at the University of California, Riverside, where she teaches medical psychology, personality, and graduate statistics. She received her B.S. from Tufts University and her Ph.D. from Harvard University. Her research on physicians' personality and the prediction of patient rapport has been supported by grants from the Massachusetts Mental Health Center, the W.K. Kellogg Foundation, and the National Institute of Mental Health. Dr. DiMatteo is the author of numerous scientific articles in medical and psychological journals.

Howard S. Friedman is Associate Professor of Psychology at the University of California, Riverside. He has also served as a visiting professor of community medicine at the University of California, San Diego, School of Medicine. Professor Friedman's research concerns social perception and face-to-face interaction, with special applications to medical settings. His emphasis is on the role of nonverbal communication. He received his A.B. from Yale University and his Ph.D. in social psychology from Harvard University.

DiMatteo and Friedman edited the volume "Interpersonal Relations in Health Care," *Journal of Social Issues,* 1979, 35(1) (whole issue).